Infective Endocarditis and Other Intravascular Infections

CURRENT TOPICS IN INFECTIOUS DISEASE

Series Editors:

William B. Greenough III
Division of Geographic Medicine
The Johns Hopkins University School of Medicine
Baltimore, Maryland

Thomas C. Merigan
Head, Division of Infectious Disease
Stanford University Medical Center
Stanford, California

The Atypical Mycobacteria and Human Mycobacteriosis
Johns S. Chapman

Infections of the Gastrointestinal Tract: Microbiology, Pathophysiology, and Clinical Features
Herbert L. DuPont and Larry K. Pickering

Coccidioidomycosis: A Text
Edited by David A. Stevens

Cytomegalovirus: Biology and Infection
Monto Ho

Infective Endocarditis and Other Intravascular Infections
Lawrence R. Freedman

A Continuation Order Plan is available for this series. A continuation order will bring delivery of each new volume immediately upon publication. Volumes are billed only upon actual shipment. For further information please contact the publisher.

Infective Endocarditis and Other Intravascular Infections

Lawrence R. Freedman, M.D.
VA Wadsworth Medical Center
UCLA School of Medicine
Los Angeles, California

PLENUM MEDICAL BOOK COMPANY
New York and London

Library of Congress Cataloging in Publication Data

Freedman, Lawrence, R.
Infective endocarditis and other intravascular infections.

(Current topics in infectious disease)
Includes index.
1. Endocarditis, Bacterial. 2. Blood-vessels—Infections. I. Title. II. Series.
[DNLM: 1. Endocarditis, Bacterial. 2. Vasculitis. WG 285 F853i]
RC685.E5F73 1982 616.1 82-12361
ISBN 978-1-4684-8210-2 ISBN 978-1-4684-8208-9 (eBook)
DOI 10.1007/978-1-4684-8208-9

Softcover reprint of the hardcover 1st edition 1982
233 Spring Street, New York, N.Y. 10013

Plenum Medical Book Company is an imprint of Plenum Publishing Corporation

To the four women I love and admire

Hanna, Julia, Leora, Rina

Acknowledgments

I wish to thank the National Institute of Allergy and Infectious Diseases (U.S.P.H.S.) for their support of my studies of intravascular infection while at Yale University, New Haven, Connecticut. I subsequently continued these investigations at the University of Lausanne, Switzerland, at the Centre Hospitalier Universitaire Vaudois, whose support was essential to the work.

At this time I am pursuing these studies under the auspices of the Veterans Administration at the VA Wadsworth Medical Center at the University of California at Los Angeles.

My thanks go to Mr. Samuel Lunenfeld (Toronto, Canada) and to Professor and Mrs. Franz Joseph (Lausanne, Switzerland) for their help and interest in this project.

To Dr. and Mrs. Bruce Rapappport and the Intermaritime Foundation (Geneva, Switzerland) I want to express deep appreciation for their commitment to medical research and education and for their friendship and generous encouragement of my research.

LAWRENCE R. FREEDMAN, M.D.
Los Angeles

Contents

Infective Endocarditis and Other Intravascular Infections

1

Introduction

The most important example of intravascular infection is infective endocarditis (IE), a common and serious disorder in man. In the past, these infections were uniformly fatal, but since the development of potent antimicrobial agents, bacteriological cure has become practical and predictable. So, for a while, it seemed that intravascular infection would diminish in importance and be relegated to the stockpile of illnesses which physicians, one or two generations earlier, used to see frequently. In recent years, however, spectacular technological advances (cardiac surgery, intravascular devices, hemodialysis), accompanied by profound social deterioration (intravenous drug usage), have provided new breeding grounds for the development of these infections. So it is that a large percentage of intravascular infections may be looked upon today as one of the diseases of medical progress and social evolution. This "progress," however, has not only contributed to the encouragement of the disease; there is another side to the coin: the same technological advances that have served to increase the frequency of infection (e.g., intravascular plastic catheters) have also led to the first simple, easily reproducible laboratory animal model for the study of the disease, thus advancing our understanding of the prophylaxis, treatment, and general biology of these infections (Figures 1 and 2). Similarly, whereas the insertion of prosthetic heart valves has created a new group of patients with endocarditis, these same surgical techniques are lifesaving to patients with endocarditis whose aortic valves have perforated.

The purpose of this presentation is to look at the problem of intravascular infection, particularly IE, giving special emphasis to how it is that our understanding and management of the disease in patients have been influenced by the experimental study of the disease in animals.

The relationship between experiment and practice is one that has been recognized by leaders in medicine for a long time. Nevertheless, I take this occasion to reemphasize it because research is currently on the firing line. In

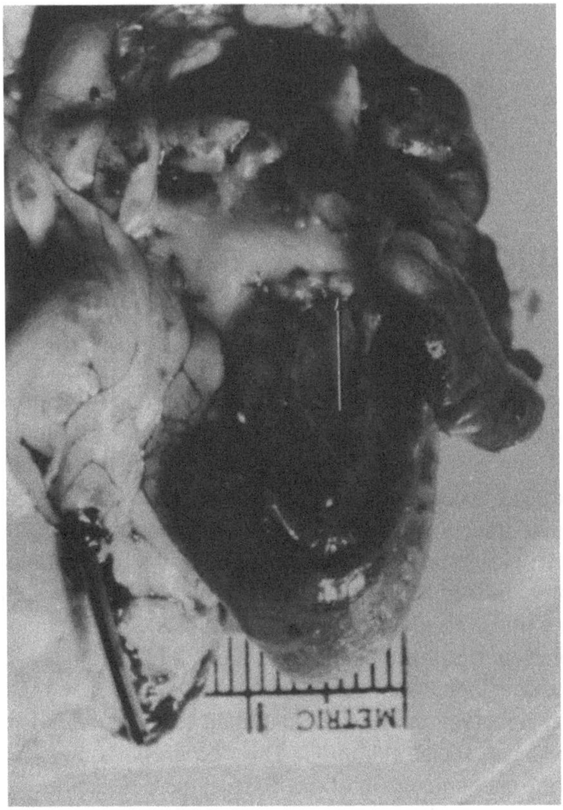

Figure 1. Small nodular sterile vegetations (NBTVs) on the tricuspid valve of a rabbit, induced by the placement of a polyethylene catheter in the venous system so that the tip lies at the entry to or within the right side of the heart. Reproduced from Garrison and Freedman[1] with permission.

fact, it will probably always be under attack. In many respects, research is to the practice of medicine as the university is to society. In both cases, the last thing that the medical or social establishment wants is to be informed that long-standing established practices are harmful or counterproductive.

There can be no separation between research and practice. The best understanding of human disease is inseparable from relevant experimental data. At the same time, the observation and treatment of disease in man impose the obligation to ask new questions in order to have better answers—in other words, to investigate. The effort to diagnose and treat intravascular infections illustrates the interdependence of experimentation and clinical medicine.

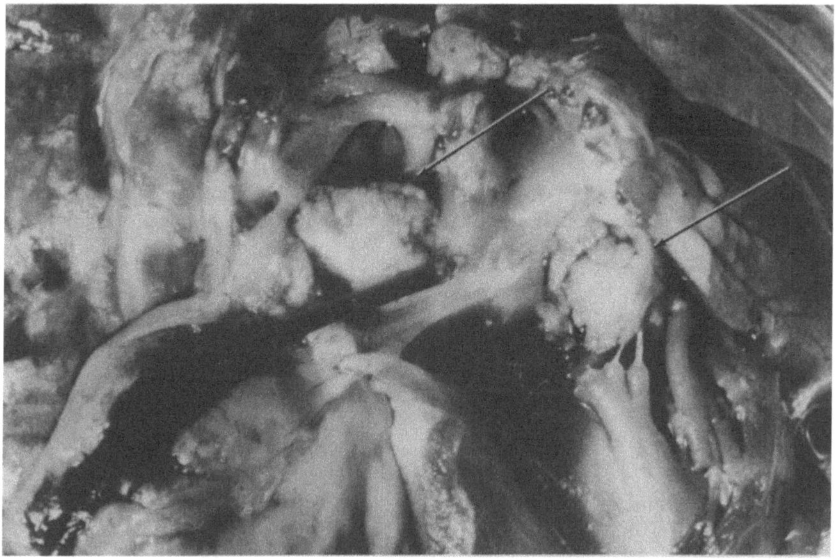

Figure 2. Vegetations in the right auricle and on the tricuspid valve after contamination of sterile vegetations (see Figure 1) with *Staphylococcus aureus*. Reproduced from Garrison and Freedman[1] with permission.

1.1. TERMINOLOGY

Intravascular infection may occur in relation to an arteriovenous or atrioventricular fistula, or it may take the form of infected thrombophlebitis, infection of an indwelling intravenous or intraarterial catheter, infection of arterial (aortic) aneurysms, infection of the heart valves or endocardium, or infection of prosthetic heart valves or vascular grafts. In contrast to other intravascular localizations, infections of the heart valves or endocardium are traditionally referred to as acute or subacute—thus the terms acute bacterial endocarditis or subacute bacterial endocarditis (endocarditis or sepsis lenta).

Although many authors still employ the terms acute and subacute bacterial endocarditis, I see no advantage in continuing this practice. The distinction was originally based on differences in clinical presentation and bacteriology. Today, however, these differences are much less clear, and the idea that subacute bacterial endocarditis is a slowly progressive and relatively benign infection due to *Streptococcus viridans,* although perhaps statistically correct, does not, in my view, give sufficient emphasis to the potential, rapidly occurring, catastrophic complications of the disorder. Thus, these terms will not be employed in this discussion; instead, all infections of the heart valves and endocardium will be referred to as infective endocarditis (IE).

REFERENCE

1. Garrison, P. K., Freedman, L. R.: Experimental endocarditis. I. Staphylococcal endocarditis in rabbits resulting from placement of a polyethelene catheter in the right side of the heart. *Yale J. Biol. Med.* **42**:394–410, 1970.

2

The Pathogenesis of Intravascular Infection

Intravascular infection is the name applied to microbial proliferation within a platelet–fibrin vegetation located within the circulatory system. The initiation of such an infection depends, in all likelihood, upon the prior establishment of a susceptible, nonbacterial thrombotic vegetation (NBTV) and dissemination via the bloodstream of microorganisms of a sort, and in a number sufficient, to attach to and multiply within the interstices of the vegetation. This sequence of events was well established 50 years ago.(1)

Despite a constellation of clinical findings which makes the diagnosis highly probable, it is the presence of constant bacteremia in the absence of a known extravascular source which stands as the hallmark of the disease.(2) In contrast to other microbial infections in which bloodstream dissemination of the infecting agent is usually episodic and related to the severity of the infection (or the inadequacy of systemic host defense mechanisms), in intravascular infections, constant bloodstream dissemination of microorganisms is a feature from the very outset despite systemic host defense mechanisms, such as polymorphonuclear leukocytes (PMN) and antibody response, which are in normal working order. This bacteremia serves, of course, as a constant source of reinfection of the original vegetation.

The constant seeding of microorganisms into the bloodstream, accompanied by the development of antibody to the causative agent, leads to the formation of circulating antigen–antibody complexes, compounds which are probably responsible for many of the clinical manifestations of the disorder.(3)

Clinically, the infection is characterized by fever and evidence for the prior existence of susceptible sterile fibrin vegetations (in the great majority of instances, a heart murmur). A wide panorama of other clinical findings in patients with intravascular infections depends upon:

1. The location of infection within the vascular system.
2. The pathogenicity of the infecting microorganisms.
3. The local invasiveness of the infection.
4. The number, size, and sites of lodgement of emboli dislodged from the infected vegetation.
5. The consequences of immune complexes in the circulation.

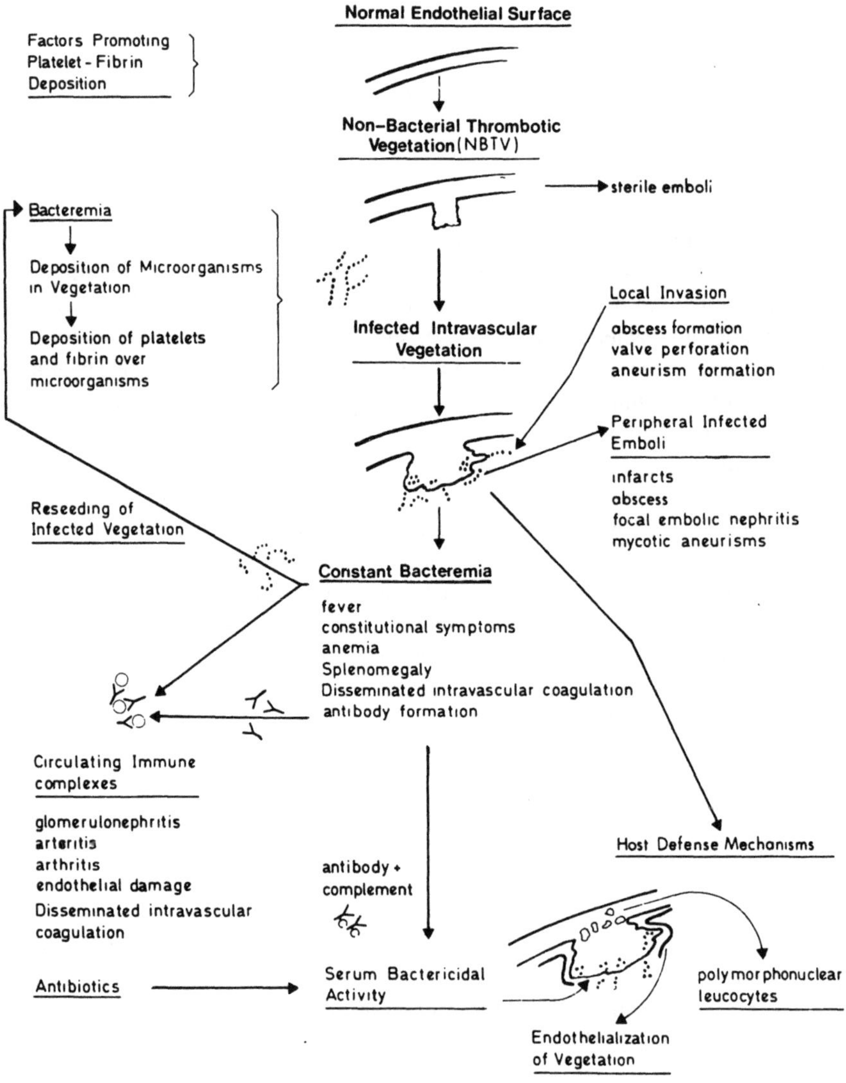

Figure 3. Pathogenesis of intravascular infection.

The treatment of intravascular infections presents particular difficulties, since PMN do not have ready access to the microorganisms embedded in the fibrin vegetation. Thus, the therapeutic problem may be looked upon as the treatment of infection in an area of localized agranulocytosis.[4] Very little is known about the host defense mechanisms which operate in these infections. The pathogenesis of intravascular infection is outlined diagramatically in Figure 3.

The disease is important clinically because it attacks patients of all ages and, if not promptly diagnosed and properly treated, may have a fatal outcome. Its frequency is difficult to determine, but there are usually at least one or two patients under treatment at a given moment in any university medical service. It is perhaps as common as patients with renal disease requiring chronic hemodialysis (50–60 cases/1,000,000 persons per year). The major difficulty in diagnosing the disease is that it is often not thought of. This is due to the generally nonspecific nature of the clinical presentation. In order to initiate proper diagnostic procedures, undertake correct treatment, and, ultimately, to prevent the disease, it is necessary to understand the biology of intravascular infections.

REFERENCES

1. Grant, R. T., Wood, J. E., Jones, T. D.: Heart valve irregularities in relation to subacute bacterial endocarditis. *Heart* **14**:247–261, 1927–1929.
2. Bennett, I. L., Beeson, P. B.: Bacteremia: A consideration of some experimental and clinical aspects. *Yale J. Biol Med.* **26**:241–262, 1954.
3. Reed, P., Williams, R. C. Jr.: Immune complexes in infectious diseases. *Adv. Intern. Med.* **22**:49–72, 1977.
4. Freedman, L. R.: Bacterial endocarditis, in: *Internal Medicine: 1976 Topics*. Louhija, A., Valtoneu, V. eds., Proceedings of the 13th International Congress of Internal Medicine, Helsinki, 1976, S. Karger, Basel, pp. 217–223, 1977.

REFERENCES

3

The Nonbacterial Thrombotic Vegetation

The normal endothelial surface is highly resistant to microbial infection, since bacteremia in normal man and animals rarely results in the establishment of intravascular infection. Rickettsial infection is probably the outstanding exception to this statement, since in these infections it would appear that normal endothelial cells are regularly colonized.[1] *Vibrio fetus* infection is often associated with a septic thrombophlebitis, but the pathogenesis of these lesions is not well understood.[2]

It is, of course, not uncommon to see inflammatory lesions of vascular structures adjacent to localized infections of any microbial origin. They are frequently seen with fungus and *Pseudomonas* infections, perhaps in the latter case due to the damaging consequences of various proteolytic toxins produced by these microorganisms.[3–5]

Prosthetic arterial grafts are often infected from without the vascular system. This may partly explain why infection of such grafts is frequently not associated with positive blood cultures.[6] In these instances, local signs of infection are evident.

The overwhelming majority (perhaps all) of intravascular infections are established on preexisting nonbacterial thrombotic vegetations (NBTVs), that is, zones of sterile platelet–fibrin vegetation formation. It is of importance to consider the factors which favor the development of these lesions, since their prevention or alteration so as to diminish their susceptibility to colonization by microorganisms offers a potential method for preventing or treating intravascular infection (Figure 4).

NBTVs have been observed clinically[7] and can be produced experimentally in two major ways: (1) by damage to the endothelial surface[8,9] or (2) by hypercoagulability.[10,11]

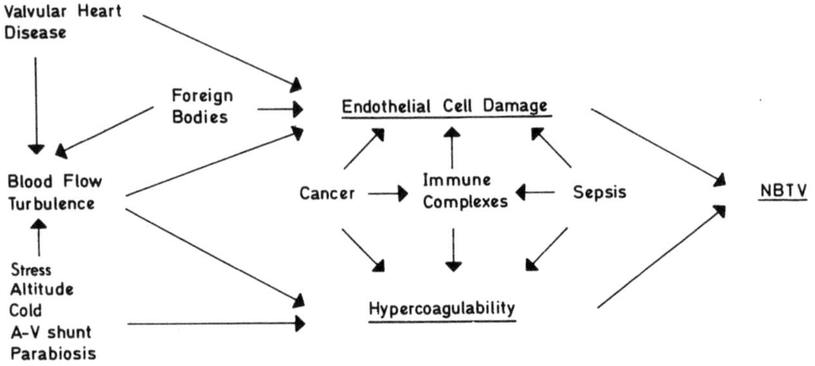

Figure 4. Pathogenesis of nonbacterial thrombotic vegetation (NBTV).

3.1. ENDOTHELIAL DAMAGE

Damage to the endothelial surface is most commonly seen and most easily understood in circumstances such as valvular heart disease[7] and indwelling catheters or prosthetic heart valves[12] (Figures 5 and 6).

In these conditions, there is valve (or endothelial) damage either by a

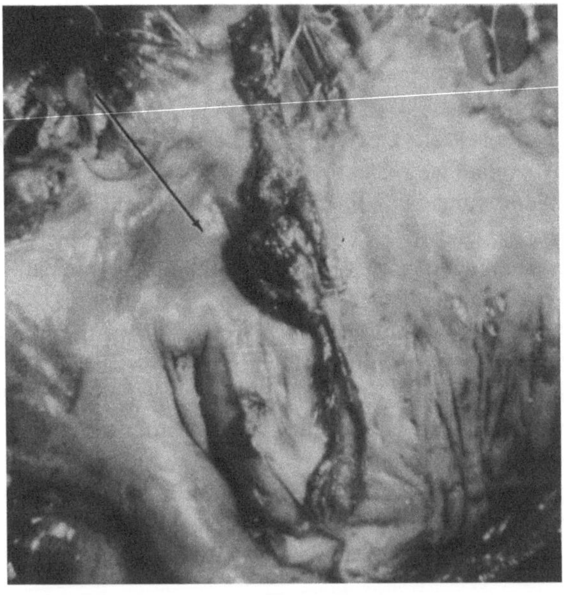

Figure 5. Vegetations (sterile) in the right ventricle several days after the placement of an intracavitary pacemaker in man.

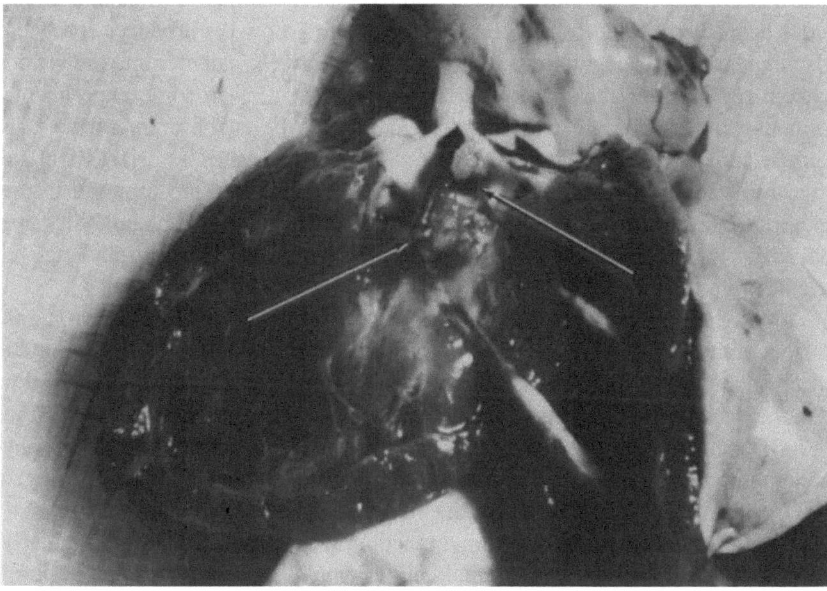

Figure 6. NBTVs on the wall of the aorta and the aortic valve 18 days after the placement of an indwelling polyethylene catheter in the left ventricle of a rabbit. Reproduced from Perlman and Freedman [77] with the permission of the *Yale Journal of Biology and Medicine*.

primary disease process such as rheumatic fever or arteriosclerosis or direct mechanical injury to endothelial cells. The release of tissue factors followed by local platelet sticking and fibrin formation is the likely pathway by which vegetations are formed.

Recent studies suggest that activated complement in the presence of polymorphonuclear leukocytes (PMN) is damaging to endothelial cells. If this mechanism is active *in vivo,* it might represent the means by which processes such as infection, immune complexes, and cancer are responsible for the development of NBTVs.[13–16]

3.2. HYPERCOAGULABILITY

Hypercoagulability in various disease states is currently a subject of great interest. The pathological consequence of hypercoagulability is the condition known as disseminated intravascular coagulation (DIC). DIC has been recognized as an important phenomenon in patients with cancer and sepsis and in association with circulating immune complexes (CICs), and is frequently associated with the formation of NBTVs.

Many states known to be associated with NBTVs probably act by the pathways of direct endothelial injury and hypercoagulability. For example, valvular heart disease and foreign bodies, by creating flow disturbances, probably also increase local coagulation. Insertion of polyethylene catheter into the venous system regularly produces NBTVs in the right heart.[12] In some experimental animals, the catheter tip was found at autopsy to be at the entry to the right auricle and not to have entered the heart cavity. Nevertheless, NBTVs of the tricuspid valve were seen in some of these animals. The presumption is that these lesions formed as a result of local turbulence and hypercoagulability produced by the presence of the catheter in the vicinity of, but not touching, the tricuspid valve.[12]

Many forms of stress have been shown to produce NBTVs; such stimuli include altitude, cold, peripheral A-V shunts, and parabiosis. It is likely that the mechanism here is also a combination of endothelial-cell damage by way of flow disturbances as well as hypercoagulability.[17] As will be discussed in Sections 3.3–3.5 cancer, immune complexes, and sepsis are capable of producing hypercoagulability as well as endothelial-cell damage, both changes leading to NBTV formation. These relations are illustrated diagrammatically in Figure 4.

In the generalized Schwartzman reaction in animals, DIC occurs regularly. Although the myocardial endothelial cells normally contain considerable fibrinolytic activity, this activity is lost during DIC, thus favoring local thrombogenesis. NBTVs are seen in 70% of experimental animals with the generalized Schwartzman reaction.[10,18] It is possible that endothelial-cell injury and hypercoagulability due to complement activation represent the common pathway responsible for NBTV production following a variety of diverse causes[13,16] (Figure 4).

A long list of the conditions which have been shown to precipitate DIC is given by Yoshikawa *et al.*[19] in their discussion of infection and DIC. Although all the conditions listed would serve as potential stimuli for the development of NBTV, this exhaustive list will not be discussed here because evidence is lacking to indicate whether in a given circumstance the lesions of NBTV occur with sufficient frequency or remain susceptible to infection for a long enough time to be important for the problem of intravascular infection.

NBTVs were found in 2.5–3.0% of autopsies of patients over the age of 60.[20] The frequency of this finding is considerably less in younger subjects, but has been described even in newborns.[21,22] When carefully looked for in one series, pathological evidence of DIC was found in 50% of autopsies of patients with NBTVs.[23] This undoubtedly underestimates the relation between these two conditions, since it is well known that DIC detectable by studies of blood coagulation may not be detectable morphologically at autopsy. Severe valve-endothelial-cell changes take place in 70% of animals undergoing the generalized Schwartzman reaction, during which all animals developed DIC.[10] NBTVs have also been described in patients believed to have thrombotic thrombocytopenic purpura.[24]

Curiously, the lesions of NBTV are found overwhelmingly on the left side of the heart and on the low-pressure side of the valves,[25] a distribution similar to that of infective endocarditis (IE) and rheumatic valvular lesions. This may be related to hypercoagulability in zones of increased turbulence.

3.3. CANCER

The lesions of NBTV are perhaps 3–5 times more frequent in patients with cancer than in patients dying of a variety of noncancerous disorders[20] (Figure 7). The reported preferential association of NBTVs with adenocarcinomas in contrast to undifferentiated tumors has stimulated the search for differences in immune responsiveness in patients with these two categories of tumors. In patients with adenocarcinomas, evidence for greater stimulation of cellular and humoral immune mechanisms has prompted the suggestion that NBTVs may be a consequence of CICs.[26] On the other hand, the relation between NBTVs and mucin-producing carcinomas and the subsequent finding of mucinous substance in intravascular thrombi and vegetations of cardiac valves has led to the view that circulating mucin may play an important role in the production of NBTVs.[27] It seems to me that there is good reason to relate NBTVs to DIC in cancer patients, but the mechanisms by which the stimulation of the hypercoagulable state takes place are conjectural.

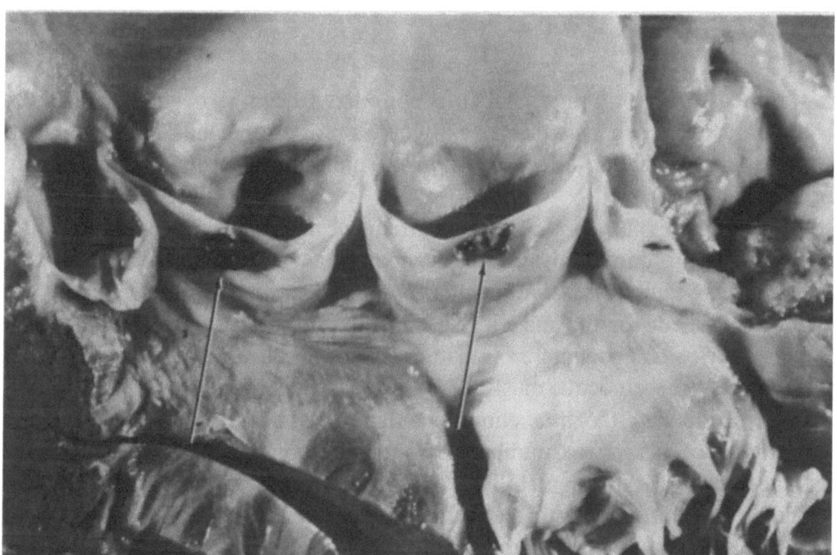

Figure 7. NBTVs on the aortic valve at autopsy in a patient with cancer.

It is frequently stated with surprise that NBTVs are often not found to be infected at autopsy.[20,28] On the other hand, if such lesions were to become infected, the patients would either have been diagnosed during life or would be classified under IE at autopsy. One study has examined the question of the frequency of IE in cancer patients as compared with general hospital populations.[29] The authors concluded that IE was not more common in cancer patients; however, their control figures were drawn from other published series, and such comparisons are difficult. For example, the age of the dying patients was not taken into consideration. In addition, the frequency of NBTVs of 0.9% in cancer patients was quite low, being about the same as one recently reported general autopsy series and one-third lower than that of another.[20,23]

It would be surprising if NBTVs were not associated with a high frequency of infection of vegetations. These lesions are ideally suited to become infected, and there is a markedly increased risk of bacteremia in patients with cancer, due to impairment of host defence mechanisms either by the primary illness or by the therapy for that illness. An examination of the microorganisms recovered from the aforementioned series of cancer patients shows that only 11% were *viridans* streptococci. Since *viridans* streptococci are the usual agents responsible for IE in the general population, this suggests that the infections seen in cancer patients were indeed different from those usually encountered in a general hospital population and seems to me to be consistent with a peculiar susceptibility of cancer patients to IE.

3.4. INFECTION

A wide variety of microbial infections have been associated with DIC. Thus, bloodstream sepsis is theoretically capable of establishing NBTVs and at the same time producing infection within the initially (even if instantaneously) sterile lesion.

In the older experimental literature, frequent mention is made of the ability to produce IE in animals by the intravenous inoculation of large numbers of bacteria. This required massive inocula, however, and the results were not sufficiently consistent for the model to be useful. Suffice it to say that bacterial inocula likely to be encountered in nature do not produce IE in animals. Thus, by inference, these inocula must not be effective in producing the lesions of NBTV. Nevertheless, the intravenous inoculation of moderate (10^6–10^7) numbers of staphylococci and large numbers of pneumococci in rabbits was regularly accompanied by hypercoagulability.[30,31] Furthermore, the lesions of DIC are commonly seen at autopsy in patients dying of staphylococcal sepsis,[32] and clinical episodes of DIC and staphylococcal (and streptococcal) sepsis are being reported with increasing frequency.[33–37]

It is interesting to speculate that the initiation of IE in drug addicts without underlying heart disease may be related to the formation of NBTVs secondary to episodes of hypercoagulability brought about by repeated intravenous injection of bacteria or perhaps other substances (?endotoxin) capable of producing the same changes in coagulation.[38] The effect of alterations in blood clotting on the natural history of IE will be discussed in Section 3.6.

Whereas it is not clear to what extent sepsis is important in the production of NBTVs, it is not unreasonable to imagine it playing a much more important role in the maintenance of an already established infected vegetation. The hypercoagulable state may, in this instance, contribute in a significant way to the rapid laying down of fibrin around bacterial colonies,[39] thereby insulating them from contact with PMN that happen to stick to the vegetation.[40] Another mechanism which might be important in fibrin deposition on infected vegetations is the generation of thromboplastin by circulating monocytes which have phagocytized bacteria.[41]

3.5. IMMUNE COMPLEXES

Immune complexes have been emphasized by Williams and others as one of the major pathogenetic mechanisms by which IE has an impact on the biology of the host.[42] It is becoming evident today that immune complexes are also able to induce the lesion of NBTV. Production of NBTVs by immune complexes is the possible consequence of two mechanisms, direct endothelial-cell (valve) injury and the hypercoagulable state. The best example of immune-complex valve damage is that of systemic lupus erythematosus (SLE), in which valve damage is said to occur almost half the time. The examination of aortic valves from two patients with SLE who developed aortic insufficiency and received a prosthetic valve replacement showed the deposition of immunoglobulins in a manner indentical to that seen in the skin and kidneys of such patients.[43] It is of considerable interest that receptors for the Fc portion of IgG are found more frequently and in greater quantities in valves on the left side of the heart than in valves on the right side of the heart.[44] These receptors may be of importance in the pathogenesis of valve damage by immune mechanisms.

Immune complexes are believed to trigger the hypercoagulable state and DIC.[42] Further evidence for the relation of immune-complex tissue injury to blood clotting comes from an examination of renal glomerular lesions. Anticoagulants are able to prevent tissue damage in immune-complex nephritis despite persistence of complexes in the circulation.[45] The morphological expression of glomerular damage induced by coagulation or by immune complexes may be indistinguishable.[45] Perhaps those patients with infective endocarditis and glomerulonephritis *without* evidence for immune-complex deposition in the glomeruli have their renal disease as a consequence of hypercoagulability.[46] CICs have been found in patients with glomerulonephritis due to severe infections without endocarditis or positive blood cultures.[47] I wonder whether such a mechanism may also account for the numerous cases of NBTV found at autopsy, frequently in association with severe infections, which cannot be attributed to the presence of cancer.[20,23]

Another circumstance in which immune complexes may be important for the formation of NBTVs is in the drug addict. Addicts have a very high rate of infection with type B hepatitis virus, which is known to produce prolonged periods in which immune complexes are found in the circulation. These "carrier" states have been associated with the development of glomerulonephritis and arteritis, and may well be responsible for the establishment of NBTVs.[42,48]

Finally, there are several reports in the older experimental literature describing the development of IE in hyperimmunized animals.[49,50,51] I wonder whether the presence of CICs may have produced NBTVs, thus permitting the development of IE after intravenous inoculation of viable bacteria in these animals.

In brief, despite the numerous clues which have been uncovered permitting the consideration of sepsis and CICs as pathogenetic mechanisms promoting the development of NBTVs, the argument remains speculative.[16] It has importance for the general biology of intravascular infections, since both these phenomena are regular findings and may be playing an important role in the maintenance of these infections.

Thus, there is a considerable body of clinical experimental evidence which provides ample reason to envision the formation of NBTVs in a wide variety of circumstances. In view of the frequency of bacteremia after hard chewing, it is a wonder that intravascular infection is not more frequent than it is.

3.6. LIMITATION OF GROWTH OF VEGETATIONS

One of the obvious questions about the development of NBTVs is: why is it that once a given stimulus for their formation exists, the vegetations do not continue to grow to gigantic proportions?

3.6.1. Embolization

There are two processes which tend to limit the size and growth of NBTVs. It is well known that pieces of the vegetation break off and may lodge anywhere in the distal arterial circulation. In the rabbit, peripheral emboli are found regularly in animals with NBTVs provoked by the presence of a polyethylene catheter in relation to the aortic valve.[77] This phenomenon is of importance clinically. MacDonald and Robbins[28] pointed out 25 years ago that such emboli contributed to or were responsible for death in 14% of instances in which such lesions were found at autopsy.

NBTV is sometimes a very early sign indicating the presence of even small cancers.[52,53] There are many reports of patient death due to the consequences of embolization from NBTVs in circumstances where the tumor was potentially curable. The volume of NBTV may become sufficient to be detected by echocardiography.[54]

It is difficult to be certain of the clinical significance of emboli in patients with NBTVs, but it is most likely that their frequency and clinical importance are underestimated. Cerebral, myocardial, and renal emboli are common, but must be carefully looked for in order to determine their true frequency.[20] Cerebral infarction is particularly frequent. In one series of 18 patients with NBTVs and cancer, 8 developed a stroke during their illness, in 5 instances as the initial manifestation of cancer.[52] In some instances of thrombotic thrombocytopenic purpura, cerebral and renal abnormalities are due to embolization from NBTVs rather than to the underlying disease process.[24] Myocardial infarction[20] and occlusion of major peripheral arteries have been described,[55] as have psychological disorders.[56]

From a review of cases reported in the literature, it is not clear to me whether anticoagulant therapy is efficacious in patients with emboli due to NBTVs. Surgical treatment has been suggested, and carried out successfully in one patient.[54] This patient is of particular interest, since he was 34 years old, had no known predisposing factor for the NBTVs, and most certainly would have been considered a patient with blood-culture-negative endocarditis were it not for the ability to examine embolic material histologically prior to the administration of antibiotics.

Studdy and Willoughby[53] have suggested criteria for a presumptive diagnosis of NBTV which seem to me to be useful and which one can hope will make possible a better evaluation of the treatment of this condition. Their criteria arc:

a) venous thrombosis accompanied by features suggesting systemic as well as pulmonary infarction;
b) progression despite anticoagulant treatment;
c) either no apparent origin for the systemic emboli or else a cardiac murmur in the presence of persistently negative blood culture.

Confirmation by echocardiography would then permit consideration of surgical treatment, assuming, of course, that such treatment was not contraindicated by the presence of associated illnesses which would render such therapy useless.

A recent study showing the frequency with which mitral-valve prolapse (MVP) is detected in young patients (<45 years of age) with transient cerebral ischemia or partial stroke is of particular interest in considering the clinical significance of NBTVs.[57] The presumption here is that there are tiny NBTVs that form and embolize from these valvular lesions, thus accounting for cerebral emboli. Careful autopsy studies have demonstrated the presence of NBTVs on the mitral valves of patients with MVP.[58] This emphasizes the importance of searching for small lesions as a possible source of IE (see Section 4.3.1).

3.6.2. Fibrinolysis, Organization, and Endothelialization

The other processes which are at work to limit the size of NBTVs are fibrinolysis, organization, and endothelialization of the vegetation. It is well known that there is constant fibrinolytic activity in the circulating blood. Stimulation of this activity by Streptokinase–Streptodornase (without antibiotic administration) was used as a treatment for experimental endocarditis nearly 25 years ago.[59] Although the vegetations seemed to be diminished in size, in the absence of antibiotic treatment, no effect on survival was seen.

These factors must be playing a very important role in the evolution of NBTVs and probably in the evolution of infected vegetations as well. In the study of experimental endocarditis in rabbits, removal of the catheter which provoked the formation of NBTVs results in prompt disappearance of the valvular lesions.[60] In addition, sterilization of an infected vegetation with antibiotics rapidly induces histological changes of healing and endothelialization.[40] The natural history of experimental right-sided streptococcal endocarditis is toward *spontaneous sterilization.*[61] Of 10 rabbits with right-sided *Streptococcus viridans* endocarditis, 1 died with infection at 34 days, but the other 9 animals, in good health, were found to have sterile vegetations 30–255 days after infection (Figure 8). In 4 of these rabbits, there were no visible vegetations, and in all

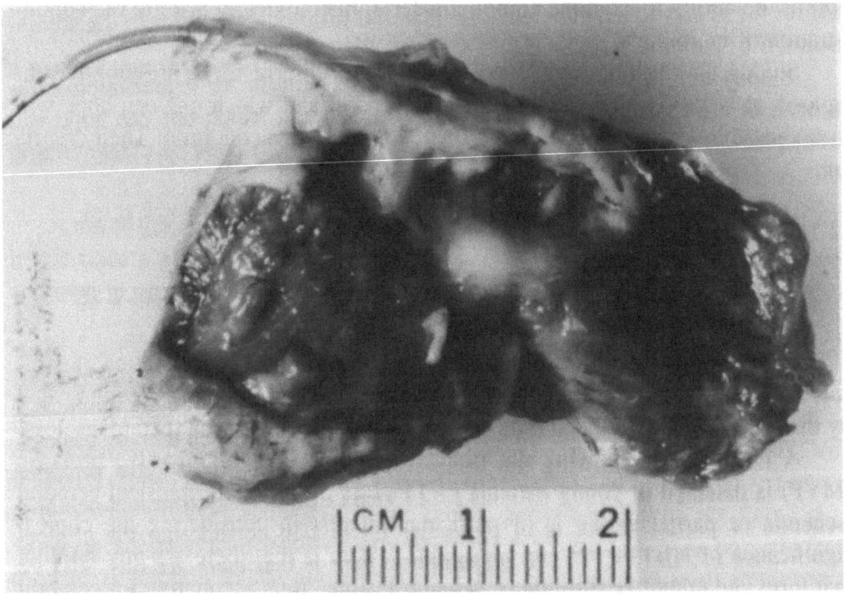

Figure 8. Spontaneous endothelialization and sterilization of a polyethylene catheter and its associated vegetations 6 weeks after placement of the catheter and initiation of infection with *Streptococcus viridans*.

animals, the catheters (used to induce NBTVs) and remaining vegetations were well endothelialized. This is a remarkable phenomenon and demonstrates that in rabbits, at least, there are active mechanisms which work not only toward limiting the size of a valvular vegetation, but also toward curing the infection, all this in the continued presence of the catheter which provoked the original NBTVs. This tendency toward spontaneous sterilization and healing of an infected vegetation was also seen within 2 weeks in staphylococcal aortic-valve infection, but only after removal of the catheter.[62]

It is evident that there must be an equilibrium between those factors tending to encourage the formation of NBTVs and those tending to limit the size of these lesions. It is likely in the rabbit that the "healing" factors take days to weeks to develop, since there is early growth of these experimental vegetations, which then seem to reach a plateau or to decrease in size.[7] Fibrinolytic activity detected in myocardial endothelial cells may play an important role in this process.[10,18]

3.7. FIBROBLASTIC PARIETAL ENDOCARDITIS WITH EOSINOPHILIA (LÖFFLER'S ENDOCARDITIS)

Löffler's endocarditis is a peculiar disease characterized by masses of thrombotic material in one or both ventricles of the heart. Patients present with clinical findings of intravascular vegetations or tumor formation: fever, petechiae, and embolic phenomena. Heart murmurs may or may not be present, and blood cultures are negative. In contrast to intravascular tumors (myxoma or endotheliosarcoma) or blood-culture-negative IE, patients with Löffler's endocarditis have an extraordinary peripheral-blood eosinophilia. It is common to find 30–60% of circulating WBC to be mature eosinophiles in the presence of a leukocytosis of 15,000–20,000 WBC/mm^3. Occasionally, the leukocytosis is marked, as high as 100,000 WBC/mm^3 with 90–95% eosinophiles—at which point the diagnosis of eosinophilic leukemia is considered. It is often not possible to distinguish this illness from eosinophilic leukemia, a condition in which endocardial thrombosis is also seen.

Judging by the recent publications concerning this disorder, it is not as rare as was once thought. And now that surgical therapy is practical for such patients, it is likely that more cases will be found.[63–66]

It has been noted that with the passage of time, the eosinophilia tends to return to normal[63] This has prompted the view that eosinophilia reflects an immune response to a specific agent or agents and that the cardiac damage itself is due to the presence of the huge number of eosinophiles. However, eosinophiles are not often identifiable in the cardiac lesions. Many believe the illness to be a stage in the development of endomyocardial fibrosis as seen in Africa.[67–69] Endocardial fibrosis with eosinophilia has been described in Hodgkin's disease, asthma, malignant melanoma, and trichinosis.[70–73] Despite considerable speculation concerning the origin of this disorder, it remains firmly, for the moment, in the category of illnesses of unknown etiology.

From the standpoint of the present discussion, Löffler's endocarditis presents several points of interest. Infection has not been described in these patients, yet infection of parietal thrombi following myocardial infarction has been described, albeit rarely.[74,75] The difference in the frequency of the two disorders could easily explain the occasional infection seen in patients with the much more common lesion of myocardial infarction.

It is curious that despite a pronounced tendency toward endocardial thrombus formation, valvular lesions are not prominent. In addition, there seems to be a predisposition for involvement of the left side of the heart.

Thus, there is something distinctly different about parietal endocarditis of unknown etiology and NBTV. Nevertheless, the presence of eosinophilia and occasional references to concomitant DIC[68,71] raise the possibility that Löffler's endocarditis is also precipitated by immunological phenomena probably linked to hypercoagulability of the blood. Subsequent studies of such patients should include investigations to examine these possibilities.

3.8. ARTERIOSCLEROSIS

NBTVs formed on ulcerated arteriosclerotic plaques in the aorta (usually at the bifurcation) are commonplace at autopsy (Figure 9). Vegetations are undoubtedly formed in relation to the endothelial damage and local flow disturbances caused by arteriosclerosis. These vegetations are of considerable interest because they so rarely become infected (see Chapter 4). Any theory of the pathogenesis of intravascular infection must take into account the relative resistance to infection of NBTVs in the aorta.

It is of some interest that there is accelerated development of arteriosclerosis in patients on chronic hemodialysis, since alternate-pathway complement activation occurs during hemodialysis.[13] A possible role for complement activation in the production of arterial lesions is suggested by its cytotoxic effect on endothelial cells in tissue culture. It has been suggested on the basis of these interesting *in vitro* studies that complement activation with resulting damage to endothelial cells may represent the common pathway by which vascular damage is produced by immune complexes, endotoxin, and organ transplantation.

3.9. NONBACTERIAL THROMBOTIC VEGETATION IN THE VENOUS SYSTEM

Thrombosis within the peripheral venous system is very common. Leg-vein thrombosis occurs frequently in the postpartum state, after surgical operations,

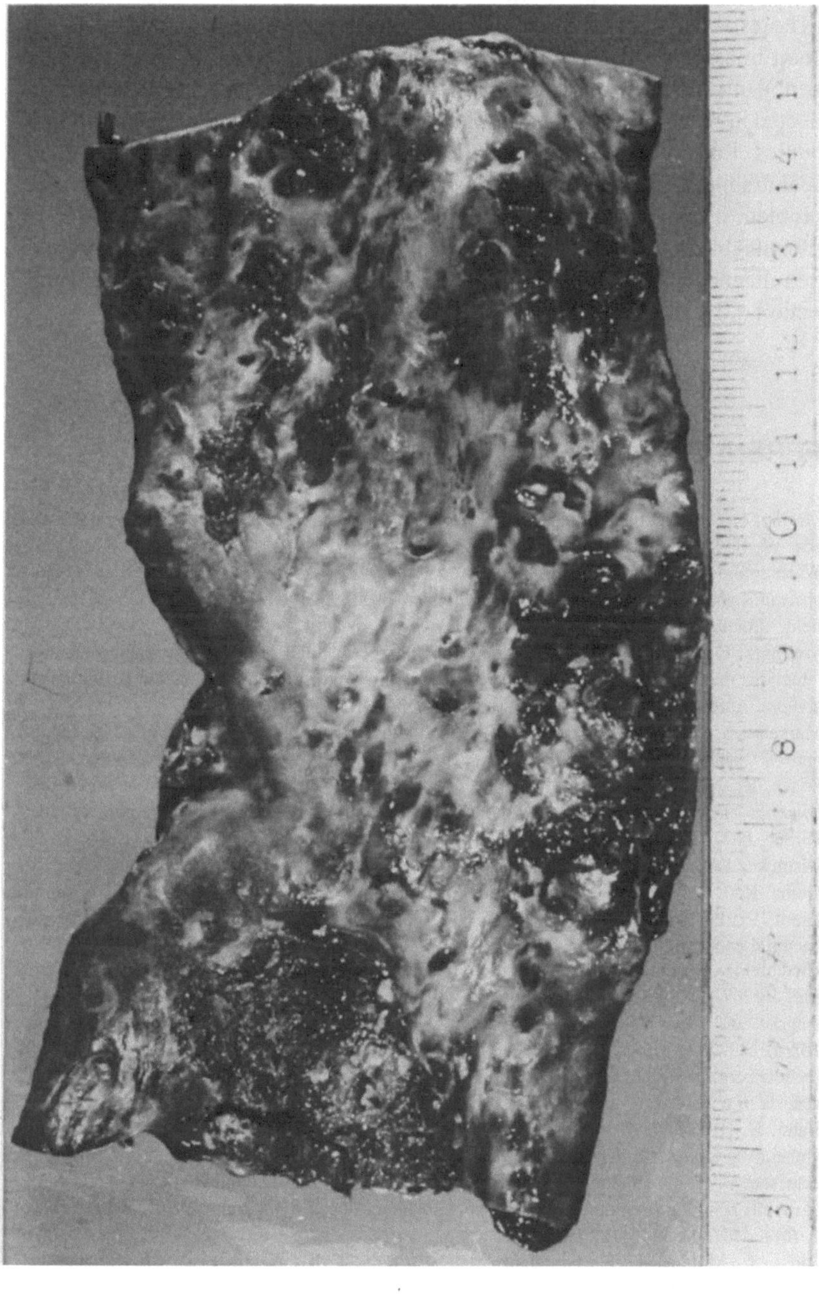

Figure 9. Atherosclerosis covered with NBTVs in the abdominal aorta at autopsy.

and in congestive heart failure. In addition, in hospital medical practice, thrombophlebitis at the site of intravenous perfusions is an everyday occurrence.

The establishment of microbial infection in the venous system, although common in association with intravenous-fluid therapy, is rare in relation to the frequency of venous thrombus formation. When it does occur, as a complication of infected intravenous catheters, resolution is often a simple matter, even without antibiotics. Rarely, septic thrombophlebitis requires antibiotic therapy and even surgical drainage, but even in these instances, cure of infection does not present the problem it does when cardiac valvular vegetations become infected. Septic thrombophlebitis may be a serious complication of total parenteral nutrition and is often diagnosed only at autopsy.[76] This subject is considered in more detail in Section 4.3.2.1f.

REFERENCES

1. Murray, E. S.: Rickettsial diseases, in: *Textbook of Medicine,* Beeson, P. B., McDermott, W., eds. W. B. Saunders, Philadelphia, p. 248, 1975.
2. Washington, J. A., II.: Bacteremia due to anaerobic, unusual and fastidious bacteria, in: *Bacteremia, Laboratory and Clinical Aspects,* Sonnenwirth, A. C., ed. Charles C. Thomas, Springfield, Illinois, pp. 47–60, 1973.
3. Saelinger, C. B., Snell, K., and Holder, I. A.: Experimental studies on the pathogenesis of infections due to *Pseudomonas aeruginosa:* Direct evidence of toxin production during *Pseudomonas* infection of burned skin tissues. *J. Infect. Dis.* **136:**555–561, 1977.
4. Margaretten, W., Nikai, H., Landing, B. H.: Significance of selective vasculitis and the "bone-marrow" syndrome in *Pseudomonas* septicemia. *N. Engl. J. Med.* **265:**773–776, 1961.
5. Soave, R., Murray, H. W., Litrenta, M. M.: Bacterial invasion of pulmonary vessels: *Pseudomonas* bacteremia mimicking pulmonary thromboembolism with infarction. *Am. J. Med.* **65:**864–867, 1978.
6. Dismukes, W.,: Discussion, in: *Infections of Prosthetic Heart Valves and Vascular Grafts,* Duma, R. J., ed. University Park Press, Baltimore, p. 265, 1977.
7. Grant, R. T., Wood, J. E., Jones, T. D.: Heart valve irregularites in relation to subacute bacterial endocarditis. *Heart* **14:**247–261, 1927–1929.
8. Hirschfelder, A. D.: The rapid formation of endocarditis "vegetations." *Johns Hopkins Hosp. Bull* **18:**267–268, 1907.
9. Angrist, A. A., Oka, M.: Pathogenesis of bacterial endocarditis. *J. Am. Med. Assoc.* **183**(4):249–252, 1963.
10. Freudenberg, N., Madreiter, H., Mittemayer, C.: Experimental investigations into the pathogenesis of endocarditis due to shock. *Beitr. Pathol* **155:**248–262, 1975.
11. Hahn, H. H., Schweid, A. I., and Beaty, M. N.: Complications of injecting dissolved methylphenidate tablets, *Arch. Intern. Med.* **123:**656–659, 1969.
12. Garrison, P. K., Freedman, L. R.: Experimental endocarditis. I. Staphylococcal endocarditis in rabbits resulting from placement of a polyethylene catheter in the right side of the heart. *Yale J. Biol. Med.* **42:**394–410, 1970.
13. Sacks, T., Moldow, C. F., Graddock, P. R., Bowers, T. K., Jacob, H. S.: Complement (c)-mediated endothelial damage: A mechanism for the accelerated atherosclerosis of hemodialysis. *Clin. Res.* **25**(4):612A, 1977.

14. Sheagren, J. N., Tuazon, C. V., Quie, P. G.: Alternate complement pathway activation by strains of *S. aureus* isolated from patients with disseminated intravascular coagulation. *Clin. Res.* **26**:526A, 1978.
15. Zimmerman, T. S., Fierer, J., Rothenberger H.: Blood coagulation and the inflammatory response. *Semin. Hematol.* **14**:391–408, 1977.
16. O'Connor, D. T., Weisman, M. H., Fierer, J.: Activation of the alternate complement pathway in *Staph. aureus* infective endocarditis and its relationship to thrombocytopenia, coagulation abnormalities and acute glomerulonephritis. *Clin. Exp. Immunol.* **34**:179–187, 1978.
17. Angrist, A., Oka, M., Nakoa, K.: Interstitial edema in valvular endocarditis. *Ann. N. Y. Acad. Sci.* **156**:480–497, 1969.
18. Becker, B. J. P.: Studies on the human mural endocardium. *Pathol. Bacteriol.* **88**:515–547, 1964.
19. Yoshikawa, T., Tanaka, K. R., Guze, L. B.: Infection and disseminated intravascular coagulation. *Medicine* **50**(4):237–258, 1971.
20. Chino, F., Kodama, A., Otake, M., Dock, D. S.: Nonbacterial thrombotic endocarditis in a Japanese autopsy sample: A review of eighty cases. *Am. Heart J.* **90**(8):190–198, 1975.
21. Oppenheimer, E. H., Esterley, J. R.: Nonbacterial thrombotic vegetations. *Am. J. Pathol.* **53**:63–81, 1968.
22. Liwnicz, B. H., Lepow, H.: Nonbacterial thrombotic endocarditis in premature child—Clinical significance and possible relationships to subvalvular hematoma. *N. Y. State J. Med.* **76**(6):912–916, 1976.
23. Kim, H. S., Suzuki, M., Lie, J. T., Titus, J. L.: Nonbacterial thrombotic endocarditis (NBTE) and disseminated intravascular coagulation (DIC)—Autopsy study of 36 patients. *Arch. Pathol. Lab. Med.* **101**:65–68, 1977.
24. Vilanova, J. R., Norenberg, M. D., Stuard, I. D.: Thrombotic thrombocytopenic purpura—systemic embolization from nonbacterial thrombotic endocarditis. *N. Y. State J. Med.* **75**:(12):2246–2248, 1975.
25. Rodbard, S.: Blood velocity and endocarditis. *Circulation* **27**:18–28, 1963.
26. Stosiek, P.: Beziehungen Zwischen Tumorimmunologie, Stromareaktion und Tumorendocarditis. *Virchows Arch. A: Pathol. Anat. Histol.* **369**:153, 1975.
27. Min, K. -W., Gyorkey, F.: Intravascular mucin and disseminated thrombosis in nonbacterial thrombotic endocarditis. *Am J. Pathol.* **86**:(2):80a–81a, 1977.
28. MacDonald, R. A., Robbins, S. L.: The significance of nonbacterial thrombotic endocarditis: An autopsy and clinical study of 78 cases. *Ann. Intern. Med.* **46**(2):255–273, 1957.
29. Rosen, P., Armstrong, D.: Infective endocarditis in patients treated for malignant neoplastic diseases: A postmortem study. *Am J. Clin. Pathol.* **60**:(2):241–250, 1973.
30. Lipinski, B., Cybulska, J., Worowski, K., Jeljaszewicz, J.: Blood clotting and fibrinolysis in experimental staphylococcal infection. *Pathol. Microbiol. (Basel)* **34**:295–304, 1969.
31. Guckian, J. C.: Coagulopathy in experimental sepsis with *Streptococcus pneumoniae* in rabbits: Effect of drug therapy and splenectomy. *J. Infect. Dis.* **134)**(2):150–157, 1976.
32. Powell, D. E. B.: Non-suppurative lesions in staphylococcal septicaemia. *J. Pathol. Bacteriol.* **82**:141–149, 1961.
33. McKeel, D.: Pemphigus vulgaris, large dose glucocorticoid therapy and staphylococcal bacteremia. *Am. J. Med.* **63**:152–160, 1977.
34. Murray, H. W., Tuazon, C. U., Sheagren, J. N.: Staphylococcal septicemia and disseminated intravascular coagulation. *Arch. Intern. Med.* **137**:844-847, 1977.
35. Case records of the Massachusetts General Hospital, B. Castleman, ed. Case 26-1971: Rapidly fatal sepsis with consumption coagulopathy in heroin addicts. *N. Engl. J. Med.* **285**(1):40–48, 1971.
36. Beylot, C., Castaing, R., Poisot, D., Bioulac, P., Cazaugade, M.: "Acral cyanosis"—Manifestation d'une coagulation intra-vasculaire disséminée au cours d'une endocardite bactérienne aigüe. *Ann. Dermatologie Syphiligr.* **101**(4):375–382, 1974.

37. Wardle, E. N., Floyd, M.: Fibrinogen catabolism study of three patients with bacterial endocarditis and renal disease. *Br. Med. J.* **3**:255–257, 1973.
38. Stimmel, B., Dack, S.: Infective endocarditis in narcotic addicts, in: *Infective Endocarditis,* Rahimtoola, S. H., ed. Grune and Stratton, New York, pp. 195–209, 1978.
39. Clumeck, N., Dereume, J. P., Hubrechts, J. M., Parmentier, R., Sternon, J.: Bacterial endocarditis, intravascular coagulation and aortic bifurcation embolism. *Acta Clin. Belg.* **31**:(5):292–294, 1976.
40. Durack, D. T.: Experimental bacterial endocarditis. iv. Structure and evolution of very early lesions. *J. Pathol.* **115**:81–89, 1975.
41. van Ginkel, C. J. W., Thörig, L., Thompson, J., Oh, J. I. H., van Aken, W. G.: Enhancement of generation of monocyte tissue thromboplastin by bacterial phagocytosis: Possible pathway for fibrin formation of infected vegetations in bacterial endocarditis. *Infect. Immun.* **25**:388–395, 1979.
42. Reed, P., Williams, R. C., Jr.: Immune complexes in infectious diseases, in: Stollerman, G. H., ed. *Advances in Internal medicine,* Vol. 22, Year Book Medical Publishers, Chicago, pp. 49–72, 1977.
43. Shapiro, R. F., Gamble, C. N., Wiesner, K. B., Castles, J. J., Wolf, A. W., Hurley, E. J., Salel, A. F.: Immunopathogenesis of Libman–Sacks endocarditis. *Ann. Rheum. Dis.* **36**:508–516, 1977.
44. Gelfand, M. C., Maclay, M., Shin, M. L., Green, I., Frank, M. M.: Binding of IgG-sensitized erythrocytes by mitral and aortic cardiac valves: A possible clue to the pathogenesis of immune valvular heart disease. *Clin. Res.* **28**:469A, 1980.
45. Kincaid-Smith, P.: Editorial review: Coagulation and renal disease. *Kidney Int.* **2**:183–190, 1972.
46. Boulton-Jones, J. M., Sissons, J. G. P., Evans, D. J., Peters, D. K.: Renal lesions of subacute infective endocarditis. *Br. Med. J.* **2**:11–14, 1974.
47. Beaufils, M., Morel-Maroger, L., Sraer, J. D., Kanfer, A., Kourilsky, O., Richet, G.: Acute renal failure of glomerular origin during visceral suppurations. *N. Engl. J. Med.* **295**:185–189, 1976.
48. Rossen, R. D., Reisberg, M. A., Singer, D. B., Schloeder, F. X., Suki, W. N., Hill, L. L., Eknoyan, G.: Soluble immune complexes in sera of patients with nephritis. *Kidney Int.* **10**:256–263, 1976.
49. Swift, H. F.: The heart in infection. *Am. Heart. J.* **3**(6):629–648, 1928.
50. Wadsworth, A. B.: A study of the endocardial lesions developing during pneumococcus infection in horses. *J. Med. Res.* **39**:279–291, 1919.
51. Wright, H. D.: The production of experimental endocarditis with pneumococci and streptococci in immunised animals. *J. Pathol. Bacteriol.* **29**:5–11, 1926.
52. Kooiker, J. C., MacLean, J. M., Sumi, S. M.: Cerebral embolism, marantic endocarditis, and cancer. *Arch. Neurol.* **33**:260–264, 1976.
53. Studdy, P., Willoughby, J. M. T.: Non-bacterial thrombotic endocarditis in early cancer. *Br. Med. J.* **1**(1):752, 1976.
54. Estevez, C. M., Corya, B. C.: Serial echocardiographic abnormalities in nonbacterial thrombotic endocarditis of the mitral valve. *Chest* **69**:801–804, 1976.
55. Delgado, G., Smith, J. P.: Gynecological malignancy associated with nonbacterial thrombotic endocarditis (NBTE). *Gynecol. Oncol.* **3**:205–209, 1975.
56. MacKenzie, T. B., Popkin, M. K.: Psychological manifestations of nonbacterial thrombatic endocarditis. *Am. J. Psychiatry* **137**:927–973, 1980.
57. Barnett, H. J. M., Boughner, D. R., Taylor, D. W., Cooper, P. E., Kostuk, W. J., Nichol, P. M.: Further evidence relating mitra-valve prolapse to cerebral ischemic events. *N. Engl. J. Med.* **302**:139–144, 1980.
58. Pomerance, A., Davies, M. J.: Strokes: A complication of mitral-leaflet prolapse (letter). *Lancet* **2**:1186, 1977.

59. Parker, B. M., Andresen, D. C., Thomas, W. A., Smith, J. R.: Effect of intravenous fibrinolytic enzymes on the vegetation of experimental bacterial endocarditis. *J. Lab. Clin. Med.* **52**:588–595, 1958.
60. Gutschik, E., Christensen, N.: Experimental endocarditis in Rabbits. 1. Technique and spontaneous course of non-bacterial thrombotic endocarditis. *Acta Pathol. Microbiol. Scand. Sect. B* **86**:215–221, 1978.
61. Freedman, L. R., Arnold, S., Valone, J.: Experimental endocarditis. *Ann. N. Y. Acad. Sci.* **236**:456–465, 1974.
62. Perlman, B. B., Freedman, L. R.: Experimental endocarditis. III. Natural history of catheter induced endocarditis after catheter removal. *Yale J. Biol. Med.* **44**:214–223, 1971.
63. Hardmeier, T., Biedermann, H. P., Winklehner, H. L.: Endocarditis parietalis eosinophilia—Are there idopathic forms? *Pathol. Microbiol.* **43**:107–113, 1975.
64. Bell, J. A., Jenkins, B. S., Webb-Peploe, M. M.: Clinical, haemodynamic, and angiographic findings in Löffler's eosinophilic endocarditis. *Br. Heart. J.* **38**:(6):541–548, 1976.
65. Binet, J. P., Pernod, J., Kermarac, J., Collette, J., Weiler, M., Bouhey, J., Bouvier, M.: Endocardite constrictive fibroblastique—A propos d'une localisée au ventricule gauche. *Arch. Mal. Coeur Vaiss.* **2**:163–168, 1977.
66. Dubost, C., Maurice, P., Gerbaux, A., Bertrand, E., Rulliere, R., Vial, F., Barillon, A., Pringent, C., Carpentier, A., Soyer, R.: The surgical treatment of constrictive fibrous endocarditis. *Ann. Surg.* **184**(3):303–307, 1976.
67. Olsen, E. G. J.: Endomyocardial fibrosis and Löffler's endocarditis parietalis fibroplastica. *Postgrad. Med. J.* **53**:538–540, 1977.
68. Olsen, E. G. J.: Löffler's endocarditis and endomyocardial fibrosis—Pathological aspects. *Pathol. Microbiol.* **43**:104–106, 1975.
69. Rüttner, J. R.: Pathology of endocarditis parietalis eosinophilica Löffler. *Pathol. Microbiol.* **43**:93–97, 1975.
70. Scott, M. E., Bruce, J. H.: Case Report: Löffler's endocarditis. *Br. Heart J.* **37**:534–538, 1975.
71. Mendes de Leon, D. E.: Eosinophilic leukaemia, Hodgkin's disease and Loeffler-type fibroplastic parietal endocarditis. *Neth. J. Med.* **19**:148–155, 1976.
72. Siebenschein, R., Siebenmann, R. E.: Parneoplastisches eosinophiles Leukämoid mit Thromboendocarditis parietalis eosinophilica bei malignem Melanom. *Schweiz. Med. Wochenschr.* **107**:1257–1265, 1977.
73. Andy, J. J., O'Connell, J. P., Daddario, R. C., Roberts, W. C.: Trichinosis causing extensive ventricular mural endocarditis with superimposed thrombosis. *Am. J. Med.* **63**:824–829, 1977.
74. Weinstein, L., Rubin, R. H.: Infective Endocarditis—1973. *Prog. Cardiovas. Dis.* **16**:239–274, 1973.
75. Chomette, G., Brocheriou, C., Delcourt, A., Agebo, M.: Les endocardites suppurées pariétales. *Ann. Med. Interne* **127**(2):83–89, 1976.
76. Goldmann, D. A., Maki, D. G.: Infection control in total parenteral nutrition. *J. Am. Med. Assoc.* **223**(12):1360–1364, 1973.
77. Perlman, B. B., Freedman, L. R.: Experimental endocarditis. II. Staphylococcal infection of the aortic valve following placement of a polyethylene catheter in the left side of the heart. *Yale J. Biol. Med.* **44**:206–213, 1971.

4

Establishment of Intravascular Infection

4.1. BACTEREMIA—THE CAPACITY TO INDUCE INFECTION

Infection of susceptible intracardiac vegetations comes about by the deposition of bacteria circulating in the bloodstream on the surface of the vegetations. This mechanism is easily demonstrable in animals, and there is no evidence to support the older suggestion that bacteria arrive in the vegetations by way of the blood supply to the valve or endocardium. Studies of the early vegetations show clearly that colonization takes place from the edge of the vegetations. With the passage of time, older colonies, often containing microbial debris with metabolically less active forms, are found at the base of the vegetations.[1–3]

The mechanism of infection of vegetations at other intravascular sites is probably similar, with the exception of prosthetic grafts of the aorta.[4] In these circumstances, local extravascular infection, undoubtedly a complication of the operative procedure, is capable of invading the graft. This explains in part why blood cultures are often negative in the presence of graft infections in man.[5]

The number of microorganisms necessary to produce infection of an intracardiac vegetation depends upon the microorganism selected and the state of infectivity of the vegetation. The influence of the stage of development and location of the vegetation is considered in Sections 4.3.1 and 4.3.2.

We have shown that the ID_{50} for three different bacteria in our laboratory was considerably different. Using rabbits with 48-hr aortic-valve vegetations produced by polyethylene-catheter placement, the ID_{50} for a strain of *Staphylococcus aureus* was $10^{3.75} \pm 0.060$, for an α-hemolytic streptococcus it was $10^{4.67} \pm 0.52$, and for *Escherichia coli* it was $10^{6.29} \pm 0.52$[6] (Figure 10). Thus, different bacteria have different capacities for initiating infection in fresh

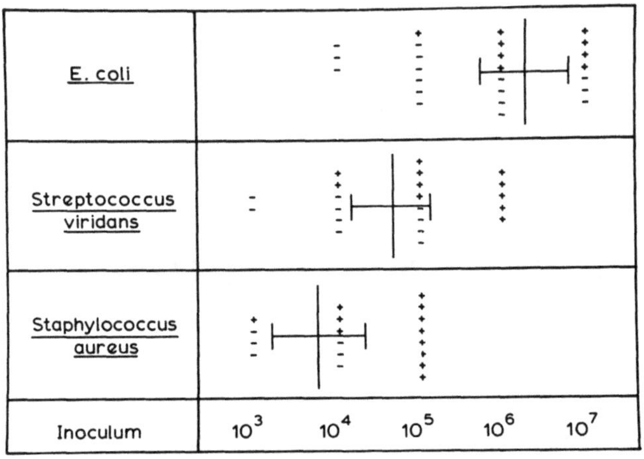

Figure 10. Number of colony-forming units (CFU) of different bacteria required to produce infection after intravenous inoculation into rabbits with NBTVs of the aortic valve. Reproduced from Freedman and Valone[6] with permission.

aortic-valve vegetations in the rabbit. In addition, the rat has proved to be more susceptible to the development of infective endocarditis (IE) than the rabbit.[7]

Durack *et al.*[8] have produced infection on the right side of the heart in rabbits with as few as 10^2–10^3 α-hemolytic streptococci inoculated intravenously (1 of 4 animals). We have produced infection on the aortic valve with the intravenous injection of 10^3 colony-forming units (CFU) of *Staph. aureus* (1 of 4 animals).[6]

Thus, a fresh endocardial vegetation is exquisitely sensitive to colonization by bacteria commonly responsible for IE [see Figures 1 and 2 (Chapter 1)]. This is of considerable importance, since, in fact, a source for bacteremia cannot be demonstrated in almost half of patients with IE.[9–11] If vegetations in man are as susceptible to infection as those in the rabbit or rat, it is obvious that the dissemination of very few bacteria would be sufficient to induce infection. Bacteremias of such magnitude occur under a wide variety of clinical circumstances (including hard chewing) and are not generally, nor would they be expected to be, accompanied by clinical signs or symptoms.

Another factor which has been noted to influence the capacity of bacteria to induce infection is their stickiness. The sticking of certain bacteria to nonbacterial thrombotic vegetations (NBTVs) depends on their ability to produce dextran.[12] Non-dextran-producing mutants of α-hemolytic streptococci are less able to induce infection of NBTVs *in vivo* and less able to stick to damaged valves *in vitro* than dextran-producing strains of the same organism[13,14] It is of interest that platelets enhance sticking of both dextran-producing and non-dextran-producing mutants *in vitro*.[15] These observations are of considerable interest, since IE in man is frequently due to dextran-producing strains of mouth streptococci, despite the simultaneous presence of non-dextran-producing strains in the blood cultures of patients after tooth extraction[12] and since platelets are important in the formation of NBTVs.[1] Stickiness may also play a role in the selection of organisms contaminating atrioventricular (A-V) shunts (see Section 4.3.2.1h).

In summary, bacteria have different capacities to induce infection of NBTVs. This is likely to be one of the factors of importance in determining the frequency of infection with different microorganisms. A study of mouth streptococci has shown that dextran production is a factor of significance in determining their ability to adhere *in vitro* to NBTVs and to induce experimental endocarditis in rabbits. In addition, it has been found that platelets are important in enhancing sticking of streptococci. This is of interest, since platelet aggregates are a major component of the NBTVs. An effort to prevent infection of experimental NBTVs by administration of an agent which prevents platelet sticking (aspirin) was, however, not successful—perhaps because the effect of aspirin in the rabbit was not sufficient to overcome the strong stimulus of trauma with a foreign body to platelet–fibrin vegetation formation, or because the number of bacteria used to induce infection was too large to be influenced by the effect of the aspirin.[16]

Recent investigations have revealed that there are other factors which are likely to play an important role in the physiopathology of intravascular infection which are related to bacterial stickiness. For example, preimmunization decreases the ability of *Streptococcus sanguis* to induce experimental IE and preformed antibody decreases the ability of *Str. sanguis* to adhere to a platelet–fibrin thrombus *in vitro*.[146] This effect does not appear to be mediated entirely by dextran. On the other hand, dextran production by bacteria *in vitro* correlates with antibiotic resistance *in vivo*.[147] The explanation for this relationship is not evident.

Subinhibitory concentrations of penicillin have been shown to decrease adherence of streptococci to fibrin–platelet clots *in vitro* and to damaged heart valves *in vivo*.[148,149,150] Teichoic acids may also be important in determining the capacity of streptococci and staphylococci to adhere to damaged heart valves.[150–153]

Susceptibility to the bactericidal properties (antibody and complement) of serum may be an additional important factor in determining the capability of different bacteria to establish IE. Durack and Beeson[17] have demonstrated in rabbits that there is a major difference in the evolution of IE due to different strains of *E. coli* according to their serum susceptibility. Bacteria sensitive to serum are rapidly destroyed after initiating infection in a cardiac vegetation, whereas those which are resistant to this effect of serum induce lasting infection.[17] Archer and Fekety[18] have shown that IE due to different strains of *Pseudomonas* is related to the bactericidal activity of serum against these strains, and Kaspar and Drutz[19] have demonstrated the same relationship with gonococci. This thesis is strengthened by the demonstration that *E. coli* sensitive to the serum bactericidal system and avirulent in normal rabbits are able to establish IE in complement-deficient rabbits.[17] On the other hand, complement-deficient mice are more susceptible to *Candida* infection than normal mice, even though *Candida* microorganisms are not susceptible to killing by antibody and complement in normal mice.[20]

The idea that bacterial aggregates due to the presence of agglutinating antibody are an important factor in the initial colonization of NBTVs[21] has not been substantiated in careful studies of the early events in IE in rabbits.[1,2]

4.2. TYPES AND SOURCE OF BACTERIA RESPONSIBLE FOR INTRAVASCULAR INFECTION

4.2.1. Infective Endocarditis

A wide variety of microorganisms are capable of producing intravascular infection in man and in experimental animals. Considerable emphasis has been given to the changing bacteriological spectrum of IE in recent years. This no doubt reflects the changing sources of bacteremia as well as the effectiveness of antibiotics and the frequency of their use for the early treatment of infections due to the pneumococcus, gonococcus, and β-hemolytic streptococcus.

4.2.1.1. Types of Bacteria

The types of bacteria responsible for intravascular infection depend on the population under study. In drug addicts, infection is usually due to staphylococci and *Pseudomonas* species.[22] Interestingly, contrary to what one would have expected, the source of staphylococci is not necessarily contamination of the material used by the addicts, but rather the staphylococci residing on the skin of such subjects.[23] Nevertheless, it is likely that contamination of material used for injection may also play a role, since "outbreaks" of endocarditis have been reported with organisms such as *Candida, Pseudomonas aeruginosa,* and *Serratia marcescens.*[22,24–26]

After cardiac surgery, infection with *Staph. epidermidis,* gram-negative bacilli, and *Candida albicans* and diphtheroids is common.[27–30] In these circumstances, the spectrum of infecting organisms will be determined by the nature of the antibiotics administered "prophylactically."[31]

Infection with more than one strain of bacterium is said to be rare; Weinstein and Rubin[32] cite a frequency of 0.28%, and Watanakunakorn,[22] after reviewing the literature, concludes that it is uncommon. On the other hand, recent reports suggest that mixed infection is much more common than was previously appreciated[33]: Mostaghim and Millard[34] recovered 76 microorganisms from 64 patients, Nager *et al.*[35] recovered 2 microorganisms in 4% of 227 cases (26% of which were culture-negative), and a similar finding was reported by Pedersen and Petersen,[36] whereas Welsby[37] found mixed infections in 7 of 91 patients.

The problem is an important one, since the knowledge of the presence of more than one infecting microorganism has considerable influence on the interpretation of antibiotic sensitivities and the level of serum bactericidal activity.[38] It is also important in any effort to localize the site of intravascular infection by cultures taken from various sites within the vascular system.[39]

It is possible that mixed infection is more frequently recognized today because of an improvement in microbiological methodology or because of the development of IE in patients (addicts, postcardiac surgery) subject to bacteremia from multicontaminated sources.

Geography is another important factor in determining the frequency of infection with certain microorganisms. It has been pointed out that in the reports of endocarditis among drug addicts, most of the *Candida* infections have come from New York City of Los Angeles. In Detroit, staphylococcus was the major organism until 1969, at which time *Pseudomonas* made its appearance.[22] In a report from the University College Hospital in Ibadan, Nigeria, among 41 culture-proven cases of endocarditis in Nigerians, only 2 were due to *Str. viridans* and 4 to *Str. faecalis,* whereas 21 were due to staphylococci.[40]

Thus, it is difficult to speak of the prevalence of different bacteria as a cause of IE without taking into consideration the characteristics of the population and the microecology to which they are exposed.

Nevertheless, it would appear that streptococci and staphylococci represent about 90% of the microorganisms responsible for IE in the general population. Group D streptococci constitute a variable proportion (about 10–20%) of the streptococci. The remaining 10% of microorganisms can be almost anything—e.g., fungi, pneumococcus, gonococcus, Q fever, *Mycobacteria,* various gram-negative bacilli, or *Hemophilus*.

4.2.1.2. Source of Infection

The source of infection in patients with IE is often unknown. This may be related to the frequent long delay between the onset of symptoms and the establishment of the diagnosis. In addition, as mentioned in Section 4.1, the number of organisms entering the bloodstream sufficient to produce infection of a susceptible vegetation may be so small as to pass unnoticed from the clinical point of view.

Another problem in trying to establish the source of infection is that many predisposing circumstances occur so frequently that it is virtually impossible to determine the rate of occurrence of the event under study in populations which do not develop IE.

For example, there is considerable controversy today concerning the relation of dental manipulations to the development of IE.[34] It is generally considered that in about 25% of patients with streptococcal endocarditis, dental procedures were recognizable as the source of bacteremia initiating infection. This estimate must be looked upon with considerable skepticism, however, since studies of this question have been retrospective and have employed widely varying criteria for establishing the relation between the suspect procedure and IE.

In a certain number of patients, there is an unequivocal association between procedure and infection.[41] Unfortunately, we are not in the habit of obtaining a history of prior dental procedures in patients with other unrelated illnesses. Nevertheless, streptococcal bacteremia is well documented after dental procedures, and recent studies in rabbits with NBTVs by McGowan and Hardie[42] and Bahn *et al.*[43] have demonstrated the ease with which streptococci introduced into the site of dental trauma induce IE. This is an interesting model and might have particular application to the effort to determine effective regimens for the prevention of IE in man.

Starkebaum *et al.*[44] have studied the duration of delay in onset of symptoms of IE after dental procedures and found that in 85% of patients in whom a relation between tooth extraction and IE was highly probable, symptoms began within 2 weeks of the extraction. About 20% had longer symptomatic incubation periods; a few did not develop symptoms until 8 weeks after extraction. Thus, even in infections due to "benign" *Str. viridans,* symptoms of IE occur promptly after the event causing bacteremia. One should be skeptical in attributing IE to an event believed responsible for provoking bacteremia when that event took place more than 2 weeks prior to the development of symptoms. Looked at from another point of view, it is important for the physician to carefully observe patients known to be at risk of developing IE for about 2 weeks after a procedure capable of producing bacteremia. It is to be hoped that this practice will shorten the 5-week median time between onset of symptoms and diagnosis. In some instances, the delay in diagnosis extended beyond 20 weeks. Unfortunately, the onset of symptoms is often so insidious that there is considerable difficulty in retrospectively determining the beginning of illness within a time span of less than 1–2 weeks.

In addition, there may be circumstances wherein infection due to indolent microorganisms might not declare itself for weeks, months, or even years after the introduction of bacteria. I am thinking especially of patients with Spitz–Holter valves (A-V shunts) and heart and aortic-graft surgery. I think that the 2-week guideline will have particular usefulness in the evaluation of the source of intravascular infections in patients not previously subjected to prosthetic cardiovascular surgery.

Sipes *et al.*,[11] as well as Everett and Hirschmann,[45] recently reviewed the sources of bacteremia potentially responsible for the initiation of IE. The list is long. Bacteremia probably does not occur in normal subjects, but it has been speculated that it may occur after normal defecation.[46] Virtually any procedure which traumatizes the normal (not to speak of diseased) epithelium in man is capable of inducing discharge of bacteria into the bloodstream (Table 1). Of particular importance as sources of infection for IE are procedures involving the oropharynx, genitourinary tract, and cardiovascular system. In hospital practice, sepsis arises commonly from contamination of intravenous infusions. This subject has recently been reviewed in detail by Maki.[47] Hornick[48] has enumerated the sources of microbial contamination associated with cardiovascular surgery. The possible sources of infection were so numerous in his study that it is a wonder that all patients with prosthetic valves do not develop endocarditis.

There is little information available which defines the risk of developing endocarditis after a procedure known to produce bacteremia. For example, blood

TABLE 1
Causes of Bacteremia

Oropharynx	
Tooth extraction	Oral irrigation devices
Gingivitis	Tonsillectomy
Dental cleaning	Nasotracheal intubation
Tooth brushing	Nasotracheal suctioning
Chewing hard candy	Rigid-tube bronchoscopy
Gastrointestinal tract	
Endoscopy	Sigmoidoscopy
Endoscopic retrograde cholangiopancreatography	Barium enema
	Liver biopsy
Genitourinary tract	
Urethral catheterization	Third stage of labor
Removal of indwelling urethral catheter	IUD
Urethral dilatation	Normal pregnancy
Cystoscopy	Induced or spontaneous abortion
Prostatectomy	Caesarian section
Prostatic massage	Uterine D & C
Menstruation	Pelvic infection
Cardiorenal system	
Peritoneal dialysis	Total parenteral nutrition
Hemodialysis	Intravenous fluids
Transvenous pacemakers	Blood products
Indwelling arterial catheters	Pooled platelet transfusions
Arterial catheter pressure transducers	A-V shunts
Cardiopulmonary bypass operations	
Indwelling intravenous plastic catheters (more than 48 hr)	
Miscellaneous	
Minor infections	Severe infections
Peridontitis	
Periapical abscess	
Tonsillitis	

cultures taken after insertion of an intrauterine device in 84 patients and after removal in 16 patients were all sterile.[49] Nevertheless, recent reports by Cobbs[50] and de Swiet *et al.*[51] make it highly likely that IE occurred under just those circumstances. De Swiet's patient died.

In a preantibiotic-era study of dental extraction in 350 "rheumatic children," 4 developed endocarditis and subsequently died.[52] Only 50% of these children had detectable postextraction bacteremia, thus putting the risk of developing endocarditis at about 2% for those patients with underlying valvular heart disease and bacteremia secondary to a dental source.

It summary, whereas staphylococci and streptococci are the most common microorganisms causing IE, the particular frequency of microorganisms in a given community can vary greatly, depending on the nature of the patient population and the frequency of procedures known to be capable of producing bacteremia. Although there are many possible sources of bacteremia, procedures involving the oropharynx, genitourinary system, and cariovascular system are particularly suspect, as well as intravenous therapy. In fact, much more information is needed as to the source of infection in patients with endocarditis. The suggestion that the great majority of infections begin symptomatically within 2 weeks of the causative bacteremia might be helpful in trying to establish the source of bacteremia.

The major problems raised by the knowledge of the ubiquitousness of bacteremia are when to administer prophylactic antibiotics and which ones to administer. As will be seen in Chapter 5, an equally difficult problem is to decide to whom to administer these antibiotics.

4.2.2. Mycotic Aneurysm

Mycotic aneurysm is seen in five clinical settings: (1) infective endocarditis; (2) trauma; (3) direct extension of adjacent infection; (4) malformations of the aorta (coarctation, patent ductus); and (5) unknown etiology (?arteriosclerosis).

The bacteria responsible for infection will obviously vary with the clinical setting.[53,54] In IE and malformations of the aorta, the bacterial spectrum is similar to that discussed in Section 4.2.1. Traumatic lesions are generally due to staphylococci, anaerobes, and gram-negative bacilli such as *Proteus, Pseudomonas,* and *E. coli*. The microorganisms implicated by direct extensions of intraabdominal or thoracic infection will depend on the nature of the original infection. Of interest is the possible occurrence of tuberculous infection of the aorta by direct extension from either vertebral osteomyelitis or caseating lymph nodes.[55]

Infections of vascular grafts are discussed in Section 4.2.3.

Of particular pertinence to the present discussion is the category *unknown etiology*. In these instances, the underlying lesion is, in all likelihood, NBTVs formed on endothelium damaged by arteriosclerosis.[56,57] Thus, the pathogenesis of these infections should be identical to that of IE. On the other hand, there are a number of curious bacteriological aspects which suggest that different pathogenetic mechanisms are involved. The single most common microorganism recovered in these infections is a *Salmonella* species, accounting for about one half of reported infections.[58,59] Occasionally, there is a documented episode of gastroenteritis preceding the development of the aneurysm, but usually the onset is insidious. The second most common agent is *E. coli,* followed by a miscellaneous group including pneumococci, staphylococci, and β-hemolytic streptococci. Despite a presumed hematogenous origin of such infections, positive blood cultures are found in only about half the patients.

It is immediately apparent from the preceding discussion that those microorganisms which spontaneously infect the lower abdominal aorta and femoral and popliteal arteries (the most common location of these infections) are precisely those microorganisms which are rarely responsible for infection of NBTVs in the heart. It would appear that the determinants of infection of NBTVs in the arterial system are different from those in the heart. There is no explanation at hand for why it is that *Salmonella* and *E. coli* seem to be able to establish infection more easily in the arterial vascular system than in the heart. In this regard, it is noteworthy that *Bacteroides fragilis* inoculated intravenously produced serious infection in atherosclerotic (cholesterol-fed) rabbits, whereas similar repeated challenges in normal rabbits were without effect.[60] Interestingly, anemia, thrombosis, and vasculitis were commonly seen in infected rabbits, and the severity of atherosclerosis was more marked in the infected group as compared with noninfected controls. These experiments might provide insight into the question as to why the bacterial spectrum of infection linked to atherosclerosis is different from that of nonatherosclerotic intravascular vegetations.

The role played by the location of the vegetation and its susceptibility to infection is considered in Section 3.

4.2.3. Vascular-Graft Infections

The general problem of infection of vascular grafts is similar in principle to that of infection of prosthetic heart valves. The operative placement of a foreign body provides an environment which is well suited to infections by a variety of different microorganisms. Staphylococci and various gram-negative bacilli account for over 80% of infections, and the mean interval between surgery and diagnosis was 27 weeks in the review of this problem presented by Liekweg *et al.*[4] This interval is much longer than would be considered acceptable to establish a relation between bacteremia and endocarditis. The difference lies in the fact that although hematogenous infection of grafts is demonstrable experimentally and is believed to occur clinically, this is by no means the usual route.

Local infection of the limb or groin is frequently implicated as the site of origin of the infecting microorganisms and in the view of some surgeons is far and away the most common source of these infections. This may explain why it is that many such infections are not associated with positive blood cultures.

4.3. SUSCEPTIBILITY OF NONBACTERIAL THROMBOTIC VEGETATION TO INFECTION

There is considerable clinical evidence which indicates that whereas any endothelial injury or NBTV may become the site of establishment of infection, there are considerable differences in susceptibility to infection depending upon the location of the lesion within the vascular system and upon its stage of development.

4.3.1. Size of Nonbacterial Thrombotic Vegetation

The question as to whether the size of the underlying vascular lesion is important in determining the susceptibility to infection is extremely important, since autopsy diagnosis and morphological study depend upon being able to find the lesion. It is evident that it is often clinically impossible to determine whether a patient with bacteremia has an infected intravascular vegetation or not. Our traditional view of the causes and consequences of IE, for example, are based on autopsy studies from the preantibiotic era. Vegetations were large and easy to find. Today, however, we are detecting bacteremia more often and patients with bacteremia are investigated at a much earlier stage of their disease than in the preantibiotic era. Furthermore, the liberal (and incorrect) use of antibiotics for virtually any febrile illness would inevitably alter the clinical course of intravascular infection. Nothing is known as to how inadequate (from the therapeutic standpoint) quantities of antibiotics may influence the size of the intravascular vegetations.

Thus, the impressive nature of visible vegetations may have deterred us from developing methods for detecting small, even microscopic, sites of intravascular infection. It is likely that such lesions exist; however, their frequency and clinical importance are unknown. Grant *et al.*[62] commented more than half a century ago that it was necessary to examine human heart valves microscopically ($\times 20$) in order to detect the lesions of NBTV which in their view served as the underlying lesion of IE. It is known that myocardial endothelial cells contain considerable fibrinolytic activity, and this might be effective in limiting the growth of vegetations under special circumstances.[63] In most experimental circumstances, infected vegetations grow rapidly to an easily visible size. That this need not always be the case, however, was seen in studies of IE in warfarinized rabbits, in which rabbits developed lethal IE without valvular vegetations visible to the naked eye.

There are several experimental studies which demonstrate that lesions of the endocardium or valve epithelium which are *invisible to the naked eye and undetectable with random microscopic sections* may serve as the seat of development of infective IE and may remain undetectable to the point where the animal has died of its infection.

It was shown by Durack *et al.*[8] that insertion of a plastic catheter in the right heart for 5 min (moving it back and forth) and then withdrawing it was sufficient, when immediately followed by an intravenous injection of 10^8 *Str. viridans,* to provoke infective endocarditis in 3 of 4 animals. Although no study was made of the rabbit endocardium immediately after catheterization, this experiment strongly suggests that a tiny, if not microscopic, endothelial lesion is all that is necessary to induce susceptibility to IE under the proper circumstances.

More to the point is a study carried out examining the effect of warfarin on the development and course of α-hemolytic streptococcus endocarditis in rabbits.[6] Anticoagulated rabbits with a plastic catheter in place in the left or right heart for 4 days showed no gross evidence of valve damage, and random sections of aortic and tricuspid valves were interpreted as normal. However, inoculation of 10^6 α-hemolytic streptoccocci regularly produced IE which was rapidly fatal in a period of 2–3 days. *Examination of the hearts of these rabbits did not reveal any gross or microscopic evidence of valve damage or infections.* One might ask how it is possible to say that these animals had IE. The argument is based on the following reasoning:

1. All blood cultures were positive 48 hr after infection, containing 10^2–10^3 CFU of α-hemolytic streptococci/ml blood. When the same number of bacteria were injected into rabbits which were warfarinized but which had not been catheterized, the blood cultures were sterile at 48 hr, and all rabbits were in good health. Furthermore, injection of lower inocula in catheterized anticoagulated rabbits did not reveal any increased susceptibility to infection.

2. Culture of the aortic valves was uniformly positive, but with a number of microorganisms lower by 2–3 logs than that found in IE in nonwarfarinized rabbits. On the right side of the heart, the valves were sterile or contained a small number of bacteria consistent with contamination by bacteria circulating in the blood. It was thought that perhaps the catheter or its contents served as the source of infection in these animals, but cultures revealed only a number of microorganisms consistent with contamination by bacteria in the blood.

These experiments were provocative from several points of view: the ability of warfarin to prevent the visible development of intracardiac vegetations as well as the hemorrhagic syndrome and increased mortality of anticoagulated rabbits with IE. These latter aspects of the experiments will be discussed later. For the immediate discussion, the point of interest is that these rabbits died of endocarditis which would not have been detected with current methods of study of endocarditis in man.

Hook and Sande[64] have observed the same phenomena in left-sided endocarditis in the rabbit and have gone on to examine the effect of penicillin in the treatment of endocarditis "without vegetations." The relation of size of the vegetation to response to antibiotic treatment is discussed in Chapter 5, and the effect of anticoagulants is considered in Sections 5.1.1 and 6.3.2.

In summary, the endothelial lesion serving as the site of development of IE may not be detectable upon gross examination and yet may be as susceptible to infection as one that is easily visible grossly. The extent to which microscopic IE (or intravascular infection elsewhere) plays a role in the clinical evolution of bacteremia is a matter of conjecture at present.

4.3.2. Localization and Frequency within the Vascular System

4.3.2.1. Clinical Data

It is difficult to talk about the frequency of intravascular infection (Table 2), since so much depends upon the criteria for diagnosis, the population under study, the availability of hemodialysis, cardiovascular surgery, the prevalence of intravenous drug usage, and other factors. In addition, much depends upon the care with which intravascular infection is sought at autopsy. I have the impression that in a general university-hospital patient population, about as many cases of endocarditis are diagnosed for the first time at autopsy as are diagnosed clinically. In Nigeria, 44% of 90 cases were first diagnosed at autopsy.[40] In patients over 60 years of age, the diagnosis is often missed clinically. In a recent series of patients diagnosed at autopsy, the diagnosis of IE was not suspected clinically in 60% of patients. In the absence of a heart murmur, IE was suspected in only 9% of patients.[75] Of course, diagnoses established exclusively at autopsy are often in patients with underlying illness complicated by prolonged intravenous (often intracardiac) infusion, in patients with impaired host defense mechanisms, or in patients treated with cortisone or potent cytotoxic agents. It is obviously necessary to define which patients one is talking about if one is to draw any meaningful conclusions about the prevalence of this infection. With these reservations in mind, I will nevertheless cite some figures from the literature which illustrate the general magnitude of the problem and the differences in susceptibility to infection in different parts of the vascular system.

Starting from the standpoint of clinical diagnosis, two recent studies cite incidence rates of 11–50 patients per million population per year.[9,37] In other terms, a perusal of recent reviews from different university hospitals indicates

TABLE 2
Estimated Risk of Developing Intravascular Infection

Subjects at risk	Estimated risk	Ref. no.
	Estimated risk of infective endocarditis	
General population	11–50 patients/million population/yr	9, 37
All hospital admissions	0.3–3.0/1000 admissions	65
All pediatric admissions	0.2–0.5/1000 admissions	66
Rheumatic heart disease (preantibiotic era)	4–7%	67
Prosthetic heart valves		
Aortic	2.2–2.7%/patient–year	68
Mitral	0.1–0.4%/patient–year	68
Drug addicts	30% within 2 years	69
Congenital heart disease		
Aortic stenosis	1.8/1000 patient–years	70
Ventricular septal defect	1.5/1000 patient–years	70
Pulmonary stenosis	0.2/1000 patient–years	70
Mitral-valve prolapse	?(8%)	71
Chronic hemodialysis	?(5%)	72
Previous IE		
Once	8–9%	11
Twice	25%	11
	Estimated risk of other intravascular infections	
Primary mycotic aneurysm (autopsy)	3 cases/50 years	73
Aortoiliac grafts	0.7–1.2%	4
Femoropopliteal grafts	1.6–5.9%	4
Ventriculo atrial shunts	27%	74

that 10–15 patients are likely to be seen per year.[10,22,34–36] Kaye[65] has estimated the frequency to be between 0.3 and 3.0 cases per 1000 hospital admissions. At the Children's Medical Center in Boston, the rate of IE has risen from 0.22/1000 hospital admissions in 1943–1952 to 0.55/1000 admissions in 1963–1972.[66]

Between 1933 and 1965, the yearly variation at the Boston City Hospital was between 15 and 44 cases for patients with IE.[22,76] This argues against a significant change in the overall frequency of infection during this period of time.

a. Mycotic Aneurysm. These figures are of particular interest, because at the same institution between 1902 and 1951, there was a careful review of cases with mycotic aneurysms. In 22,792 autopsies, the diagnosis of mycotic aneurysm was made only 9 times, and only 3 or 4 of these cases would fit into the category of mycotic aneurysm of unknown etiology, that is, engrafted on arteriosclerotic vegetations without trauma, adjacent infection, or malformation of the aorta.[73]

This, from an institution renowned for its interest in the study of bacteremia and other infectious diseases. To my mind, this is a dramatic demonstration of the differences in susceptibility to infection of intracardiac vegetations as compared to intravascular vegetations in relation to arteriosclerosis of the aorta.

b. Rheumatic Heart Disease. In patients with rheumatic heart disease in the preantibiotic era, according to the review by Kerr,(67) between 4 and 7% of patients with rheumatic heart disease developed IE. IE was the cause of death in 20–30% of rheumatic-heart-disease patients. In the analysis by Watanakunakorn,(22) there has been no decrease in the risk of developing IE since the introduction of antibiotics. Of course, there has been a significant change in prognosis.

c. Prosthetic Heart Valves. All analyses of the frequency of valve involvement in infection in rheumatic heart disease have shown the mitral valve to be most frequently involved, followed by the aortic, pulmonary, and tricuspid valves.(22) This progression follows the frequency with which the various valves are involved by the rheumatic process [and curiously by NBTVs in cancer and disseminated intravascular coagulation (DIC); it is also consistent with the left-heart predominance of endocardial lesions in Löffler's endocarditis]. It is thus difficult to judge from these data whether IE is more likely to occur on a *diseased valve* on the left side of the heart as compared with the right side.

Some notion of the difference in susceptibility to infection of the two sides of the heart is obtained by reference to the frequency of infection following the *placement of prosthetic heart* valves. In the Mayo Clinic series of 4586 patients who received prosthetic valves and were followed for from 6 months to 10 years, infections developed on 1.3% of aortic valves, 0.61% of mitral valves, and in none of 275 valves placed on the right side of the heart.(75) Surgery is shorter and simpler on the right side of the heart, and so these figures may reflect merely less opportunity for perioperative contamination in patients with right-heart-valve operations. On the other hand, since two thirds of the infections occurred more than 2 months after operation, these are probably the most convincing clinical data demonstrating an increased susceptibility of left-heart lesions to IE as compared with comparable lesions of the right heart.

It is of some interest that in patients with prosthetic heart valves, infection occurs 2–3 times more commonly on the aortic prosthesis than on the mitral prosthesis.(68,77,78) This difference is apparent in patients with Starr–Edwards valves as well as in patients receiving Hancock bioprosthetic heterografts.(68) The reason for the difference in susceptibility to infection within the left side of the heart is not understood. The problem has not been studied in animals. That this difference is in contrast to the frequency of valve involvement in patients with rheumatic heart disease confirms the impossibility of drawing conclusions about susceptibility to infection in circumstances (rheumatic heart disease) in which there is an unequal distribution of the underlying lesion giving rise to the increased susceptibility to infection.

It has become common practice to separate infections of prosthetic valves into those occurring early, within 1–2 months of operation, and those occurring late, after 1–2 months. The division is arbitrary. In general, there are higher frequencies of infection with staphylococci, fungi, and gram-negative microorganisms in the early postoperative period. This is to be expected, since infections in the early postoperative period occur at the time that patients receive prophylactic antibiotics effective against streptococci.

Of greater interest is the fact that this preponderance of staphylococci, fungi, and gram-negative bacteria persists even in late prosthetic-valve endocarditis (PVE). The explanation for this is not clear, but it is possible that microorganisms introduced into the bloodstream at the time of operation or in the early postoperative period do not become manifest until much later.[79–81] *Candida* infection of prosthetic valves is known to be capable of lying dormant for prolonged periods of time (>6 months).[82]

A strong argument in favor of this thesis is a study of an outbreak of *Staph. epidermidis* PVE due to operating-room contamination.[80] There was a clustering of the time of operation and diagnosis, the interval between the two varying from 11 days to 20 months (mean: 4 months). Thus, in this study of PVE, in which it is possible to be reasonably certain that infection of the prosthesis occurred early, 7 of the 10 patients would have to be classified as late PVE. A similar observation was made in an outbreak of *Staph. epidermidis* endocarditis in 6 patients receiving porcine valve xenografts. In this instance, 4 of the 6 patients would be classified as "late" endocarditis, the longest interval between surgery and diagnosis of infection being 25 months.[83]

Early PVE is decreasing in frequency, due probably to improvements in operative technique and postoperative management and perhaps also to more effective suppression of early manifestations of valve infections by antibiotics. Overall, the frequency of early PVE has fallen from 2.53 to 0.75%.[81] In recent publications from some centers, the rates are even lower, 0.4%, and zero in 800 patients.[68,84] In the face of these lower rates of early PVE, a recent analysis of linearized rates of PVE (percentage per patient–year) revealed rates of infection of aortic-valve prostheses of 2.2–2.7% and of mitral-valve prostheses of 0.1–1.4% for heterografts and Starr–Edwards valves, respectively.[68] This level of risk has persisted over about 10 years of follow-up and emphasizes the continued susceptibility of prosthetic valves to intravascular infection.

d. Congenital Heart Disease. Congenital heart disease represents fertile ground for the development of IE. In the preantibiotic era, these patients were at least as susceptible to the development of IE as patients with rheumatic disease. All types of congenital heart disease have been associated with IE. It is difficult to say whether one lesion is more susceptible to infection than another, since the reported data are presented in terms of the role of infection causing the death of patients with a particular defect. The figures cited by Kerr[67] report IE as the cause of death in 20–40% of deaths due to congenital abnormalities of the aortic valve, interventricular septal defect, tetralogy of Fallot, and patent ductus arteriosus. In patients with pulmonary stenosis, about 15% of deaths were due to infection; in coarctation of the aorta, just over 10%; and in intraatrial septal defects, virtually zero.[67]

On the other hand, recent studies of the natural history of congenital heart disease provide data which clearly support the previous finding of increased risk of developing IE in the left heart as compared to the right heart. The incidence of IE in patients with aortic stenosis (1.8/1000 patient–years) or ventricular septal defect (1.5/1000 patient–years) was significantly higher than in patients with pulmonary stenosis (0.2/1000 patient–years).[70] Whereas there was a 5-fold decrease in the risk of developing IE after surgical repair of ventricular septal defect, the risk was not changed after prosthetic-valve placement for repair of aortic stenosis.

e. Aortoiliac Grafts. The rate of infection of aortoiliac grafts varies from 0.7 to 1.2%. It is higher for aortofemoral and femoropopliteal grafts (1.6–5.9%). It is hard to compare these figures with those for infection of prosthetic heart valves, since local infection plays a much more important role in aortoiliac grafts.[4]

Thus, although the data for rheumatic heart disease are unsatisfactory, clinical evidence from long-term follow-up of children with congenital heart disease and from the postoperative course of surgical patients shows that the risk of developing IE is greater with lesions in the left side than in the right side of the heart, and that infections are still less frequent in the thoracic aorta, and rare indeed in the bifurcation of the aorta. It is noteworthy also that, as referred to earlier, NBTVs were found at autopsy more frequently on the left side of the heart than on the right, irrespective of the mechanism.

f. Venous System. As mentioned in Section 3.9, although infections of NBTVs of the venous system do occur and may be of a most serious nature, they must be rare indeed relative to the trauma and frequent sterile thrombotic lesions provoked daily in the course of normal hospital medical practice. On the other hand, total parenteral nutrition has been associated with a rate of septicemia of 7–72%, and some instances of septic thrombophlebitis have been discovered only at autopsy.[85] The relative resistance of NBTVs in the venous system to infection is reflected in the relative ease of treatment of such infections when they do occur.[86]

g. Drug Addicts. For obvious reasons, the estimation of the risk of developing IE among drug addicts is difficult and of little utility. It is clear, however, that IE is a common complication of drug usage. The majority (about three fourths) of reported patients have no underlying heart disease, and about half the infections involve the tricuspid valve.[22] It has become evident, however, that the localization of infection in drug addicts depends upon the infecting microorganism. Three reports have emphasized that staphylococcal infection affects primarily the tricuspid valve, whereas enterococcal infection affects principally the left side of the heart.[26,87,88] The prognosis of right-sided heart infection has been consistently better than that of left-heart infection. This difference in prognosis is clearly illustrated in a series of addicts with *S. marcescens* endocarditis: 12 of 13 patients with aortic- or mitral-valve involvement died, whereas 5 of 6 patients with tricuspid-valve involvement survived.[25] It is evident that conclusions concerning the efficacy of any medical or surgical program of treatment should consider right-heart infections separately from those of the left heart.

The pathogenesis of IE in drug addicts remains a mystery. There is no good explanation for why it is that this population is susceptible to infection at all and why staphylococci establish infection predominantly on the right side of the heart whereas group D streptococci do so mainly on the left. The mechanisms that seem worthy of consideration include NBTV formation secondary to localization of foreign bodies on heart valves[89] or to circulating immune complexes due to repeated injection of foreign material, or perhaps resulting from the known high frequency of hepatitis B infection in this population. Alternatively, it is possible that the repeated intravenous injections of foreign material or certain bacteria provoke a hypercoagulable state with consequent NBTV formation or perhaps activate the complement system, thus provoking endothelial damage.[90,91] The source of bacterial contamination has already been considered (see Section 4.2.1.2). The frequency of local skin and subcutaneous abscesses in this population may also be important. Some of these patients develop mycotic aneurysms in the vicinity of injection sites. Drug addicts with prosthetic valves (as treatment for previous IE) who continue intravenous drug use have a 30% chance of developing IE within about 2 years.[69]

h. Ventriculoatrial Shunts. Ventriculoatrial shunts are at high risk of becoming infected. Schoenbaum *et al.*[74] reported the development of infection in 27% of shunted patients. About three fourths of infections were apparent within 4 months of operation. This fact, together with the predominance of *Staph. epidermidis* (Baird–Parker subgroup S II A) as the infecting microorganism (50% of infections) and *Staph. aureus* as the second most common microoorganism (25%), are strong arguments in favor of local contamination as the predominant source of infection. The predominance of a specific subgroup of *Staph. epidermidis* is of interest because of the capacity of this microorganism to produce a mucoid substance which might be protective against the lytic action of lysosyme and which may enhance sticking of bacteria to smooth surfaces.[92,93]

i. Hemodialysis. Regularly dialyzed patients are also at risk of developing IE. Goodman *et al.*[94] reported 2 such patients among 47 in a chronic dialysis program. Leonard *et al.*[95] presented 9 examples of this problem and reviewed an additional 18 reported cases. On the average, 20 months elapsed between the onset of dialysis and endocarditis, and the majority of patients (20/27) were not known to have prior heart diseases. This complication of hemodialysis occurs in patients with peripheral A-V shunts or cannulas. Whereas the pathogenesis of infection in patients with shunts was originally thought to be due to the formation of NBTVs in association with increased aortic output,[94] the development of IE in patients with cannulas has prompted the suggestions that these infections are more closely related to the pathogenesis of infections as seen in drug addicts.[95] Cannula and fistula infections commonly preceded the development of endocarditis. Of the 4 patients with *Staph. aureus* infection, 2 patients were diagnosed as having right-sided endocarditis, and the other 2 had severe coronary-artery disease. Experimental studies in rabbits confirm this view of the pathogenesis of intravascular infections in patients with A-V shunts.[96]

Whereas staphylococcal endocarditis is predominantly right-sided in addicts (in the absence of underlying heart disease), left-sided infection is more common in dialyzed patients. Perhaps this is due to the accelerated arteriosclerosis known to occur in regularly dialyzed patients.[90] However, there are so many differences between a patient on chronic hemodialysis (antibody production, coagulation mechanisms) and a drug addict that one must exercise caution in proposing an explanation for what appears to be an interesting difference in localization of infection.

j. Infections in the Neonate. There appears to be a remarkable increase in the frequency of IE in the neonate.[97–99] Infection is usually on the right side of the heart and is often associated with evidence of DIC. It is very difficult to diagnose during life. Most authors attribute the recent appearance of so many reported cases to the vigorous diagnostic and resuscitative measures (involving right-heart catheterization via the umbilical vein and parenteral nutrition) currently being applied to newborn infants, although NBTVs due to hemodynamic factors and congenital malformations may also play an important role.[100,101]

k. Infections in the Aged. Almost all discussions of IE comment on the fact that the mean age of patients today is higher than it was in the preantibiotic era. This may be a consequence merely of the general aging of the population. The location of infection within the heart (and the responsible bacteria) seem quite comparable to those in younger patients.[22,75]. Although the prognosis is excellent when the disease is recognized, 60% of patients in a recent series were recognized only at autopsy.[75,102]

One of the interesting aspects of the recent interest in IE in the elderly is that one no longer can find mention of lesions of arteriosclerotic or degenerative heart disease as the site of infection. Despite the rather frequent finding of "degenerative" lesions in autopsy populations without IE, in a recent series of IE in patients over 60 years of age, 38 hearts were examined at autopsy, and only 1 carried the label of "senile calcific aortic stenosis."[75] This is a rather interesting finding, and makes one wonder whether the rarity of infection of aortic arteriosclerotic lesions has something to do with the arteriosclerotic process rather than with its location at the bifurcation of the aorta.

l. Mitral-Valve Prolapse. Mitral-valve prolapse (MVP) has recently been recognized as a lesion serving as the basis for the development of IE.[103] Among 62 patients, follow-up of 9–22 years revealed the development of IE in 5.[104] It is estimated that at least one third of patients with IE and mitral regurgitation have MVP.[105] One can only wonder what this lesion was called in earlier autopsy series and how many patients with this disorder were clinically considered to have rheumatic heart disease. In fact, it is curious that evidence of preceding streptococcal infection was found in 60% of children with MVP but in only 7% of control children with congenital heart disease.[106] The dilemma created by the recognition of MVP is that it has been detected in from 5 to 21% of subjects in routine surveys of healthy young women[105] and in children.[107]

The propensity for NBTV formation in patients with MVP is evident. MVP was found in 40% of patients less than age 45 with transient cerebral ischemia or partial stroke.[108,109] On the other hand, it is important to recognize that IE in subjects with MVP may not be due to infected vegetations located on the surface of the mitral valve.[154] In certain instances of MVP associated with rupture of chordae tendineae, the infected lesion may be established in the left auricle in a thrombotic vegetation resulting from the endothelial "trauma" of a regurgitant jet stream.

Is it necessary to consider antibiotic prophylaxis prior to procedures known to produce bacteremia in all healthy young women with MVP? This subject is under considerable discussion and is discussed further in Section 5.1.5. MVP is considered by some to represent a *forme fruste of Marfan's syndrome,* another condition known to be associated with a significant risk for developing IE.[110-113]

m. Miscellaneous. A wide variety of miscellaneous underlying lesions and disease states have been associated with the development of intravascular infection and endocarditis: severe burns,[114] syphilitic aortitis,[65] Transvenous pacemaker,[115,116] Plastic catheters in the right heart,[117–119] Amyloidosis,[75] Myocardial infarction,[120] Avulsed papillary muscle tip,[121] Idiopathic hypertrophic subaortic stenosis,[122] Traumatic rupture of aortic valve,[123] Foreign body in the heart,[124] Acromegaly,[125] Cogan's syndrome,[126] and calcified mitral annulus fibrosus.[127]

n. Summary. In summary, consideration of the clinical patterns of intravascular infection leads to the conclusion that the left side of the heart is more susceptible to infection than the right and that infections within the aorta are less common than those in the right heart. Furthermore, when the aorta does become involved, there is a peculiar susceptibility to *Salmonella* and *E. coli* infections, microorganisms rarely recovered from patients with IE. NBTVs in the venous system rarely become infected by the hematogenous route. A considerable number of experimental studies which illuminate these observations in man are discussed in the following section.

4.3.2.2. Experimental Findings

Although several experimental models of IE have been proposed in the past, it was only recently that a simple, reproducible small animal model was developed, which has permitted extensive laboratory studies of IE.(128)

It had been observed that indwelling intravenous catheters served as a frequent source of sepsis in hospitalized patients.(118) It was reasoned from this clinical study that placing a plastic catheter in the vena cava of the rabbit and contaminating it with bacteria would lead to the establishment of an infected intravascular vegetation and continuous bacteremia. This would then simulate IE and permit a study of constant bacteremia and its immunological consequences in the laboratory.(128)

Catheters were thus placed, via a peripheral vein, in the inferior vena cava (IVC) of the rabbit and filled with 10^2 *Staph. aureus* bacteria. Surprisingly, nothing happened. A venous thrombus was seen around the catheter and attached to the IVC, and viable bacteria were recovered from the catheter, but blood cultures remained sterile, evidence of metastatic infection did not develop, the heart was normal, and the rabbits remained in good health. Going back to the original series of patients, it was recognized that one had developed streptococcal endocarditis of the right heart in vegetations provoked by an indwelling central venous catheter (Figure 11). It was decided, therefore, to repeat the rabbit experiments, but this time to advance the tip of the catheter to within the right heart. With the use of the same technique employed for the IVC experiments, it was observed that within a few days after placement of the catheter, the rabbits regularly developed IE with bacteremia and metastatic infection. It was evident that it was *much easier to induce infection in the right heart than in the IVC*. By inserting catheters through the carotid or femoral artery, it was shown that one could produce in any part of the heart or aorta NBTVs which could then be infected either by contaminating the catheters with microorganisms or, as first carried out by Durack and Beeson, by the intravenous inoculation of microorganisms.(129–131)

The natural history of infections on the two sides of the heart was different. Infections of the aortic valve with staphylococci or streptococci (or other bacteria) were usually fatal within 10–14 days. Streptococcal infections of the right side of the heart, on the other hand, were rarely fatal and in fact had a natural history which evolved toward spontaneous sterilization of the lesion, despite the continued presence of the catheter responsible for originally inducing the NBTVs [see Figure 8 (Chapter 3)]. There was, however, an important mortality from staphylococcal infection of the right heart (5 of 13 animals dead) within 18 days. Thus, staphylococcal infection seemed to be more virulent than streptococcal infection on the right side of the heart.(6,8,128)

On the left side of the heart, the findings were reversed. When the catheter was removed 24 hr before intravenous inoculation of streptococci, infection

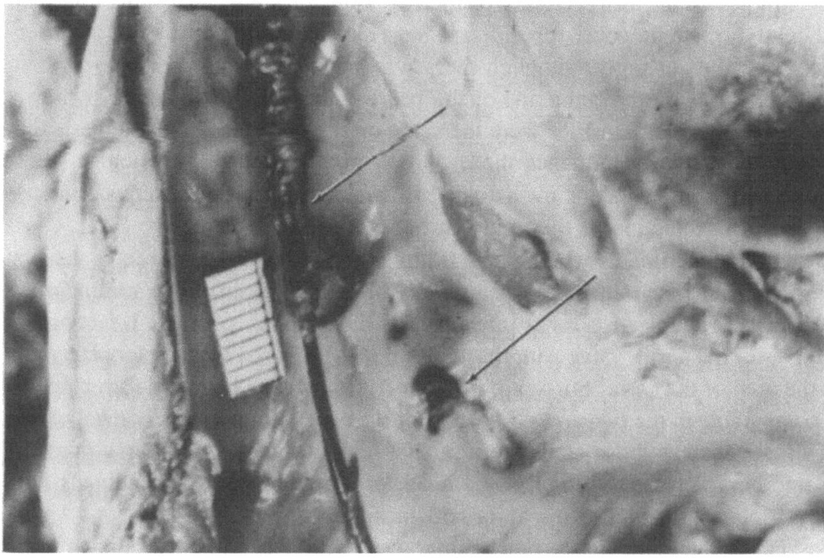

Figure 11. Autopsy photograph of the right auricle of a patient with a central venous catheter *in situ*. Vegetations infected with *Str. viridans* are seen wrapped around the catheter and attached to the right auricle. This is the human conterpart of the rabbit model for the production of IE [see Figures 1 and 2 (Chapter 1)].

occurred uniformly in all animals: 9 of 13 died within 1 week, and 3 of the remaining 4 animals were infected. With left-sided staphylococcal infection, however, the removal of the catheter after initiation of infection markedly changed the evolution of the infection: within 2 weeks, only 3 of 14 animals died and 8 were found to have sterilized their lesions at autopsy. Sterilization was seen even more commonly when the same catheter was removed after staphylococcal infection was established in the right side of the heart. Thus, whereas both staphyloccoccal and streptococcal infections were more virulent on the left side of the heart than on the right side, staphylococci were relatively more virulent than streptococci in right-heart infection, whereas the reverse was found in left-heart infections.[129]

To further study the difference between infections in the right and left sides of the heart, vegetations were induced simultaneously on the two sides of the heart, and α-hemolytic streptococci (or *E. coli*) were injected intravenously. After 48 hr, the number of bacteria recovered from the right side of the heart was found to be several hundred times less than the number recovered from the left side.[6,132] Similar differences were also noted with *C. albicans* infection.[133] This provided additional evidence that the biology of infection on the two sides of the heart is different.

Studies of the *susceptibility* of the two sides of the heart to infection with α-hemolytic streptococci or *Bacteroides* have not demonstrated a difference.[6,134] Interestingly, although there was a lower density of *Bacteroides* in the vegetations on the right side of the heart at the onset of infection, within a few days, bacterial densities were the same on the two sides. This suggests that oxygen tension may influence the evolution of *Bacteroides* infection in IE. If this is an important factor for aerobes, it cannot explain the difference in susceptibility to infection of the right heart and the IVC.

Other experiments which make it unlikely that the difference in O_2 tension (and other chemical attributes of arterial and venous blood) plays an important role in the biology of aerobic infection are those which compare infections of NBTVs of the aortic valve with those of NBTVs localized by catheter placement in the arch of the aorta. Susceptibility to infection with α-hemolytic streptococci is comparable in the two areas, but most of the aortic lesions are sterilized within 14 days, whereas those of the aortic valve remain infected with large numbers of microorganisms, resulting in the death of many animals. The animals with intravascular infection of the aorta remain in good health.[131]

These experiments fit remarkably well with the inferences drawn from clinical observation of the distribution of infection within the vascular system, namely, that host defense mechanisms are active with increasing effectiveness in the right heart, aortic arch, and IVC. The nature of the host defense is unknown, but it is probably cellular and can be inhibited by dexamethasone.[131] Host defense mechanisms are least effective in infections of the left heart (aortic valve). It would seem important to take these host defense mechanisms into consideration when evaluating the efficacy of antibiotics in man.

As discussed in Section 4.1, fresh intracardiac NBTVs are susceptible to infection in the following order: staphylococci, streptococci, *E. coli* (see Figure 10).

Experiments testing the relative susceptibility of right- and left-heart vegetations to intravenous inocula of streptococci or *Bacteroides* have not shown differences. That the problem is complicated, however, is illustrated by experiments demonstrating that susceptibility of NBTVs in different locations to different bacteria may change according to the age of the vegetations under study. In addition, removal of the catheter from the left side of the heart between 8 and 14 days prior to challenge with α-hemolytic streptococci showed a significant decrease in susceptibility to infection when studies were carried out 48 hr after bacterial challenge.[6] This rapid decrease in susceptibility of aortic lesions to infection was noted a century ago.[62]

It is obviously dangerous to try to go too far in comparing disease in man with disease in rabbits. These experiments in rabbits show that the factors which determine the susceptibility of NBTVs in infection in different parts of the vascular system change with aging of the vegetation and that bacterial challenge under these conditions may have different consequences for different bacteria.

They are consistent, however, with the distribution of IE in different intravascular locations in man, and they may further provide insight into the peculiar distribution of staphylococci in the right heart and streptococci in the left heart of drug addicts.

Beyond the question of susceptibility to infection, there is good evidence that the evolution of IE in the rabbit is different in the two sides of the heart. As already mentioned, left-heart infection with staphylococcal or streptococcal infection with the catheter left in place is rapidly fatal. In the right heart, however, streptococcal infection *heals spontaneously,* whereas there is significant mortality associated with staphylococcal infection (although less than in left-heart infections).

It is quite possible that in man, right-heart infection occurs as commonly as left-heart infection, but depending upon the microorganism, may heal spontaneously or heal with a quantity of antibiotics which would not be considered sufficient for left-heart infections. The same could be true of microbial infections of ulcerated plaques in the aorta. The good response to treatment of drug addicts with right-sided endocarditis has already been commented upon.[25,26]

The fascinating aspect of these experiments relates not only to whether or not they are a true reflection of the human condition, but also to the fact that they demonstrate that there are host defense mechanisms at work which can be shown to be remarkably different in effectiveness in vegetations separated by only a few millimeters (aortic valve vs. arch of the aorta). This subject is explored in more detail in Chapter 7.

Another factor which contributes to the peculiar biology of IE has to do with the physics of flow from high-pressure to low-pressure areas within the vascular system.[21,144] Rodbard[144] demonstrated about 20 years ago that bacteria adhere more readily to vessel walls located downstream from an orifice separating a high-pressure source from a low-pressure sink (the Venturi effect). This has been taken to explain the localization of infected vegetations in IE in man. This explanation has served also to explain the rarity of IE in circumstances (such as atrial septal defects) in which pressure differences on two sides of an orifice are not marked.

In view of recent experimental work in rabbits, (cited above), it has been shown that the natural history of intravascular infection is different in different parts of the vascular system despite an equal ability of bacteria to adhere in the different locations studied. Thus, it does not seem likely that the bacterial sticking due to the Venturi effect is an adequate explanation for these differences in the natural history of infection.

It seems more likely to me that the arguments of Rodbard, which do provide good correlations for the clinical frequencies of intravascular infection, are more pertinent to the establishment of NBTVs. If the Venturi effect were important in the pathogenesis of NBTVs by virtue of an increased tendency to local coagulation of the blood, the clinical correlations would remain equally valid. This hypothesis would nevertheless leave unanswered the questions concerning the nature of the antibacterial host defense mechanisms effective in combating intravascular infections.

Finally, it is worth noting that endocarditis is a common cause of considerable financial loss in dairy cows in Hokkaido, Japan. Curiously, the disease occurs predominantly in the *right side* of the heart.[145] Unfortunately, but understandably, there are few bacteriological observations in this remarkable disease in cows.

4.3.3. Pathology of Thrombotic Vegetation

4.3.3.1. Sterile Lesions

Hirschfelder[135] pointed out 75 years ago that the fresh vegetation which formed on the traumatized aortic valve of the dog was composed of platelets and fibrin. Grant *et al.*[62] referred to the microscopic thrombotic lesions in man which they considered to be the underlying lesion of IE as platelet thrombi without signs of an inflammatory reaction. Similar lesions have been found on about one third of prolapsed mitral valves.[109] The careful anatomical study by Durack[1] of vegetations produced by the presence of a plastic catheter in the left heart of the rabbit fully confirms these earlier views. Durack estimated that the major portion of the early lesion was made up of platelets. No collagen was identified. After 3–4 days, the vegetations were progressively covered by endothelium. The catheter was buried under smooth endothelium after 2 weeks. Vegetations progressively decreased in size. Healed infected or noninfected lesions examined after weeks or months are frequently impossible to identify by gross inspection of valve surfaces. Removal of the catheter provoking the formation of NBTVs on the aortic valve in rabbits resulted in disappearance of vegetations within about 10 days.[136]

4.3.3.2. Infected Lesions

In the experimental animal, it is possible to identify bacteria on the surface of the vegetation 30 min after their inoculation (in huge numbers 10^{10}) intravenously[1,2] by scanning-electron-microscopic studies. Microrganisms stick to the surface of the vegetation and seem to be trapped in the meshwork of platelets and fibrin.[1,2,137] At 24 hr, bacterial colonies were surrounded (packaged) by strands of fibrin (Figure 12). After 24 hr, vegetations were larger, there was multiplication of bacteria within them, and the appearance of layers of fibrin and bacteria were interpreted as evidence for reseeding of the vegetation from the bloodstream (Figure 13). Leukocytes were rarely seen within the fully developed vegetation, and those few that were seen were effectively separated from

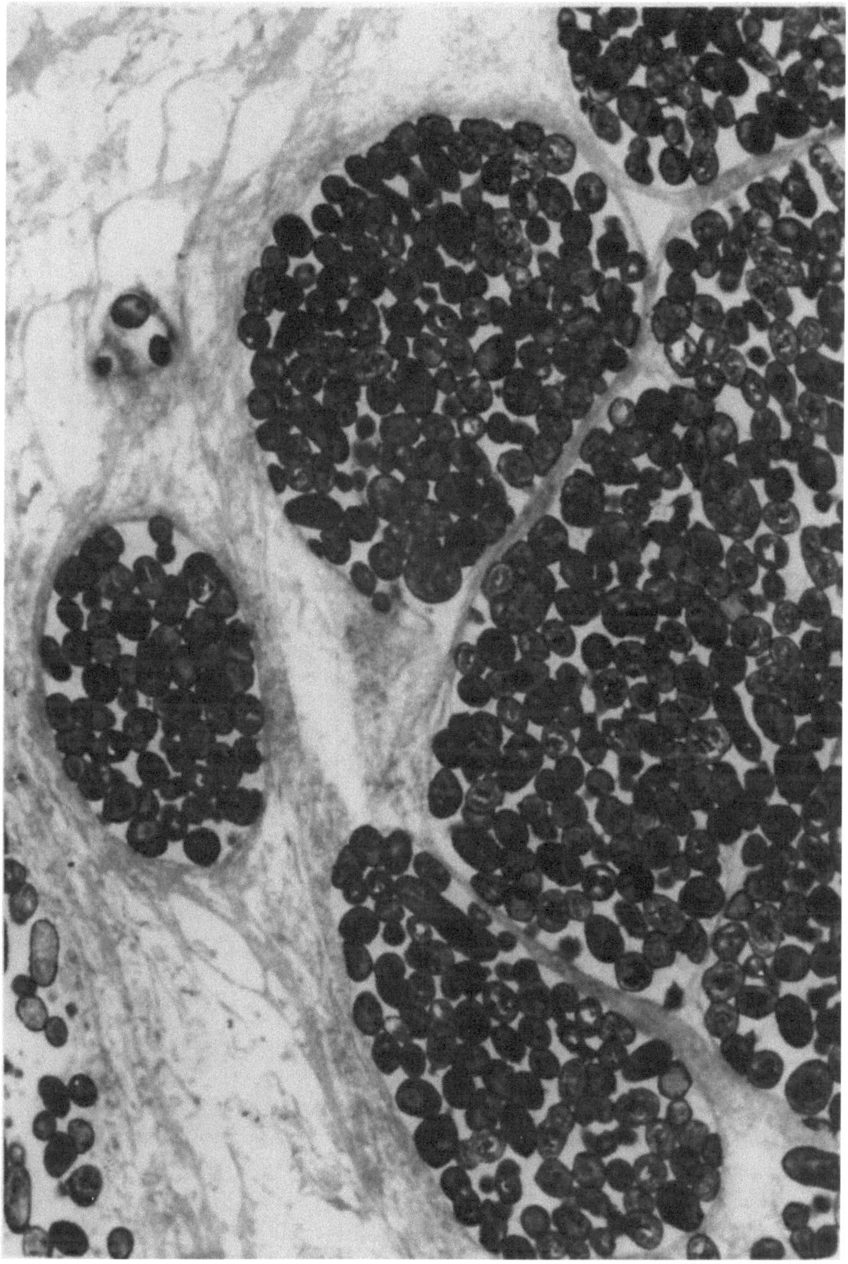

Figure 12. Electron micrograph of colonies of streptococci encapsulated by layers of fibrin in a tricuspid vegetation 24 hr after intravenous injection of *Str. sanguis* into a rabbit with NBTVs. ×7800. This photograph was given to me by Dr. David Durack to whom I am most grateful. Reproduced from Durack[1] with permission.

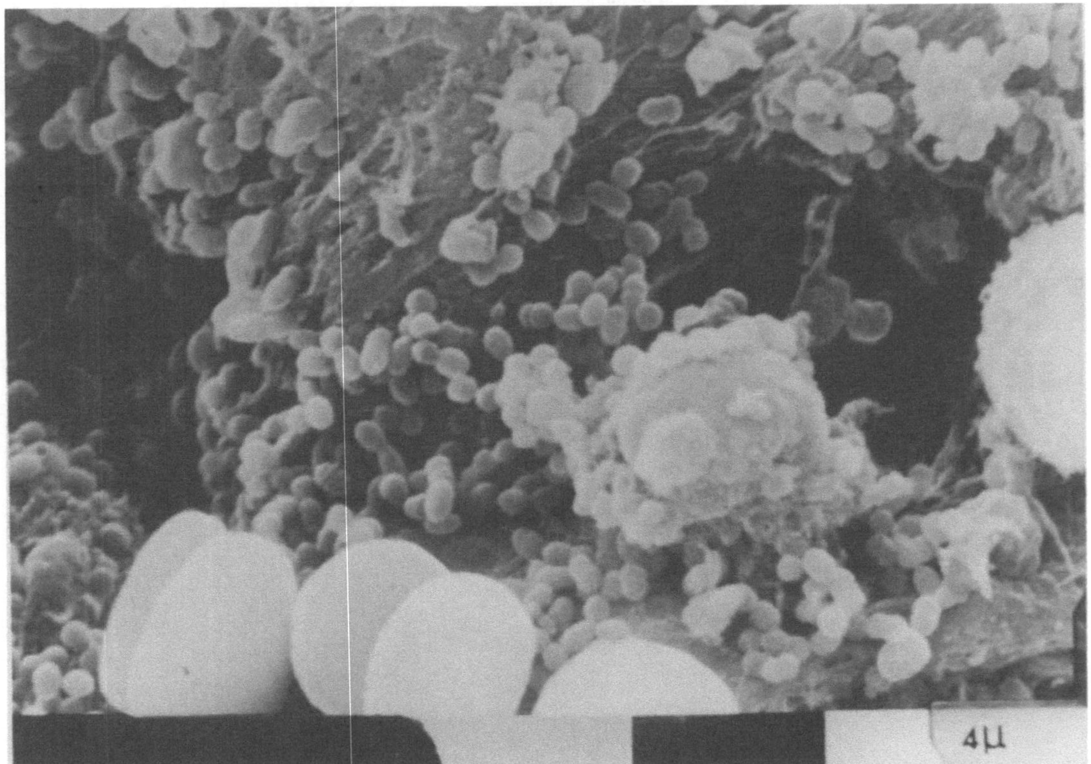

Figure 13. Scanning electron micrograph of a vegetation on the aortic valve of a rabbit 3 days after infection of NBTVs by the intravenous injection of *Str. mitior*. The round smooth objects are erythrocytes; the shaggy cells are leukocytes. Streptococci cover the fibrin surface. This photograph was given to me by Dr. D.A. McGowan, to whom I am most grateful.

bacteria by the layer of fibrin encasing the bacteria (Figure 14). Study of human heart valves removed at operation reveals identical structures of vegetations and similar trapping of microorganisms in the fibrin mesh of the vegetation.[138]

After 24 hr, older, deeper-situated bacterial colonies contained debris and spaces, indicating death of bacteria within these colonies.

Healing consists of progressive endothelialization of the surface of the vegetation, phagocytosis of bacterial debris, and calcification and fibroblastic organization.[139,140] Durack[1] observed a covering of the surface of infected vegetations with elongated mononuclear cells as little as 6 hr after administration of penicillin.

The interest of these recent, elegant studies of the development and evolution of the infected vegetation is that they provide good evidence for four phenomena in IE that have received little consideration:

1. The quantitative importance of platelets in the underlying NBTV. In this regard, it has been possible to detect infected vegetations in rabbits by cardiac imaging after the intravenous administration of indium-111-labeled platelets.[141] Labeled polymorphonuclear leukocytes were not detectable in vegetations with this technique. It is also of considerable interest that platelets greatly facilitate the sticking of streptococci to fibrin clots *in vitro*.[74] But thrombocytopenia does not decrease sticking of streptococci to established NBTVs.[142]

2. The importance of reseeding of the vegetation as a reason for persistence of infection. The phenomenon of reseeding and its importance in the maintenance of infection was demonstrated by the prevention of sterilization of IE of the tricuspid valve in rabbits, even after removal of the catheter, in the presence of concomitant IE of the aortic valve.[131]

3. The "natural death" of bacteria in the center of colonies wrapped up in bundles of fibrin, as a factor working toward sterilization (?strangulation) of infection.

4. The rapidity with which still-infected lesions are "endothelialized" with monocytes after antibiotic treatment. This is a fascinating phenomenon and suggests that such "endothelialization" is prevented either quantitatively, by the number of viable bacteria in a vegetation, or qualitatively, by the rate at which bacteria are able to produce the factor which prevents this covering. This process is perhaps related to the ability of rabbits to spontaneously sterilize right-sided steptococcal endocarditis, since the density of CFU of bacteria in these lesions is generally 2 logs lower than that of lesions on the left side of the heart, which are not sterilized spontaneously.

Recent studies with *Str. faecalis* in rabbits have demonstrated that bacteria which produce proteolytic enzymes provoke vegetations which are smaller and more friable and embolize more easily than bacteria which do not produce these enzymes.[143] The fatal outcome of infection is more rapid in animals infected with proteolytic strains.

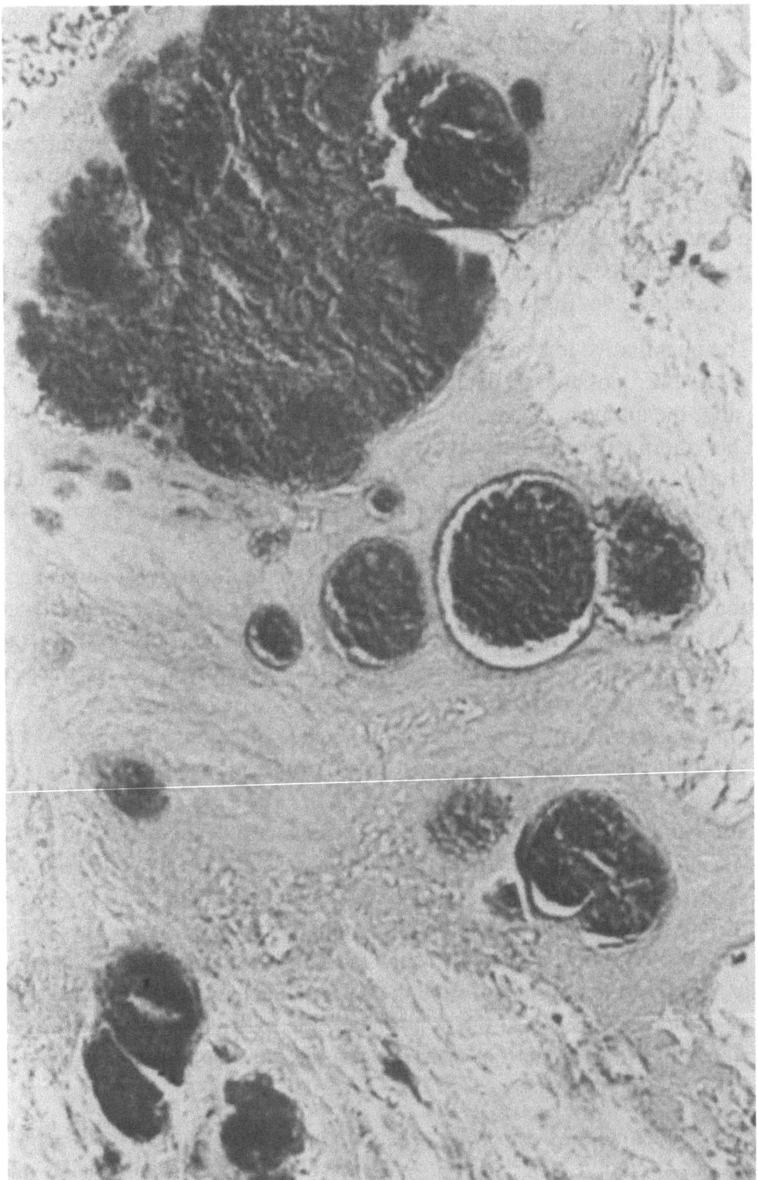

Figure 14. High-powered light-microscopic view of a vegetation from the aortic valve of a rabbit infected with *Str. intermedius* 14 days previously. Note the dark colonies of masses of bacteria. No cells are evident in the vicinity of the bacterial colonies.

REFERENCES

1. Durack, D. T.: Experimental bacterial endocarditis. IV. Structure and evolution of very early lesions. *J. Pathol.* **115:**81–89, 1975.
2. Durack, D. T., Beeson, P. B.: Experimental bacterial endocarditis. II. Survival of bacteria in endocardial vegetations. *Br. J. Exp. Pathol.* **53:**50–53, 1972.
3. Archer, G. L.: Experimental endocarditis, in: *Infections of Prosthetic Heart Valves and Vascular Grafts,* Duma, R. J., ed. University Park Press, Baltimore, pp. 43–59, 1977.
4. Liekweg, W. G., jr., Levinson, S. A., Greenfield, L. J.: Infections of vascular grafts: Incidence, anatomic location, etiologic agents, morbidity, and mortality, in: *Infections of Prosthetic Heart Valves and Vascular Grafts,* Duma, R. J., ed. University Park Press, Baltimore, pp. 239–251, 1977.
5. Dismukes, W.: Discussion, in: *Infections of Prosthetic Heart Valves and Vascular Grafts,* Duma, R. J., ed. University Park Press, Baltimore, p. 265, 1977.
6. Freedman, L. R., Valone, J.: Experimental endocarditis. *Prog. Cardiovasc. Dis.* **22:**169–180, 1979.
7. Heraief, E., Glauser, M., Freedman, L. R.: Vancomycin prophylaxis of streptococcal endocarditis in rats, in: *Current Chemotherapy and Infectious Disease,* Proceedings of the 11th International Congress of Chemotherapy and 19th Interscience Conference on Antimicrobial Agents and Chemotherapy, American Society of Microbiology, Washington, D.C., pp. 911–913, 1980.
8. Durack, D. T., Beeson, P. B., Petersdorf, R. G.: Experimental bacterial endocarditis. III. Production and progress of the disease in rabbits. *Br. J. Exp. Pathol.* **54:**142–151, 1973.
9. Critten, J., Waldvogel, F. A.: Endocardites bactériennes: Aspects cliniques, bactériologiques et facteurs de pronostic. *Schweiz. Med. Wochenschr.* **107**(21)(Suppl. 5)**:**1–26, 1977.
10. Pelletier, L. L., Petersdorf, R. G.: Infective endocarditis: A review of 125 cases from the University of Washington hospitals: 1963–1972. *Medicine* **56**(4)**:**287–313, 1977.
11. Sipes, J. N., Thompson, R. L., Hook, E. W.: Prophylaxis of infective endocarditis: A reevaluation (review and bibliography). *Annu. Rev. Med.* **28:**371–391, 1977.
12. Editorial: Bacterial stickiness. *Lancet* **1:**716–717, 1974.
13. Scheld, W. M., Guerrant, R. L., Sande, M. A.: Bacterial adherence in the pathogenesis of endocarditis. *Clin. Res.* **25:**57A., 1977.
14. Ramirez-Ronda, C. H.: Adherence of *Streptococcus mutans* to normal and damaged canine aortic valves. *Clin. Res.* **25:**382A, 1977.
15. Scheld, W. M., Sande, M. A.: Bacterial adherence in the pathogenesis of endocarditis. *Clin. Res.* **25:**492A, 1977.
16. Levison, M. E., Carrizosa, J., Tanphaichitra, D., Schick, P. K., Rubin, W.: Effect of aspirin on thrombogenesis and on production of experimental aortic valvular *Streptococcus viridans* endocarditis in rabbits. *Blood* **49**(4)**:**645–650, 1977.
17. Durack, D. T., Beeson, P. B.: Protective role of complement in experimental *Escherichia coli* endocarditis. *Infect. Immun.* **16**(1)**:**213–217, 1977.
18. Archer, G., Fekety, F. R., Jr.: Experimental endocarditis due to *Pseudomonas aeruginosa.* I. Description of a model. *J. Infect. Dis.* **134:**1–7, 1976.
19. Kaspar, R. L., Drutz, D. J.: Perihepatitis and hepatitis as complications of experimental endocarditis due to *Neisseria gonorrhoeae* in the rabbit. *J. Infect. Dis.* **136**(1)**:**37–42, 1977.
20. Morelli, R., Rosenker, L. T.: Role of complement during experimental candida infection in mice. *Infect. Immun.* **3:**521–523, 1971.
21. Weinstein, L., Schlesinger, J. J.: Pathoanatomic, pathophysiologic and clinical correlations in endocarditis. *N. Engl. J. Med.* **291:**832–837, 1122–1126, 1974.

22. Watanakunakorn, C.: Changing epidemiology and new aspects of infective endocarditis, in: *Advances in Internal Medicine*, Stollerman, G. H., ed. Year Book Medical Publishers, Chicago, pp. 21–47, 1977.
23. Tuazon, C. U., Sheagren, J. N.: Staphylococcal endocarditis in parenteral drug abusers: Source of the organism. *Ann. Intern. Med.* **82**(6):788–790, 1975.
24. Noriega, E. R., Rubenstein, E., Simberkoff, M. S., Rahal, J. J., Jr.: Subacute and acute endocarditis due to *Pseudomonas cepacia* in heroin addicts. *Am. J. Med.* **59**:29–36, 1975.
25. Mills, J., Drew, D.: *Serratia marcescens* endocarditis: A regional illness associated with intravenous drug abuse. *Ann. Intern. Med.* **84**(1):29–35, 1976.
26. Reiner, N. E., Gopalakrishna, K. V., Lerner, P. I.: Enterococcal endocarditis in heroin addicts. *J. Am. Med. Assoc.* **235**(17):1861–1863, 1976.
27. Wilson, W. R., Jaumin, P. M., Danielson, G. K., Giuliani, E. R., Washington, J. A., II, Geraci, J. E.: Prosthetic valve endocarditis. *Ann. Intern. Med.* **82**(6):751–756, 1975.
28. Arnett, E. N., Roberts, W. C.: Prosthetic valve endocarditis. *Am. J. Cardiol.* **38**(3):281–292, 1976.
29. Anderson, D. J., Bulkley, B. H., Hutchins, G. M.: A clinopathologic study of prosthetic valve endocarditis in 22 patients: Morphologic basis for diagnosis and therapy. *Am. Heart J.* **94**(3):325–332, 1977.
30. Petheram, I. S., Boyce, J. M. H.: Prosthetic valve endocarditis: A review of 24 cases. *Thorax* **32**:478–485, 1977.
31. Schaffner, W.: Antibiotic prophylaxis in valvular replacement surgery, in: *Infections of Prosthetic Heart Valves and Vascular Grafts*, Duma, R. J., ed. University Park Press, Baltimore, pp. 313–321, 1977.
32. Weinstein, L., Rubin, R. H.: Infective Endocarditis—1973. Prog. Cardiovas. Dis., 239–274, 1973.
33. Saravolatz, L. D., Burch, K. H., Quinn, E. L., Cox, F., Madhavan, T., Fischer, E.: Polymicrobial infective endocarditis: An increasing clinical entity. *Am. Heart J.* **95**(2):163–168, 1978.
34. Mostaghim, D., Millard, H. D.: Bacterial endocarditis: A retrospective study. *Oral Surg. Oral Med. Oral Pathol.* **40**(2):219–234, 1975.
35. Nager, F., Pfisterer, M., Rothlin, M., Kappenberger, L.: Epidemiologie und Klinik der infectiösen Endokarditis. *Schweiz. Med. Wochenschr.* **105**(44):1421–1428, 1975.
36. Pedersen, F. K., Petersen, E. A.: Bacterial endocarditis at Blegdamshospitalet in Copenhagen, 1944–1973. *Scand J. Infect. Dis.* **8**:99–105, 1976.
37. Welsby, P. D.: Infective endocarditis—A retrospective study. *Practitioner* **218**:382–387, 1977.
38. Bergogne-Berezin, E. N., Lambert-Zechovsky, J. -P.: Les endocardites à germes associés. *Med. Mal. Infect.* **6**(8):283–286, 1976.
39. Pazin, G. J., Peterson, K. L., Griff, F. W., Shaver, J. A., Ho, M.: Determination of site of infection in endocarditis. *Ann. Intern. Med.* **82**(6):746–750, 1975.
40. Falase, A. O., Jaiyesimi, F., Iyun, A. O., Attah, E. B.: Infective endocarditis—Experience in Nigeria. *Trop. Geogr. Med.* **28**:9 15, 1976.
41. Durack, D. T., Littler, W. A.: Failure of "adequate" penicillin therapy to prevent bacterial endocarditis after tooth extraction (letter). *Lancet* **2**:846–847, 1974.
42. McGowan, D. A., Hardie, J. M.: Production of bacterial endocarditis in prepared rabbits by oral manipulation. *Br. Dental J.* **137**(4):129–131, 1974.
43. Bahn, S. L., Bitterman, P., Ross, D., Bahn, A. N.: Induction of experimental endocarditis by mucosal injection of oral streptococci (IADR Abstract L 405). *J. Dent. Res.* **54**:L101, 1975.
44. Starkebaum, M., Durack, D., Beeson, P. B.: The "incubation period" of subacute bacterial endocarditis. *Yale J. Biol. Med.* **50**:49–58, 1977.

45. Everett, E. D., Hirschmann, J. V.: Transient bacteremia and endocarditis prophylaxis: A review. *Medicine* **56**(1):61–77, 1977.
46. Weinstein, L.: Chemoprophylaxis for bacterial endocarditis. *N. Engl. J. Med.* **292:**427, 1975.
47. Maki, D. G.: Sepsis arising from extrinsic contamination of the infusion and measures for control, in: *Microbiological Hazards of Infusion Therapy,* Philipps, I., Meers, P. D., d'Arcy, P. F., eds. MTP Press, Lancaster, pp. 99–143, 1976.
48. Hornick, R. B.: Source of contamination in open heart surgery, in: *Infections of Prosthetic Heart Valves and Vascular Grafts,* Duma, R. J., ed. University Park Press, Baltimore, pp. 81–99, 1977.
49. Everett, E. D., Reller, L. B., Droegemueller, W., Guez, B. E.: Absence of bacteremia after insertion or removal of intrauterine devices. *Obstet. Gynecol.* **47:**207, 1976.
50. Cobbs, C. G.: IUD and endocarditis. *Ann. Intern. Med.* **78:**541, 1973.
51. de Swiet, M., Ramsay, I. D., Rees, G. M.: Bacterial endocarditis after insertion of intrauterine contraceptive device (case report). *Br. Med. J.* **117:**76, 1975.
52. Toran, L. M.: Rheumatic fever in its relation to dental disease. *N. Y. J. Dent.* **14:**107, 1944.
53. Mundth, E. D., Darling, R. C., Alvarado, R. H., Buckley, M. J., Linton, R. R., Austen, W. G.: Surgical management of mycotic aneurysms and the complications of infection in vascular reconstructive surgery. *Am. J. Surg.* **117:**460–470, 1969.
54. Anderson, C. B., Butcher, H. R., Ballinger, W. F.: Mycotic aneurysms. *Arch. Surg.* **109:**712–717, 1974.
55. Felson, B., Akers, P. V., Hall, G. S., Schreiber, J. T., Greene, R. E., Pedrosa, C. S.: Mycotic tuberculous aneurysm of the thoracic aorta. *J. Am. Med. Assoc.* **237:**1104–1108, 1977.
56. Bennett, D. E.: Primary mycotic aneurysms of the aorta. *Arch. Surg.* **94:**758–765, 1967.
57. Cliff, M. M., Soulen, R. L., Finestone, A. J.: Mycotic aneurysm—A challenge and a clue. *Arch. Intern. Med.* **126:**977–982, 1970.
58. Zak, F. G., Strauss, L., Saphra, I.: Rupture of diseased large arteries in the course of enterobacterial *(Salmonella)* infections. *N. Engl. J. Med.* **258:**824–828, 1958.
59. McNally, E. M., Kennedy, R. J., Grace, W. R.: *Salmonella infantis* infection of a pre-existent ventricular aneurysm. *Am. Heart J.* **68:**540–548, 1964.
60. Klusteld, D. M., Allison, M. J., Gerszten, E., Dalton, H. P.: Systemic *Bacteroides* Infections in atherosclerotic rabbits. Abstracts of the Annual Meeting of the American Society for Microbiology, 1976, p. 14, abstract B20.
61. Szilaggi, E.: Discussion, in: *Infections of Prosthetic Heart Valves and Vascular Grafts,* Duma, R. J., ed. University Park Press, Baltimore, p. 283, 1977.
62. Grant, R. T., Wood, J. E., Jones, T. D.: Heart valve irregularities in relation to subacute bacterial endocarditis. *Heart* **14:**247–261, 1927–1929.
63. Becker, B. J. P.: Studies on the human mural endocardium. *Pathol. Bacteriol.* **88:**541–547, 1964.
64. Hook, E. W. III., Sande, M. A.: Role of the vegetation in experimental streptococcus viridans endocarditis. *Infect. Immun.* **10**(6):1433–1438, 1974.
65. Kaye, D.: Definitions and demographic characteristics, in: *Infective Endocarditis,* Kaye, D., ed. University Park Press, Baltimore, pp. 1–10, 1976.
66. Johnson, D. H., Rosenthal, A., Nadas, A. S.: A forty-year review of bacterial endocarditis in infancy and childhood. *Circulation* **51:**581–588, 1975.
67. Kerr, A.: *Subacute Bacterial Endocarditis.* Charles C. Thomas, Springfield, Illinois, 1955.
68. Rossiter, S. J., Stinson, E. B., Over, P. E., Miller, D. C., Schapira, J. N., Martin, R. P., Shumway, N. E.: Prosthetic valve endocarditis. *J. Thorac. Cardiovasc. Surg.* **76**(6):795–803, 1978.
69. Welton, D. E., Young, J. B., Gentry, W. O., Raizner, A. E., Alexander, J. K., Ghahine, R. A., Miller, R. R.: Recurrent infective endocarditis—Analysis of predisposing factors and clinical features. *Am. J. Med.* **66:**932–938, 1979.

70. Gersony, W. M., Hayes, C. J.: Bacterial endocarditis in patients with pulmonary stenosis, aortic stenosis of ventricular septal defect. *Circulation Suppl. I* **56**(2):I84–I87, 1977.
71. Allen, H. Harris, A., Leatham, A.: Significance and prognosis of an isolated late systolic murmur: A 9 to 22 year follow-up. *Br. Heart J.* **36**:525, 1974.
72. Lavelle, K. J., Dentino, M. M.: Surgical treatment of infective endocarditis in hemodialysis patients. *Clin. Nephrol.* **9**(1):6–10, 1978.
73. Parkhurst, G. F., Decker, J. P.: Bacterial aortitis and mycotic aneurysm of the aorta. *Am. J. Pathol.* **31**:821–835, 1955.
74. Schoenbaum, S. C., Gardner, O., Shillito, J.: Infections of cerebro-spinal fluid shunts: Epidemiology, clinical manifestations and therapy. *J. Infect. Dis.* **131**(5):543–552, 1975.
75. Thell, R., Martin, F. H., Edwards, J. E.: Bacterial endocarditis in subjects 60 years of age and older. *Circulation* **51**(1):174–182, 1975.
76. Finland, M., Barnes, M. W.: Changing etiology of bacterial endocarditis in the antibacterial era: Experience at Boston City Hospital 1933–1965. *Ann. Intern. Med.* **72**:341, 1970.
77. Wilson, W. R.: Prosthetic valve endocarditis: Incidence, anatomic location, cause, morbidity, and mortality, in: *Infections of Prosthetic Heart Valves and Vascular Grafts,* Duma, R. J., ed. University Park Press, Baltimore, pp. 3–16, 1977.
78. Kloster, F. E.: Infective prosthetic valve endocarditis, in: *Infective Endocarditis,* Rahimtoola, S. H., ed. Grune & Stratton, New York, pp. 291–305, 1978.
79. Freedman, L. R.: Endocarditis updated. *Dis. Month* **26**:1–71, 1979.
80. Hammond, G. W., Stiver, H. G.: Combination antibiotic therapy in an outbreak of prosthetic endocarditis caused by *Staphylococcus epidermidis*. *Can. Med. Assoc. J.* **118**(5):524–530, 1978.
81. Watanakunakorn, C.: Prosthetic valve infective endocarditis. *Prog. Cardiovasc. Dis.* **22**:181–192, 1979.
82. Galgiani, J. N., Stevens, D. A.: Fungal endocarditis: Need for guidelines in evaluating therapy—Experience with two patients previously reported. *J. Thorac. Cardiovasc. Surg.* **73**(2):293–296, 1977.
83. Downham, W. H., Rhoades, E. R.: Endocarditis associated with porcine valve xenografts. *Arch. Intern. Med.* **139**:1352–1362, 1979.
84. Newsom, S. W. B.: Antibiotic prophylaxis for open heart surgery. *J. Antimicrob. Chemother.* **4**:389–394, 1978.
85. Goldmann, D. A., Maki, D. G.: Infection control in total parenteral nutrition. *J. Am. Med. Assoc.* **223**(12):1360–1364, 1973.
86. Iannini, P. B., Crossley, K.: Therapy of *Staphylococcus aureus* bacteremia associated with a removable focus of infection. *Ann. Intern. Med.* **84**(5):558–560, 1976.
87. Banks, T., Fletcher, R., Ali, N.: Infective endocarditis in heroin addicts. *Am. J. Med.* **55**:444–451, 1973.
88. Riad El-Khatib, M., Wilson, F. M., Lerner, A. M.: Characteristics of bacterial endocarditis in heroin addicts in Detroit. *Am. J. Med. Sci.* **271**(2):197–201, 1976.
89. Hahn, H. H., Schweid, A. I., Beaty, H. N.: Complications of injecting dissolved methylphenidate tablets. *Arch. Intern. Med.* **123**:656–659, 1969.
90. Sacks, T., Moldow, C. F., Graddock, P. R., Bowers, T. K., Jacob, H. S.: Complement (c)-mediated endothelial damage: A mechanism for the accelerated atherosclerosis of hemodialysis. *Clin. Res.* **25**(4):612A, 1977.
91. Sheagren, J. N., Tuazon, C. V., Quie, P. G.: Alternate complement pathway activation by strains of *S. aureus* isolated from patients with disseminated intravascular coagulation. *Clin. Res.* **26**:526A, 1978.
92. Bayston, R.: Serological investigations in children with colonized Spitz–Holter valves. *J. Clin. Pathol.* **25**:718–720, 1972.

93. Bayston, R., Penny, S. R.: Excessive production of mucoid substance in *Staphylococcus* SIIA: A possible factor in colonization of Holter shunts. *Dev. Med. Child. Neurol. Suppl.* **27**:25–28, 1972.
94. Goodman, J. S., Crews, H. D., Ginn, H. E., Koenig, M. G.: Bacterial endocarditis as a possible complication of chronic hemodialysis. *N. Engl. J. Med.* **280**(16):876–877, 1969.
95. Leonard, A., Raij, L., Shapiro, F. L.: Bacterial endocarditis in regularly dialyzed patients. *Kidney Int.* **4**:407–422, 1973.
96. Lane, T. W., Abrutyn, E.: Induction and prevention of experimental arteriovenous fistula infections. *Antimicrob. Agents Chemother.* **16**:638–640, 1979.
97. Blieden, L. C., Morehead, R. R., Burke, B., Kaplan, E. L.: Bacterial endocarditis in the neonate. *Am. J. Dis. Child.* **124**:747–749, 1972.
98. Symchych, P. S., Krauss, A. N., Winchester, P.: Endocarditis following intracardiac placement of umbilical venous catheters in neonates. *J. Pediatr.* **90**(2):287–289, 1977.
99. Edwards, K., Ingall, D., Czapels, E., Davis, A. T.: Bacterial endocarditis in 4 young infants: Is this complication on the increase? *Clin. Pediatr.* **16**:607–609, 1977.
100. Oppenheimer, E. H., Esterly, J. R.: Nonbacterial thrombotic vegetations: Occurrence in neonate, infant and child, and relation to valvular lesions in cardiac defects. *Am. J. Pathol.* **53**:63–81, 1968.
101. Liwnicz, B. H., Lepow, H.: Nonbacterial thrombotic endocarditis in premature child. *N. Y. State J. Med.* **76**:912–916, 1976.
102. Tan, J. S., Watanakunakorn, C., Terhune, C. A., Jr.: *Streptococcus viridans* endocarditis: Favorable prognosis in geriatric patients. *Geriatrics* **28**:68–73, 1973.
103. Devereux, R. B.: Mitral valve prolapse. *Am. J. Med.* **67**:729–731, 1979.
104. Allen, H., Harris, A., Leatham, A.: Significance and prognosis of an isolated late systolic murmur: A 9 to 22 year follow-up. *Br. Heart J.* **36**:525, 1974.
105. Corrigall, D., Bolen, J., Hancock, E. W., Popp, R. L.: Mitral valve prolapse and infective endocarditis. *Am. J. Med.* **63**:215–222, 1977.
106. Tamer, D., Wolff, G., Ferrer, P., Gelbaud, H., Garcia, O.: Streptococcal antibodies in mitral valve prolapse. *Clin Res.* **28**:14A, 1980.
107. Weinstein, A. J., McHenry, M. C.: Bacterial endocarditis in a patient with mitral valve prolapse. *Arch. Intern. Med.* **139**:1191–1192, 1979.
108. Barnett, H. J. M., Boughner, D. R., Taylor, D. W., Cooper, P. E., Kostuk, W. J., Nichol, P. M.: Further evidence relating mitral-valve prolapse to cerebral ischemic events. *N. Engl. J. Med.* **302**:139–144, 1980.
109. Pomerance, A., Davies, M. J.: Strokes: A complication of mitral-leaflet prolapse (letter). *Lancet* **2**:1186, 1977.
110. Read, R. C., Thal, A. P., Wendy, V. E.: Symptomatic valvular myxomatous transformation (the Floppy valve syndrome): A possible forme fruste of the Marfan syndrome. *Circulation* **37**:897–910, 1965.
111. Soman, V. R., Breton, G., Herdhkowitz, M., Mark, H.: Bacterial endocarditis of mitral valve in Marfan syndrome. *Br. Heart J.* **36**:1247–1250, 1974.
112. Dowling, J. N., Lee, W. S., Sacco, R. J., Ho, M.: Endocarditis caused by *Neisseria mucosa* in Marfan's syndrome. *Ann. Intern. Med.* **81**:641–643, 1974.
113. Hammer, D., Leier, C. V., Baba, N., Vasko, J. S., Wooley, C. F., Pinnel, S. R.: Altered collagen composition in a prolapsing mitral valve with ruptured chordae tendineae. *Am. J. Med.* **67**:863–866, 1979.
114. Baskin, T. W., Rosenthal, A., Pruitt, B. A.: Acute bacterial endocarditis: A silent source of sepsis in the burn patient. *Ann. Surg.* **184**(5):618–621, 1976.
115. Garcia, R., Hakimi-Naini, M.: Bacterial endocarditis and incarceration of a transvenous pacemaker. *Henry Ford Hospital Med. J.* **23**:135–140, 1975.

116. Zeller, N. H., Lusk, R. H., Palmer, D. L.: Nonsurgical cure of endocarditis associated with a pacemaker. *Arch. Intern. Med.* **135**:580–581, 1975.
117. Watanakunakorn, C., Baird, I. M.: *Staphylococcus aureus* bacteremia and endocarditis associated with a removable infected intravenous device. *Am. J. Med.* **63**:253–256, 1977.
118. Smith, H., Freedman, L. R.: Prolonged venous catheterization as a cause of sepsis. *N. Engl. J. Med.* **276**:1229–1233, 1967.
119. Green, J. F., Fitzwater, J. E., Clemmen, T. P.: Septic endocarditis and indwelling pulmonary artery catheters. *J. Am. Med. Assoc.* **233**:891–892, 1975.
120. Chomette, G., Brocheriou, C., Delcourt, A., Agebo, M.: Les endocardites suppurées pariétales. *Ann. Med. Interne* **127**(2):83–89, 1976.
121. Satterwhite, T. K., McGee, Z. A., Schaffner, W., Friesinger, G. C., Mishu, M., Collins, R. D.: Infection of an avulsed papillary muscle tip simulating bacterial endocarditis. *Am. Heart J.* **86**:107–111, 1973.
122. Habibzadeh, M. A., Curd, G. W., Zeller, N. H.: Subacute bacterial endocarditis (SBE) superimposed on idiopathic hypertrophic subaortic stenosis (IHSS)—A case report with special emphasis on prophylactic antibiotic therapy. *Ariz. Med.*, October 1976.
123. Morgan, M. G., Glasser, S. P., Sanusi, I. D.: Bacterial endocarditis—Occurrence on a traumatically ruptured aortic valve. *J. Am. Med. Assoc.* **233**:810–811, 1975.
124. Markowitz, S. M., Szentpetery, S., Lower, R. R., Duma, R. J.: Endocarditis due to accidental penetration of foreign bodies. *Am. J. Med.* **60**:571–576, 1976.
125. Jugdutt, B., Basualdo, C., Freeman, H., Crockford, P.: Acromegaly, the systolic click and group D streptococcal endocarditis. *Chest* **69**:690–692, 1976.
126. Bernhardt, D., Veltmann, G., Dörwald, R., Huth, F.: Cogan-Syndrom bei Angiitis von Hirnnerve, Aortitis, Endokarditis und Glomerulonephritis. *Dtsch. Med. Wochenschr.* **101**(10):373–377, 1976.
127. Hollenberg, B., Gross, S.: Endocarditis—involving calcified mitral annulus fibrosus. *N. Y. State J. Med.* **79**(10):1578–1580, 1979.
128. Garrison, P., Freedman, L. R.: Experimental endocarditis. I. Staphylococcal endocarditis in rabbits resulting from placement of a polyethylene catheter in the right side of the heart. *Yale J. Biol. Med.* **42**:394–410, 1970.
129. Perlman, B. B., Freedman, L. R.: Experimental endocarditis. III. Natural history of catheter induced endocarditis after catheter removal. *Yale J. Biol. Med.* **44**:214–223, 1971.
130. Durack, D. T., Beeson, P. B.: Experimental bacterial endocarditis. I. Colonization of a sterile vegetation. *Br. J. Exp. Pathol.* **53**:44–49, 1972.
131. Francioli, P., Freedman, L. R.: Streptococcal infection of endocardial and other intravascular vegetations in rabbits: Natural history and effect of dexamethasone. *Infect. Immun.* **24**:483–491, 1979.
132. Freedman, L. R., Arnold, S., Valone, J.: Experimental endocarditis. *Proc. N. Y. Adad. Sci.* **236**:456–465, 1974.
133. Freedman, L. R., Johnson, M. L.: Experimental endocarditis. IV Tricuspid and aortic valve infection with *Candida albicans* in rabbits. *Yale J. Biol. Med.* **45**:163–175, 1972.
134. Carrizosa, J., Tanphaichitra, D., Levison, M. E.: Experimental *Bacteroides fragilis* endocarditis in rabbits. *Infect. Immun.* **15**(3):871–873, 1977.
135. Hirschfelder, A. D.: The rapid formation of endocarditic "vegetations." *Johns Hopkins Hosp. Bull.* **18**:267–268, 1907.
136. Gutschik, E., Christensen, N.: Experimental endocarditis in rabbits. 1. Technique and spontaneous course of non-bacterial thrombotic endocarditis. *Acta Pathol. Microbiol. Scand. Sect. B* **86**:215–221, 1978.
137. McGowan, D. A.: Lactobacillus infective endocarditis. *Proc. R. Soc. Med.* **70**:584, 1977.
138. McGowan, D. A.: Scanning electron microscopy of heart-valve vegetations. *Lancet* **2**:822, 1977.

139. Moore, R. A.: The cellular mechanism of recovery after treatment with penicillin. I. Subacute bacterial endocarditis. *J. Lab. Clin. Med.* **31**(12):1279–1293, 1946.
140. McGeown, M. G.: Bacterial endocarditis: An experimental study of healing. *J. Pathol. Bacteriol.* **67**:179–186, 1954.
141. Riba, A. L. Thakur, M. T., Gottschalk, A., Andriole, V. T., Zaret, B. L.: Imaging experimental infective endocarditis with indium-111-labeled blood cellular components. *Circulation* **59**(2):336–343, 1979.
142. Durack, D. T., Beeson, P. B.: Pathogenesis of infective endocarditis, in: *Infective Endocarditis*, Rahimtoola, S. H., ed. Grune and Stratton, New York, pp. 1–53, 1978.
143. Gutschik, E., Möller, S., Christensen, N.: Experimental endocarditis in rabbits. 3. Significance of the proteolytic capacity of the infecting strains of *Streptococcus faecalis*. *Acta Pathol. Microbiol. Scand. Sect. B* **87**:353–362, 1979.
144. Rodbard, S.: Blood velocity and endocarditis. *Circulation* **27**:18–28, 1963.
145. Lacuata, A. Q., Nakamura, Y., Hirose, T.: Electrocardiographic and echocardiographic findings in four cases of bovine endocarditis. *J. Am. Vet. Med. Assoc.* **176**:1355–1365, 1980.
146. Scheld, W. M., Thomas, J. H., Sande, M. A.: Influence of preformed antibody on experimental *Streptococcus sanguis* endocarditis. *Infect. Immun.* **25**:781–785, 1979.
147. Pulliam, L., Inokuchi, S., Hadley, W. K., Mills, J.: Effects of penicillin (PCN) tolerance and Dextran production by viridans streptococci on PCN therapy in experimental endocarditis. 20th Interscience Conference on Antimicrobial Agents and Chemotherapy, September 1980, Abstr. No. 276.
148. Ramírez-Ronda, C. H., Gutiérrez, J.: Decreased adherence (AD) of *S. sanguis* to damaged heart valves by subinhibitory concentrations of penicillin *in vitro*. *Clin. Res.* **28**:377A, 1980.
149. Neuhaus, E., Lowy F., Chang, D., Horne, D., Tomasz, A., Steigbigel, N.: Penicillin (P) tolerant (T) *S. viridans:* effect of P on host-bacterial interaction. 20th Interscience Conference on Antimicrobial Agents and Chemotherapy, September 1980, Abstr. No. 356.
150. Bernard, J. -P., Francioli, P., Glauser, M. P.: Vancomycin prophylaxis of experimental *Streptococcus sanguis*. Inhibition of bacterial adherence rather than bacterial killing. *J. Clin. Invest.* **68**:1113–1116, 1981.
151. Ramírez-Ronda, C. H., Gutiérrez, J.: Effect of antiteichoic acid serum (ATAS) on the adherence (AD) of *S. aureus* (SA) CR-100 to damaged heart valves in-vitro. *Clin. Res.* **28**:377A, 1980.
152. Ramírez-Ronda, C. H., Gutiérrez, J., Bermúdez, R. H.: Effects of teichoic acids (TA) on adherence (AD) of *S. sanguis* (SS), *S. mutans* (SM), and enterococci (EC) to damaged heart valves in-vitro. *Clin. Res.* **28**:377A, 1980.
153. Ramírez-Ronda, C. H., Gutiérrez, J., Bermúdez, R. H.: Effect of teichoic acids (TA) on adherence (AD) of staphylococci (S) to heart valves *in-vitro*. *Clin. Res.* **28**:377A, 1980.
154. Ringer, M., Feen, D. J., Drabkin, M. S.: Mitral valve prolapse: Jet stream causing mural endocarditis. *Am. J. Cardiol.* **45**:383–385, 1980.

5

Prophylaxis of Intravascular Infection

5.1. INFECTIVE ENDOCARDITIS

There is considerable debate concerning the indications for administering antibiotics with the goal of preventing IE. There is also uncertainty as to how much of which antibiotics should be administered in those instances where it is evident that prophylaxis should be given.

The reasons for the current controversy are agreed upon by everyone. They are: the lack of information indicating the effectiveness of antibiotic prophylaxis of IE in man and the likelihood of being able to prevent only a small percentage of the total cases of IE.

Even assuming that it were possible to predict the nature of the potential infecting microorganism and that one were able to administer prophylactically antibiotics which were 100% effective, the facts that only about 50% of patients with IE know of the prior existence of heart disease and that in only about 50% (this is probably an overestimation) it is possible to identify a specific preceding event serving as the source of bacteremia reduce the population in which antibiotic prophylaxis could be effective to about 25% of total cases.[1]

Nevertheless, IE is potentially so dangerous an illness that despite these statistical limitations, it is reasonable to administer prophylactic antibiotics when subjects known to be at risk are subjected to procedures known to be likely to provoke bacteremia. It is important not to conclude from all our uncertainties that there is no reason at all to administer prophylactic antibiotics. There is good and ample evidence showing that many patients develop IE under circumstances in which prophylactic antibiotics, shown to be effective in animal studies, would theoretically have been capable of preventing infection in man. The problem is to define which patients undergoing which procedures should receive which antibiotics.

5.1.1. Anticoagulants

Referring to the diagram describing current views of the pathogenesis of IE [Figure 3 (Chapter 2)], it is evident that there are several potential points at which intervention might be effective in preventing intravascular infection. Since the formation of a platelet–fibrin thrombus is thought to be the underlying endocardial lesion, anticoagulants administered in such a way as to prevent the development of such a thrombus might be expected to be useful. Studies in rabbits which have prevented the formation of a grossly visible thrombus, associated with the trauma produced by a plastic catheter, have not been effective in preventing infection of the microscopic traumatic valvular injury.[2,3] Indeed, the combination of anticoagulation and untreated IE is rapidly lethal in animals and equally dangerous in man.[2–5] Aspirin was ineffective in preventing thrombus formation and the establishment of infection.[6]

Administration of warfarin after the formation of the initial nonbacterial thrombotic vegetation (NBTV) but before the inoculation of the test microorganism was ineffective in preventing colonization with *Streptococcus sanguis* but, interestingly, was effective in decreasing susceptibility to *Staphylococcus epidermis* infection.[7,8] Penicillin, begun 24 hr after *Str. sanguis* infection, tended to sterilize the lesions, but did not prevent death of the animals.[7] The only glimmer of hope to come from these studies was the finding of Hook and Sande[3] that penicillin treatment (started 2–3 days after infection) was more effective in sterilizing the "minilesions" of anticoagulated rabbits than the fully developed vegetations in nonanticoagulated rabbits. It is possible that penicillin begun before infection of these animals would be much more effective. At present, anticoagulants have no place in the management of patients with IE, except when necessary for other reasons and when given in association with, and preferably after the institution of, effective antibiotic therapy. In patients with prosthetic-valve endocarditis (PVE), discontinuing anticoagulants seems to be more dangerous than continuing them, in the presence of effective antibiotic therapy.[9]

5.1.2. Bacterial Sticking

Another possible point of attack is to interfere with the ability of bacteria to stick to NBTVs. Study is being directed to the factors which promote this sticking (see Section 4.1), but for the present, aside from the interesting decreased colonization of vegetations by *Staph. epidermidis* in anticoagulated rabbits, there is yet no clear path to a useful therapeutic development from these studies. Induction of thrombocytopenia in rabbits with established NBTVs did not prevent the establishment of infection with *streptococci*.[10] Increasing fibrinolytic activity with Streptokinase was effective in decreasing the number of streptococci in vegetations, but this effect may have been due to loss of bacteria from the vegetation due to a change in its structure, rather than to decreased sticking.[10]

From the practical point of view, the only currently available approach in man is to prevent bacteremia or to alter the environment in such a way as to inhibit the multiplication of microbes which deposit on a vegetation. Antibiotics would appear to be suitable agents to accomplish both these tasks. It is of considerable interest that antibiotics have also been shown to act prophylactically by inhibiting bacterial sticking to vegetations (see Section 4.1).

The potential sources of bloodstream invasion by microorganisms and the underlying conditions increasing susceptibility to IE were discussed in Section 4.2.1. It remains only to establish some rational approach to the use of antibiotics. But there are several obstacles to the establishment of such an approach:

1. It is not known precisely which microorganisms are potential pathogens in a given host.

2. Although we can get some idea of how much of certain antibiotics are necessary to prevent experimental infection in the laboratory, we do not have comparable data in man.

3. Techniques of noninvasive cardiological investigation have so advanced that large numbers of persons who would previously have been considered normal are now found to have cardiac valvular abnormalities which make them potential candidates for developing IE.

5.1.3. Microorganisms

Reference to the types of microorganisms recovered from the bloodstream of subjects undergoing procedures involving the oropharynx indicates that prophylaxis in these patients should be directed against *non-group D α-hemolytic streptococci*. Although a variety of microorganisms may circulate in the bloodstream after procedures involving the gastrointestinal tract, *group D streptococci* present the greatest threat for the development of infection. The same is true of the normal genitourinary tract. Of course, in the presence of urinary infection, bacteremia arising from this source may be related to the organism already known to be in residence.[11] Bacteremia arising from cardiovascular procedures depends on the source of contamination of the procedure. The risk of miscellaneous infections will also vary according to the microorganism responsible for infection (Table 3).

Although there is a general consensus concerning the bacteria for which one should administer prophylactic antibiotics, it is not clear which procedures

TABLE 3
Target Bacteria for the Establishment of Antibiotic Regimens to Prevent Infective Endocarditis and Procedures Giving Rise to Their Bloodstream Dissemination

A. Streptococci (nonenterococcal, non-group A)
  Arising from:
    Dental procedures likely to result in gingival bleeding
    Surgery or instrumentation of the respiratory tract, including bronchoscopy
B. Penicillin-resistant streptococci (nonenterococcal, non-group A)
  Arising from:
    Dental and respiratory-tract procedures in patients receiving (1) oral penicillin for rheumatic-fever prophylaxis or (2) parenteral carbenicillin
C. Enterococci
  Likely to arise from:
    Surgery or instrumentation of the urinary tract
    Surgery of the lower digestive tract or gallbladder
    Gynecological infections
  Less likely to arise from:
    Upper gastrointestinal endoscopy
    Percutaneous liver biopsy
    Proctoscopy, sigmoidoscopy, barium enema
    Pelvic examination, uterine dilitation and curettage
    Uncomplicated insertion or removal of an intrauterine device
D. Staphylococci
  Arising from:
    Contamination during cardiac surgery
    Drainage of staphylococcal abscesses

constitute a reasonable risk. There is agreement that prophylaxis should be given for any dental procedure except for chewing and tooth brushing and that oral irrigation devices should be avoided by susceptible patients.[12,13] Any oropharyngeal surgery as well as surgery of the gastrointestinal and genitourinary tracts also constitute indications for prophylaxis in susceptible patients. The patient should also be protected before instrumentation of the urinary tract. There is no unanimity of opinion concerning bronchoscopy, gastrointestinal-tract endoscopy, barium enema, liver biopsy, pelvic examination, uterine dilatation and curettage, or insertion of an intrauterine device.[14–22] As mentioned earlier, bacteremia has not been documented after insertion of an IUD, but IE has been!

5.1.4. Choice of Antibiotics

The choice and quantity of antibiotics are difficult to establish. A series of recent experiments by Durack, Petersdorf, and Pelletier and their co-workers in the rabbit model cast doubt on the efficacy of current accepted recommendations.[23-28] These experiments have been critized, however, as not being sufficiently comparable to the situation in man to serve, in themselves, as reason to change the current recommendations.[29] On the other hand, Durack and Littler[30] have commented on failures of the currently recommended programs. These reported failures represent very few patients, but reporting failures has never been a popular pastime, and notification is not obligatory; thus, it is difficult to judge the magnitude of the problem.

The American Heart Association, stimulated by these experimental studies, has recently changed its recommendations for antibiotic prophylaxis of IE. These recommendations are reprinted in their entirety in the Appendix.[31]

Although the mechanism of action of prophylactic antibiotics might appear self-evident at first glance, the understanding of the mechanism has proved to be considerably more complicated. In a study by Durack and Petersdorf,[23] antibiotics which were capable of "total kill" were believed necessary to be effective. It was shown that in the rabbit model, antibiotics administered 30 min after intravenous inoculation of test organisms were as effective as those administered 30 min before, thus making it unlikely that in these studies antibiotics have an effect upon bloodstream clearance or sticking of bacteria to the NBTVs. The fact that antibiotics effective within 30 min of the inoculation of test bacteria were ineffective after a delay of 6 hr provided evidence that the metabolic state of the bacteria in the vegetation is important in determining their susceptibility of antibiotics.[32] Consistent with this view was the demonstrated ineffectiveness of bacteriostatic antibiotics.[25] On the other hand, *Candida* endocarditis, in the same rabbit model, was effectively prevented by an agent, 5-fluorocytosine (5-FC), considered predominantly bacteriostatic.[33] The prophylactic efficacy of 5-FC was remarkable in view of its ineffectiveness in treating *Candida* IE in the rabbit.[34]

It was next pointed out that the effectiveness of prophylactic antibiotics is influenced by the inoculum used to provoke infection: the lower the inoculum, the more effective the antibiotic.[26] Thus, erythromycin, ineffective in preventing IE provoked by an inoculum of 10^8 streptococci, was very effective when the inoculum was reduced to 10^5 streptococci. This effect of inoculum has also been noted in the prevention of *Str. intermedius* in IE rats with a bactericidal antibiotic, vancomycin.[35] The effect of inoculum may be related to a decreased number of persisting colonies of lower inoculum,[23] but under certain circumstances, antibiotics may alter bacterial clearance from the bloodstream and sticking, effects which are perhaps not evident when using higher inocula.

Even more puzzling is the observation that the removal of the catheter employed to induce the NBTVs markedly increased the effectiveness of prophylactic antibiotics.[35] It is difficult to know in what way the presence of a foreign body could influence the action of an antibiotic, particularly in a lesion which is supposed to be devoid of a significant number of polymorphonuclear leukocytes (PMN). On the other hand, it is possible that PMN do play a role in the early phases of infection, immediately after the intravenous inoculation of bacteria, which is not apparent later, when fibrin bands effectively isolate the bacteria from PMN [see Figure 3 (Chapter 2)]. A role for macrophages in the delivery of streptococci to NBTVs was described by Durak, but has not been confirmed by others.(36–38)

Thus, investigations of the mechanism of antibiotic activity in preventing IE in rabbits raise several questions touching the effect of antibiotics and the way in which a foreign body interferes with antibiotics and host defense mechanisms which, in the long run, may have biological and clinical importance far beyond that relating only to the question of the prevention (and treatment) of IE.

Recently, antibiotic regimens given for the prophylaxis of IE in man have been examined to see whether the serum levels of bactericidal activity achieved were comparable to those shown to be associated with effective prophylaxis in the rabbit model.(39–41) It is difficult to compare these studies because it has been shown that the ability to prevent enterococcal IE in rabbits is not predictable from *in vitro* sensitivity tests.(28) Furthermore, the methods for determining *in vitro* sensitivity and for estimating serum inhibitory and bactericidal activity were either not comparable or not described in sufficient detail to permit comparisons.(28,39,40) As described in Section 9.2, the lack of standardization of these methods is a major problem in comparing results of different laboratories.

5.1.5. Choice of Subjects

It is not easy to decide which subjects should receive antibiotic prophylaxis (Table 4). There is general agreement that any patient with acquired or congenital heart disease (except uncomplicated secundum atrial septal defect) and IHSS should be protected. At particularly high risk of developing second or third infections are patients with a history of IE. The risk is estimated to be 8–9% for second and 25% for third infections in these subjects.(42) Patients with the MVP syndrome pose a difficult problem; there is no question but that there is a risk of developing IE. Indeed, one third of IE in patients with mitral regurgitation is believed attributable to MVP. The problem is that between 5 and 21% of "normal," healthy young women are believed to have this valve abnormality.(43) The American Heart Association believes that such patients should receive prophylaxis.

Routine cardiac catheterization carries a low risk and is not considered an indication for the use of prophylactic antibiotics.

There are other circumstances in which the risk is small but not negligible, such as patients with surgically corrected patent ductus arteriosus and surgically corrected ventricular septal defect. The risk is probably greater in patients with permanent cardiac pacemakers and ventriculoatrial shunts for relief of hydrocephalus. I would be inclined to administer prophylactic antibiotics to the latter two groups of patients.

TABLE 4
Classification of Patients as Candidates for Antibiotic Prophylaxis by Reason of Risk of Developing Infective Endocarditis

A.	Very high risk
	Previous IE (even without current evidence of heart disease)
	Heart-valve prosthesis
	Coarctation of the aorta
	Indwelling vascular catheter (left side of the heart)
B.	High risk
	Rheumatic and other acquired valvular heart disease
	Congenital heart disease: ventricular septal defect, tetrology of Fallot, aortic stenosis, complex cyanotic heart disease, patent ductus arteriosus, systemic–pulmonary artery shunts
	Idiopathic hypertrophic subaortic stenosis (IHSS)
	Mitral-valve prolapse (MVP) with mitral insufficiency
	Marfan's syndrome
	Indwelling vascular catheters (right side of the heart)
	Renal dialysis with A-V shunt appliance
	Ventriculoatrial shunts for hydrocephalus
C.	Low risk
	Indwelling transvenous cardiac pacemakers
	Congenital pulmonary stenosis
	MVP without mitral insufficiency

When the decision is made to administer prophylactic antibiotics, they should be begun about 1–2 hr before the procedure and continued for no more than 1–2 days, in order to avoid having the patient colonized with resistant strains of bacteria. Furthermore, judging from animal studies, bacteriostatic antibiotics such as tetracycline are probably ineffective.[25]

Finally, although extraction of healthy teeth was once recommended so as to avoid the development of IE, cases of *Str. viridans* IE have been reported in edentulous persons, probably related to poorly fitting dentures. Thus, this approach is not recommended.[44]

Most important is the need to inform patients after placement of a prosthetic valve that they are at least at the same risk of developing IE as they were before operation.[45] Many of these patients believe that the operation has eliminated this risk and promptly develop IE after a tooth extraction without having received prophylactic antibiotics.

It is rather interesting that coronary-artery surgery does not seem to represent a significant risk for the development of IE. I am tempted to compare this to the general difficulty seen in animals in maintaining infection of NBTVs located in extracardiac intravascular sites.[46]

In Table 5, the antibiotic regimens for the prevention of the most common causes of IE are described according to the relative risk of developing IE. The

TABLE 5
Recommendations for Antibiotic Prophylaxis of Infective Endocarditis According to Predicted Infecting Bacterium and Relative Patient Risk[a]

Patient risk	Nonenterococcal, non-group A Streptococci: Penicillin-sensitive	Nonenterococcal, non-group A Streptococci: Penicillin-resistant	Enterococci, Bacteremia: Likely	Enterococci, Bacteremia: Less likely	Staphylococci
Very high	D/G	F/G	F/G	F/G	H/G
High	A or B/C or E	—/C	F/G	—	H/G
Low[b]	B/C or E	—/C	F/G	—	H/G

[a] The capital letters A–H denote the antibiotic regimens described in Table 6. That following the slash is recommended in case of penicillin allergy.
[b] There is considerable uncertainty concerning the need to recommend antibiotic prophylaxis in low-risk patients (Table 4).

antibiotic recommendations are those of the American Heart Association, but limited to a treatment period of 48 hr (Table 6).

It is worth emphasizing that since there is uncertainty as to the efficacy of antibiotic prophylaxis in man, it is difficult to advocate one recommendation for antibiotic prophylaxis rather than another. On the other hand, the experimental data have provided a reference point for recommendations in man. Of the utmost importance is the recording of cases of IE believed to have occurred despite the administration of prophylactic antibiotics. Such cases may be recorded by contacting the American Heart Association National Center in Dallas, Texas.

Other aspects of the controversy over antibiotic prophylaxis for IE include the high cost of various questionably necessary but expensive medications, the inconvenience of intravenous medications, and its effect on the frequency with which antibiotic prophylaxis is carried out at all.[42,47–49] The latter argument can be summarized by asking whether it is better from a public-health standpoint to recommend more effective antibiotics which because of inconvenience are given less frequently or more convenient but (perhaps) less effective antibiotics which are administered more frequently. In short, the issue is complicated and not likely to be resolved without the collection of more data in man.

5.2. PROSTHETIC-VALVE SURGERY

The general consensus is that all cardiovascular surgeons give prophylactic antibiotics to patients undergoing placement of prosthetic heart valves, and probably also aortic grafts, and yet there is no evidence to indicate that antibiotics

TABLE 6
Antibiotic Regimens for the Prophylaxis of Infective Endocarditis

Antibiotic	Dosage	Schedule
A. Aqueous crystalline penicillin G	1,000,000 U	I.M. ½–1 hr prior to procedure
mixed with		
Procaine penicillin G	600,000 U	
then		
Penicillin V	500 mg P.O.	Every 6 hr × 8
B. Penicillin V	2.0 g P.O.	½–1 hr prior to procedure
then	500 mg P.O.	Every 6 hr × 8
C. Erythromycin	1.0 g P.O.	1½–2 hr prior to procedure
then	500 mg P.O.	Every 6 hr × 8
D. A + Streptomycin	1.0 g I.M.	½–1 hr prior to procedure
then		
Penicillin V	500 mg P.O.	Every 6 hr × 8
E. Vancomycin	1.0 g I.V. during ½–1 hr	½–1 hr prior to procedure
then		
Erythromycin	500 mg P.O.	Every 6 hr × 8
F. Aqueous crystalline penicillin G	2,000,000 U I.M. or I.V.	½–1 hr prior to procedure (applies to all of F through Streptomycin 1.0 g I.M.)
or		
Ampicillin	1.0 g I.M. or I.V.	
plus		
Gentamicin	1.5 mg/kg [not to exceed 80 mg] I.M. or I.V.	
or		
Streptomycin	1.0 g I.M.	
then		
If Gentamicin:	repeat every 8 hr × 2	
If Streptomycin:	repeat every 12 hr × 2	
G. Vancomycin	1.0 g I.V. during ½–1 hr	½–1 hr prior to procedure
plus		
Streptomycin	1.0 g I.M.	May be repeated in 12 hours
H. β-Lactamase-resistant penicillin		
or		
Cephalosporin antibiotics[a]		

[a] Employed in prosthetic valve surgery (see Section 5.3).

under these circumstances are useful. The studies that have been carried out indicate that there is no difference in the frequency of valve infection, but patients receiving antibiotics developed infections resistant to the antibiotics administered prophylactically, whereas those infections developing in patients not receiving prophylactic antibiotics were sensitive to usual antibiotics.[50,51]

The logical conclusion in the face of such data would seem to me to be *not* to administer prophylactic antibiotics. Indeed, perhaps a large part of the reason that post-valve-surgery infection is so difficult to manage, and has such a high mortality, may be precisely because these infections are resistant to many of the most useful antibiotics. The difficulty is that no one is willing to withhold antibiotics from such patients. Many physicians say that they just could not *not* administer penicillin, knowing that patients were at risk of developing pneumococcal endocarditis. When it became obvious that staphylococci were the major bacteriological risk after valve surgery, prophylaxis evolved imperceptibly but uniformly to a penicillinase-resistant penicillin. Today, with the rising frequency of infections due to gram-negative bacilli and fungi, recommendations are changing to add gentamicin to the semisynthetic penicillin.

There has been a progressive fall in the frequency of early PVE in recent years.[52,53] Whether this is due to improvements in surgical techniques, postoperative management, or prophylactic antibiotics is impossible to determine.

Concomitantly, as the period of observation of operated patients continues, more patients are being seen with late PVE. Curiously, although there are increasing numbers of patients being seen with late PVE due to the usual kinds of streptococci, there is a predominance of infection with staphylococci, gram-negative bacteria, and fungi which suggests that some cases of late PVE are patients whose intravascular vegetations (or foreign bodies) are contaminated early but in whom signs and symptoms of infection do not appear until several months, perhaps several years later.[52,53] There is good epidemiological evidence to support this viewpoint.[54]

In general, current practice is to limit the use of prophylactic antibiotics to immediately before and after surgery and to continue for a total of 48 hr.[52,53] In one hospital (Papworth regime), "loading" doses of cloxacillin, benzylpenicillin, and gentamicin are given intramuscularly with the premedication with an intravenous booster at the end of cardiopulmonary bypass. For the next 48 hr, 1,000,000 U benzylpenicillin and 500 mg cloxacillin are given every 6 hr intravenously, as well as gentimicin, according to age, weight, and renal function, at the same intervals. Use of this program for a period of 4 years in more than 800 open-heart procedures has been associated with a complete absence of early PVE.[55]

Obviously, there are great difficulties in evaluating the effectiveness of prophylactic antibiotics in prosthetic-valve surgery. The problem of differentiating improvements in operative and postoperative techniques from effects of antibiotics has already been mentioned. It is necessary to add to this list the episodic (outbreak) nature of many examples of operative or postoperative infection as well as the fact that many patients with late PVE are examples of failure of antibiotic prophylaxis administered at the time of operation.[54]

5.3. VASCULAR GRAFTS

The arguments for and against the use of prophylactic antibiotics in vascular-graft procedures have recently been summarized by Szilagyi and Elliott.[51] The problem is similar to that of prosthetic-valve surgery, the major difference being that local wound infection is thought to play a much greater role in initiating vascular-graft infection than in initiating PVE. The consequences are the same—catastrophic; therefore, the desire to avoid these infections is equally great in both circumstances. As a consequence, prophylactic antibiotics are generally employed in femoral grafting procedures, where the risk of local infection is highest. The antibiotic chosen is generally a penicillinase-resistant penicillin. On the other hand, it is felt that prophylactic antibiotics are not necessary for patients with vascular grafts undergoing oropharyngeal procedures. The attitude after genitourinary-tract instrumentation is less clear.

Experiments in dogs with aortic grafts and rabbits with A-V fistulae have demonstrated the efficacy of prophylaxis regimens under circumstances in which the test strain of bacteria, administered intravenously, is susceptible to the antibiotics employed.[51,56] The difficulty, of course, as in the case of prosthetic-valve surgery, is that there are always potential pathogens in the environments which are resistant to the antibiotics chosen for prophylactic use.

REFERENCES

1. Kaplan, E. L., Rich, H., Gersony, W., Manning, J.: A collaborative study of infective endocarditis in the 1970's—Emphasis on infections in patients who have undergone cardiovascular surgery. *Circulation* **59**(2):327–335, 1979.
2. Freedman, L. R., Valone, J.: Experimental endocarditis. *Prog. Cardiovasc. Dis.* **22**:169–180, 1979.
3. Hook, E. W., III, Sande, M. A.: Role of the vegetation in experimental *Streptococcus viridans* endocarditis. *Infect. Immun.* **10**(6):1433–1438, 1974.
4. Petch, C. P.: Anticoagulants in bacterial endocarditis (letter). *Br. Med. J.* **3**:502, 1973.
5. Bailey, I. K., Richards, J. G.: Infective endocarditis in a Sydney teaching hospital—1962–1971. *Aust. N. Z. J. Med.* **5**:413–420, 1975.
6. Levison, M. E., Carrizosa, J., Tanphaichitra, D., Schick, P. K., Rubin, W.: Effect of aspirin on thrombogenesis and on production of experimental aortic valvular *Streptococcus viridans* endocarditis in rabbits. *Blood* **49**(4):645–650, 1977.
7. Thompson, J., Eulderink, F., Lemkes, H., van Furth, R.: Effect of warfarin on the induction and course of experimental endocarditis. *Infect. Immun.* **14**(6):1284–1289, 1976.
8. Thorig, L., Thompson, J., Eulderink, F.: Effect of warfarin in the induction and course of experimental *Staphylococcus epidermis* endocarditis. *Infect. Immun.* **17**(3):504–509, 1977.

9. Wilson, W. R., Geraci, J. E., Danielson, G. K., Thompson, R. L., Spittell, J. A., Jr., Washington, J. A., II, Giuliani, E. R.: Anticoagulant therapy and central nervous system complications in patients with prosthetic valve endocarditis. *Circulation* **57**(5):1004–1007, 1978.
10. Durack, D. T., Beeson, P. B.: *Pathogenesis of Infective Endocarditis in Infective Endocarditis*, Rahimtoola, S. H., ed. Grune and Stratton, New York, pp. 1–53, 1978.
11. Marier, R., Valenti, A. J., Madri, J. A.: Gram-negative endocarditis following cystoscopy. *J. Urol.* **119**:134–137, 1978.
12. Kaplan, E. L., Anderson, R. C.: Infective endocarditis after use of dental irrigation device (letter). *Lancet 2*:610, 1977.
13. Drapkin, M. S.: Endocarditis after the use of an oral irrigation device (technical note). *Ann. Intern. Med.* **87**(4):455, 1977.
14. de Swiet, M., Ramsay, I. D., Rees, G. M.: Bacterial endocarditis after insertion of intrauterine contraceptive device (case report). *Br. Med. J.* **117**:76, 1975.
15. Kahn, H. S., Tyler, C. W.: IUD and endocarditis (letter). *Ann. Intern. Med.* **79**(1):134, 1973.
16. Sobrero, A. J., Lane, M. E.: IUD and endocarditis (letter). *Ann. Intern. Med.* **79**(1):134, 1973.
17. Fleming, H. A.: Antibiotic prophylaxis against infective endocarditis after delivery. *Lancet* **1**:144–145, 1977.
18. Labrosse, H., Bouvet, A.: Endocardite maligne chez une femme porteuse d'un stérilet. *Gaz. Med. Fr.* **85**(37):4469–4472, 1978.
19. Stang, J. M., Weinstein, L.: Chemoprophylaxis for bacterial endocarditis (letters). *N. Engl. J. Med.* **297**(8):427–428, 1975.
20. Ward, R. L.: Endocarditis complicating ulcerative colitis (letter). *Gastroenterology* **75**(5):1189–1190, 1977.
21. Meyer, G. W.: Prophylaxis of infective endocarditis during gastrointestinal procedures: Report of a survey. *Gastrointest. Endosc.* **25**(1):1–2, 1979.
22. Munster, A. M., Weiner, J., Gibson, G.: Prophylactic antibiotics in surgery. *J. Am. Med. Assoc.* **241**(7):717–718, 1979.
23. Durack, D. T., Petersdorf, R. G.: Chemotherapy of experimental streptococcal endocarditis. I. Comparison of commonly recommended prophylactic regimens. *J. Clin. Invest.* **52**:592–598, 1973.
24. Durack, D. T., Pelletier, L. L., Petersdorf, R. G.: Chemotherapy of experimental streptococcal endocarditis. II. Synergism between penicillin and streptomycin against penicillin-sensitive streptococci. *J. Clin. Invest.* **53**(3):829–833, 1974.
25. Southwick, F. S., Durack, D. T.: Chemotherapy of experimental streptococcal endocarditis. III. Failure of a bacteriostatic agent (tetracycline) in prophylaxis. *J. Clin. Pathol.* **27**:261–264, 1974.
26. Pelletier, L. L., Durack, D. T., Petersdorf, R. G., Nielson, K.: Chemotherapy of experimental streptococcal endocarditis. IV. Further observations on prophylaxis. *J. Clin. Invest.* **56**:319–330, 1975.
27. Pelletier, L. L., Petersdorf, R. G., Nielson, K.: Chemotherapy of experimental streptococcal endocarditis. V. Effects of duration of infection and retained intracardiac catheter on response to treatment. *J. Lab. Clin. Med.* **87**:692–702, 1976.
28. Durack, D. T., Starkebaum, M. K., Petersdorf, R. G.: Chemotherapy of experimental endocarditis. VI. Prevention of enterococcal endocarditis. *J. Lab. Clin. Med.* **90**(1):171–179, 1977.
29. Cohen, P. S., Maguire, J. H., Weinstein, L.: Infective endocarditis caused by gram-negative bacteria: A review of the literature 1945–1977. *Prog. Cardiovasc. Dis.* **22**:205–242, 1980.
30. Durack, D. T., Littler, W. A.: Failure of "adequate" penicillin therapy to prevent bacterial endocarditis after tooth extraction (letter). *Lancet* **2**:846–847, 1974.
31. Kaplan, E. L., Anthony, B. F., Bisno, A., Durack, D. T., Houser, H., Millard, H. D., Sanford, J., Shulman, S. T., Stillerman, M., Taranta, A., Wenger, N.: AHA Committee Report: Prevention of bacterial endocarditis. *Circulation* **56**(1):139A–143A, 1977.

32. Durack, D. T., Beeson, P. B.: Experimental bacterial endocarditis. II. Survival of bacteria in endocardial vegetations. *Br. J. Exp. Pathol.* **53**:50–53, 1972.
33. Demierre, G., Freedman, L. R.: Candida endocarditis in rabbits: Prophylaxis with 5-fluorocytosine (10th International Congress of Chemotherapy, Zurich, 1977). *Curr. Chemother.* **1**:217–219, 1978.
34. Sande, M. A., Bowman, C. R., Calderone, R. A.: Experimental *Candida albicans* endocarditis: Characterization of the disease and response to therapy. *Infect. Immun.* **17**(1):140–147, 1977.
35. Heraief, E., Glauser, M., Freedman, L. R.: Vancomycin in prophylaxis of streptococcal endocarditis in rats (11th International Congress of Chemotherapy and 19th Interscience Conference on Antimicrobial Agents and Chemotherapy, Boston, 1979). *Curr. Chemother.* **1**:911–913, 1980.
36. Durack, D. T., Beeson, P. B., Petersdorf, R. G.: Experimental bacterial endocarditis. III. Production and progress of the disease in rabbits. *Br. J. Exp. Pathol.* **54**:142–151, 1973.
37. Thörig, L., Thompson, J., Eulderink, F., van Furth, R.: The role of host factors in the pathogenesis of bacterial endocarditis. *Neth. J. Med.* **22**(5):174–175, 1979.
38. Gillett, R., McGowan, D. A.: The reprocessing of scanning electron microscope specimens for conventional transmission electron microscopy, and its use in confirming bacterial colonization on heart valves in experimental bacterial endocarditis. *J. Dent. Res.* **58**:1267, 1979.
39. Murillo, J., Standiford, H. C., Tatem, B. A., Caplan, E. S., Calia, F. M.: Parenteral prophylaxis against enterococcal endocarditis. *Am. J. Med. Sci* **277**(2):195–200, 1979.
40. Thompson, M. E., Vickers, R. M., Pazin, G. A., Lyon, J. A.: Antibiotic levels achieved during bacterial endocarditis prophylaxis. *Circulation* **60**(4):11–37, 1979.
41. Shanson, D. C.: High-dose oral amoxycillin for preventing endocarditis. *Br. Med. J.* **280**:446, 1980.
42. Sipes, J. N., Thompson, R. L., Hook, E. W.: Prophylaxis of infective endocarditis: A reevaluation (review or bibliography). *Annu. Rev. Med.* **28**:371–391, 1977.
43. Corrigall, D., Bolen, J., Hancock, E. W., Popp, R. L.: Mitral valve prolapse and infective endocarditis. *Am. J. Med.* **63**:215–222, 1977.
44. Goodman, J. S., Kolhouse, J. F., Koenig, M. G.: Recurrent endocarditis due to *Streptococcus viridans* in an "edentulous" man. *South. Med. J.* **66**(3):352–358, 1973.
45. Gersony, W. M., Hayes, C. J.: Bacterial endocarditis in patients with pulmonary stenosis, aortic stenosis or ventricular septal defect. *Circulation Suppl. I* **56**(2):184–187, 1977.
46. Francioli, P., Freedman, L. R.: Streptococcal infection of endocardial and other intravascular vegetations in rabbits: Natural history and effect of dexamethasone. *Infect. Immun.* **24**:483–491, 1979.
47. Kaye, D.: New guidelines for preventing endocarditis. *Drug Ther.*, Nov. 1977, pp. 26–46.
48. Petersdorf, R. G.: Antimicrobial prophylaxis of bacterial endocarditis—Prudent caution or bacterial overkill? *Am. J. Med.* **65**:220–223, 1978.
49. Brooks, S. L.: Survey of compliance with American Heart Association guidelines for prevention of bacterial endocarditis. *J. Am. Dent. Assoc.* **101**:41–43, 1980.
50. Schaffner, W.: Antibiotic prophylaxis in valvular replacement surgery, in: *Infections of Prosthetic Heart Valves and Vascular Grafts*, Duma, R. J., Ed. University Park Press, Baltimore, pp. 313–321, 1977.
51. Szilagyi, D. E., Elliott, J. P.: Antibiotic prophylaxis in vascular grafting, in: *Infections of Prosthetic Heart Valves and Vascular Grafts*, Duma, R. J., ed. University Park Press, Baltimore, pp. 323–342, 1977.
52. Rossiter, S. J., Stinson, E. B., Oyer, P. E., Miller, D. C., Schapira, J. N., Martin, R. P., Shumway, N. E.: Prosthetic valve endocarditis. *J. Thorac. Cardiovasc. Surg.* **76**(6):795–803, 1978.
53. Watanakunakorn, C.: Prosthetic valve infective endocarditis. *Prog. Cardiovasc. Dis.* **22**:181–192, 1979.

54. Hammond, G. W., Stiver, H. G.: Combination antibiotic therapy in an outbreak of prosthetic endocarditis caused by *Staphylococcus epidermis*. *Can. Med. Assoc. J.* **118**(5):524–530, 1978.
55. Newsom, S. W. B.: Antibiotic prophylaxis for open heart surgery. *J. Antimicrob. Chemother.* **4**:389–394, 1978.
56. Lane, T. W., Abrutyn, E.: Induction and prevention of experimental arteriovenous fistula infections. *Antimicrob. Agents Chemother.* **16**:638–640, 1979.

6

Consequences of Intravascular Infection

6.1. ESTABLISHING THE DIAGNOSIS

The clinical features of intravascular infection are secondary to its biology. However, particularly in the early phase, the symptoms are nonspecific, and diagnosis will depend to a considerable degree upon the patient's appreciation of his symptoms and the physician's alertness to the diagnostic possibility. In addition, some important biological consequences may not contribute to clinical symptomatology.

For these reasons, this chapter deals first with the clinical presentation from the standpoint of establishing the diagnosis and then considers the biological consequences of intravascular infection, whether or not they contribute to clinical symptomatology. Chapter 7 considers the host defense mechanisms which develop in response to infection, and Chapters 8 through 11 deal with, respectively, the problem of when and how to treat these infections, indices of effectiveness of treatment, outcome of treatment, and complications of treatment itself.

6.1.1. Clinical Presentation of Infective Endocarditis

It is evident from the preceding discussion that there are many circumstances under which susceptibility to intravascular infection is increased. A wide variety of microorganisms are capable of establishing infection. Thus, the probability of intravascular infection producing a particular symptom will depend upon the underlying cause of the nonbacterial thrombotic vegetation (NBTV), its location within the vascular system, the infecting microorganism, the duration and complications of intravascular infection, any associated underlying illness, and any medications the patients might be taking which either influence host defense mechanisms or alter the characteristics of the infection itself. The nonspecificity and variability of the mode of onset of infective endocarditis (IE) are evident in the description given by Libman and Friedberg[1] some 40 years ago:

> The onset of the disease is usually insidious. As a rule, the patient is known to have suffered from a cardiac lesion which has been well compensated. He may be up and around long after the disease has begun. The first symptoms are variable and often difficult to determine because of their slow development. Most often there is lassitude or weakness, anorexia and a low grade fever. The patient may complain of undue fatigue toward evening and an unwonted desire to go to sleep early. Often the beginning of the disease may be dated more accurately from the time of appearance of the latter symptom than from that of the onset of fever. The patient may complain of vague and diffuse pains such as occur with a "grippal" infection. This may lead to his temperature being taken and the discovery of an endocarditis.
>
> Sometimes the patient first consults his physician because of a loss of weight. A careful review of the patient's history may reveal a respiratory or other febrile infection from which the patient seemed to recover but after which he never returned to a state of good health or complete apyrexia. At times the patient suffers from an acute rheumatic episode with fever and arthritis, which symptoms merge imperceptibly into a complicating bacterial endocarditis. The symptoms of the disease may seem to develop insidiously after an operative procedure or after childbirth. Almost any symptom of the disease may be its first manifestation, particularly cardiac weakness, urinary symptoms, pulmonary symptoms, headache, vertigo or digestive disturbances.
>
> Occasionally there is a sudden onset, characterized by a sharp elevation of temperature with or without chills or by evidences of embolism of one of the cerebral, visceral or peripheral arteries. Thus the onset may occur acutely with hemiplegia, local paralysis of an extremity, embolism of the retinal artery or sharp pain in the abdomen or lumbar region due to a splenic or renal infarction.

As long ago as 1951, Friedberg was cited[2] as advocating

> making a diagnosis of bacterial endocarditis in any patient with valvular heart disease who runs fever for more than a week if no other cause can be found, even though the other clinical features of the disease are absent.

It is generally held that the clinical criteria for the diagnosis of IE have undergone considerable change in recent times.[3] This is exemplified by the statement of Weinstein and Rubin[4] that if one were to use the diagnostic criteria of 25–30 years ago, one would not suspect the diagnosis in at least 90% of cases.

It is important to emphasize that the change in diagnostic criteria refer not to a fundamental change in the nature of the disease or in the nature of these criteria, but rather to a decreased frequency of certain findings at the time the patient is first admitted to the hospital. This is probably because physicians see patients and consider the possibility of IE at a much earlier stage in the evolution of the disease today than was the case previously. Thus, the clinical features of the disease, which depend upon the duration of infection and the consequent ability to establish an immunological response (emboli, anemia, clubbing of the fingers, splenomegaly, petechiae, Osler and Janeway lesions, glomerulonephritis) are less frequent today when the diagnosis is established than in the preantibiotic era.

Another reason for an apparent difference in the clinical features of IE in the preantibiotic era and today is that there has been a change in the way the features of the illness are analyzed. In the past, emphasis was put on findings that were detectable either at what was presumed to be the onset or at any time during the long evolution of the illness, whereas today, one should distinguish the signs and the symptoms at the onset of infection from those present upon admission to the hospital (at the time of diagnosis) and from those which occur subsequent to the onset of antibiotic treatment. These simple distinctions are of obvious importance for establishing the source of infection (and the evaluation of prophylaxis), for improving our capacity for early diagnosis, and finally for evaluating the effectiveness of antibiotic therapy.

6.1.1.1. Delay in Diagnosis

Delay in diagnosis will, of course, influence the nature of the clinical presentation. It is the rule today for symptoms to have been present before hospitalization for more than 4 weeks in about 50% of patients and for more than 3 months in about 20% of patients.[5] Infections due to staphylococci and enterococci tend to be associated with shorter intervals between the onset of symptoms and hospitalization than infections with *viridans* streptococci. The overlap is of such a magnitude, however, that this distinction is not useful clinically.

Delay in diagnosis will, of course, vary from patient to patient depending on his concern about symptoms which might seem to be no more serious than those of the "flu." Physicians, on the other hand, might be responsible for delay in diagnosis when they focus narrowly on symptoms such as vomiting or weight loss.

6.1.1.2. Gastrointestinal Symptoms

It is common for patients to come to the physician with gastrointestinal symptoms. Recently, a woman undergoing a thorough 2-week surgical investigation, for persistent vomiting, was subsequently found to have IE. Patients with IE are often sent to the hospital to search for a possible cancer of the GI tract.

There are several reasons that patients with IE should develop GI symptoms. Aside from the anorexia and weight loss associated with any severe illness, there is the possibility of emboli to the GI tract or abdominal symptoms resulting from emboli to the gallbladder, liver, spleen, or kidneys, common findings at autopsy.[6-9] Rarely, emboli to the spleen may be responsible for splenic rupture or may serve as the source of recurrent infection.[7–10] In addition, congestion of the liver secondary to the recent onset of heart failure may also present predominantly as abdominal discomfort.

It is of some interest that there appears to be an association of carcinoma of the colon and IE due to *Streptococcus bovis*.[11–14] Intestinal carriage rates of *Str. bovis* are increased in patients with colon carcinoma.[11] This association is important, since the colon carcinoma has often been asymptomatic at the time of treatment of the endocarditis. It is clearly indicated to carry out a radiological investigation of the intestine (as well as sigmoidoscopy) in any patient with *Str. bovis* endocarditis. Whether this association represents an increased susceptibility of patients with intestinal cancer to *Str. bovis* bacteremia or whether the carriage of *Str. bovis* is related to the development of intestinal cancer is not known (see Section 8.5.12).

6.1.1.3. Alcoholism and Cirrhosis

Alcoholism and cirrhosis tend to predispose to the development of IE, the rates being about twice those in a noncirrhotic population.[15] There is a tendency toward an increased risk of infection with gram-negative bacilli and perhaps pneumococci,[15,16] most likely related to the increased risk of bacterial infection (pneumonia and gram-negative sepsis) in these patients.[15,17]

6.1.1.4. Neuropsychiatric Symptoms

Neuropsychiatric symptoms are also very common (as high as 50% in some series) in the early symptomatic phase of IE and are commonly misinterpreted, resulting in delay in the diagnosis of IE.[18] It has been emphasized that in the elderly, mental change may be the most prominent feature of the symptom complex of the patient with IE.[18] In some instances, the diagnosis of IE has been established only after the patient has already received electroshock for his presumed psychiatric illness.[19]

Aside from headache and "organic or toxic brain syndrome," the central nervous system (CNS) symptoms range from those of transient ischemic episodes preceding hemiplegia, choreiform movements, to meningoencephalitis, sterile or purulent meningitis, brain abscess or cerebral hemorrhage, or aneurysm. Any of the cranial nerves may be involved.

In the majority of instances, the presence of CNS symptomatology does not alter the management or treatment of IE except in those instances where it is indicated to perform surgical drainage of a brain abscess or where the possibility of a mycotic aneurysm exists. Spinal-fluid findings are variable and depend upon the underlying lesion and the infecting microorganism.[20–22,220]

6.1.1.5. Heart Murmurs

Whereas in most series of patients with IE, heart murmurs are detectable in about 90% of patients upon admission to the hospital,[23] in a recent series of patients over 60 years of age, a heart murmur was absent in about one fourth of patients.[24] In this elderly population, the clinical diagnosis was suspected in only 40% of the whole series and in only 9% of those without a heart murmur. It was recently recommended that "bacterial endocarditis should be suspected in any elderly patient who has not been feeling well."[25] In an addict population, IE is often established on normal heart valves or on the right side of the heart, both circumstances being likely not to give rise to heart murmurs.

6.1.1.6. Heart Failure

Signs and symptoms of heart failure are present in about one third of patients at the time of hospital admission. This may be a consequence of the presence of infection in a patient with underlying heart disease, valve perforation, conduction defects secondary to emboli in the myocardium or valve-ring abscess formation, or myocardial infarction. Dyspnea and hemoptysis may also result from pulmonary emboli secondary to right-heart infection.[26]

6.1.1.7. Fever

In the preantibiotic era, fever was said to be present in about 99% of patients, although afebrile periods in the evolution of infection were well documented. Today, fever is frequently absent both as a presenting complaint and as a sign upon admission to the hospital. In three recent general-hospital series, about 25–30% of patients were afebrile (<100.5°F and <38°C).[5,23,27]

6.1.1.8. Skin and Embolic Manifestations, Septic Complications, Mycotic Aneurysms, and Splenomegaly

Skin manifestations (petechiae, Osler and Janeway lesions), embolic manifestations, septic complications, mycotic aneurysms, and splenomegaly have been described in varying percentages in recent analyses, usually being found in 20–40% of patients at the time of hospital admission.[4,5,23,27,28] In the preantibiotic era, these findings were about twice as frequent at the time of hospital admissions. The pathogenesis and consequences of these lesions are discussed in later sections.

6.1.1.9. Glomerulonephritis

Glomerulonephritis with renal insufficiency is relatively uncommon today, occurring in 0–15% of patients, whereas hematuria is seen frequently, in about 50% of patients. In general terms, these findings were also about twice as common in the preantibiotic era.

6.1.1.10. Clubbing of the Fingers

Clubbing of the fingers was a virtually universal finding in patients before antibiotics, whereas it is rare today (0–10%). I cannot recall having seen a patient who developed clubbing of the fingers as a consequence of IE in the past 10 years. This is a good indication of the fact that we recognize endocarditis much earlier today than previously.

6.1.1.11. Musculoskeletal Complaints

On the other hand, musculoskeletal complaints, e.g., myalgia, arthralgia, and back pain, as well as mono- and polyarthritis, are noted frequently in intravascular infections, perhaps in 30–40% or more of patients. These complaints are of particular interest because they may lead to mistaken diagnoses of acute rheumatic fever or, when combined with appropriate skin lesions, acute vasculitis or temporal arteritis.[29–33,221] Several patients with biopsy-proven arteritis and rheumatic syndromes have been treated with corticosteroids (until the proper diagnosis was established by blood culture)—interestingly, without seeming to have an adverse effect on the evolution of the infection.[34–36] Septic arthritis and disk-space infections have also been noted in the past several years as modes of presentation of patients with IE.[37–41]

6.1.1.12. Disseminated Intravascular Coagulation

Occasionally, the clinical presentation of IE has been overshadowed by clinical and laboratory features of disseminated intravascular coagulation (DIC).[42-51] Associated skin lesions include those of petechiae, purpura fulminans, and acral cyanosis.

6.1.1.13. Thrombotic Thrombocytopenic Purpura

In one report, the presentation was typical of thrombotic thrombocytopenic purpura.[52] Infecting organisms associated with these coagulation abnormalities have included *Aspergillus* species, *Str. viridans*, group B streptococci, and *Staphylococcus aureus*, the latter being the most frequent.

6.1.1.14. Anemia

Anemia is a common finding in the majority of patients with IE at the time of hospitalization and obviously may play a significant role in contributing to the general state of fatigue and breathlessness of the patient.[4,5,23,27,28]

6.1.1.15. Previous Heart Disease

A history of previous heart disease or prior cardiac surgery is, of course, very important in raising the possibility of IE. Any patient with a prosthetic heart valve who develops a new murmur, valvular dysfunction, heart failure, or embolic disease should be suspected of having IE. It has been pointed out also that sudden bleeding in prosthetic-valve (or any) patients who up to then had been well controlled with Dicumarol should be looked upon as a sign of possible intravascular infection.[53]

6.1.2. Mycotic Aneurysm (Primary)

The other category of intravascular infection of major importance is primary infection of major arteries [not secondary to IE (mycotic aneurism)]. The clinical presentation of these patients is almost always pain in the region of the aneurysm and fever. Diagnosis, once suspected, should be pursued vigorously, since rupture of such an aneurysm is almost always fatal.

6.1.3. Infection in Peripheral Veins

Infection in peripheral veins may be relatively difficult to diagnose. Septic thrombophlebitis after prolonged catheterization requiring surgical drainage may produce local signs of inflammation, but may be relatively silent, to be discovered only at autopsy.

Of course, the suspicion of infection of the extracardiac vascular system is greatly increased by a history of previous vascular grafts and by hospital procedures associated with venous catheterization. Total parenteral nutrition is particularly notorious for its ability to produce catheter-associated infections.

In brief, there is no substitute for a high index of suspicion. I do not know what percentage of the time the diagnosis of intravascular infection is suspected and finally discarded, but even if one has to take blood cultures in 10 or 20 patients in order to make the diagnosis once, this is a small price to pay to establish the diagnosis of potentially curable disease which, if undiagnosed or diagnosed too late, results in permanent disability or death.

There is little use in tabulating all the possible symptoms of intravascular infection and assigning percentage figures. It is difficult to think of a symptom complex that could not be attributable to intravascular infection. What is important to bear in mind is that patients with such infections may be afebrile or not have an audible heart murmur, but it must be exceptionally rare that both these signs are absent.

6.1.4. Clinical Diagnosis

The clinical diagnosis depends on finding the causative organism in the bloodstream. In a certain percentage of patients thought to have IE (5–20%), blood cultures are reported as negative. In extracardiac intravascular infection, the percentage of negative cultures is about 50% and should not deter treatment if the diagnosis is probable clinically or demonstrable arteriographically.

The clinical and laboratory manifestations of intravascular infections will be discussed from the standpoint of their diagnostic usefulness under the headings of prolonged bacteremia, host responses to bacteremia, local invasion, and peripheral emboli.

6.2. PROLONGED BACTEREMIA

6.2.1. Blood Culture

The diagnosis of intravascular infection is usually made indirectly, since the site of infection is, in most instances, inaccessible to direct examination. The infrequent occasions when direct access is possible include infections of peripheral venous thrombi, arterial emboli, and atrioventricular (A-V) fistulae or shunts. Diagnosis in these instances is facilitated by radiological studies (arteriography) and local surgical access, thus permitting combined histological and bacteriological examination.

In instances when direct access is not possible—the great majority of the time—the diagnosis of intravascular infection depends upon the isolation of the causative agent from the bloodstream.

Considerable emphasis has been given to the prolonged nature of bacteremia in IE. It has been clearly demonstrated in IE that when microorganisms are recovered from the bloodstream, there may be variation in the concentration of microorganisms in the blood, but their presence is constant over long periods of time.[54–56] Unfortunately, intravascular infections are not the only type of infections to be accompanied by prolonged shedding of microorganisms into the bloodstream; thus, this finding is not pathognomonic of intravascular infection. For example, patients with agranulocytosis, osteomyelitis, liver and renal abscesses (often in diabetics or alcoholics), and leprosy, as well as infection due to microorganisms which survive intracellularly (*Salmonella*, meningococci,

Brucella, Listeria, viruses), are also associated with "prolonged" discharge of microorganisms into the bloodstream. Other, less common infections also associated with prolonged bacteremia include tularemia, plague, glanders, melioidosis, anthrax, Haverhill fever, rat bite fever, Weil's disease, histoplasmosis, and bartonellosis.[57] In addition, this phenomenon may be associated with other severe infections, but the clinical indications for prompt effective antibiotic therapy usually make it impossible to observe the duration of bacteremia.

Thus, whereas prolonged shedding of microorganisms into the bloodstream is a characteristic feature of intravascular infection, it is not found exclusively with these types of infection. Furthermore, there is no generally accepted definition of "prolonged."

On the other hand, the duration of bacteremia, although of considerable theoretical interest, nowadays rarely if ever plays a role in establishing the clinical diagnosis of endocarditis. The usual clinical problem is that of a patient whose clinical or laboratory findings lead the physician to suspect the diagnosis of intravascular infection. Aerobic and anaerobic blood cultures are taken and any local lesions (emboli, shunts) examined bacteriologically. Because of the constancy of bacteremia in endocarditis, 3–5 blood-culture pairs (aerobic and anaerobic) taken over a few hours are sufficient to establish the presence of bacteria in the circulation. It is distinctly uncommon, but not unknown, to obtain positive blood cultures after the first 3–5 negative ones in patients previously untreated with antibiotics. Antecubital venous blood is as satisfactory as arterial blood for culture, since there is a minimal loss of bacteria from the bloodstream as it traverses the capillary beds in the arms.[54] This may not hold for fungal infections, in which arterial blood cultures may be advantageous (see Section 8.5.8).

It is not uncommon for several days or, in rare instances, even weeks to pass before the presence of a microorganism in the blood cultures is evident. The pertinent question is obvious—how long does one wait before starting antibiotic therapy? This problem is discussed in Section 8.1.

There is considerable variation from one patient to another in the number of microorganisms found in the bloodstream. Some patients have hundreds of microorganisms per milliliter of blood, whereas the majority with endocarditis have fewer than 30, and some have sterile blood cultures.[58,59] Factors which may be responsible for these quantitative differences include: (1) the site of infection; (2) the nature of the infecting agent; (3) the available culture techniques; (4) the prior administration of antibiotics; (5) uremia; and (6) the so-called "bacteria-free" stage of IE.

6.2.1.1. Site of Infection

The site of infection in IE has long been known to influence the ability to recover the infecting agent in blood cultures. Even though the lung is probably a relatively poor bacterial filter (although very little is known about this), bacterial infection of the right side of the heart has been reported to be accompanied by an inability to culture bacteria from the bloodstream.[60,61]

Quantitative studies of infected vegetations in rabbits have consistently demonstrated that bacterial densities are about 2 logs higher in the left side of the heart than in the right.[62–64] These experiments, carried out with *Str. viridans*, *Escherichia coli*, and *Candida albicans* as test organisms, would easily account for the presence of fewer circulating bacteria with right-heart infections, resulting in the more frequent finding of negative blood cultures.

Comparison of the density of bacteria in vegetations infected with *Bacteroides fragilis* in rabbits shows a similar difference in the concentration of bacteria at the onset of infection (3 days). However, at 5 days, the density of bacteria was the same on the two sides of the heart, and the tricuspid vegetations had become about twice as large as those on the aortic valve. The authors suggest that the relatively low oxygen tension on the right side of the heart favored the growth and development of these vegetations infected with anaerobic bacteria.[65]

Although oxygen tension may play an important role in the evolution of infection with anaerobic bacteria, this does not explain the fact that the natural history of vegetations infected with aerobic bacteria may be different depending upon their location within the vascular system. Differences are seen between infections in different parts of the arterial or venous side of the circulation. For example, infections of arterial vascular prostheses frequently do not give rise to positive blood cultures.[66] These clinical studies are in accord with experimental studies (see Section 4.3.2.2) in rabbits, which demonstrate that streptococcal infections of aortic-arch vegetations contain many fewer bacteria than simultaneously infected vegetations located on the aortic valve.[67] Similarly, many fewer bacteria are recovered from infected vegetations in the inferior vena cava as compared with infections in the right side of the heart.[67]

It has been observed clinically that blood cultures are likely to be negative in streptococcal infections of the right heart, but that blood cultures are generally positive when the right-heart infection is due to staphylococci.[68] This would be consistent with the experimental data discussed earlier in Section 4.5.2.2, which showed that staphylococci were more virulent than streptococci on the right side of the heart, whereas the reverse was the case on the left side.[63] As already mentioned, the finding of staphylococcal infection principally on the right side of the heart (with positive blood cultures) and streptococcal infections principally on the left side is consistent with these experimental observations.

6.2.1.2. Nature of the Infecting Agent

The nature of the infecting agent is important in determining its ability to be detected in the bloodstream. It goes without saying that certain microorganisms with special growth characteristics (e.g., *Brucella*, *pseudomonas*, cell-wall-deficient forms) will be recovered from cultures only if attention has been directed to their *in vitro* growth requirements.(58,59,68–75) Cell-wall-deficient bacterial forms have been identified in histological sections of damaged aortic valves in patients with unequivocal IE and negative blood cultures.(76)

The problem is of a different nature in fungal endocarditis. Positive blood cultures may be unusual or even rare in patients and experimental animals with left-sided fungal endocarditis, even though *in vitro* cultivation of these microorganisms is not difficult.(77–80)

The number of colony-forming units of *Candida*(77) or *Aspergillus*(79) per gram of infected vegetations in animals is considerably less than that usually found for bacteria. This would easily explain the absence of positive blood cultures, but it is difficult to know how to interpret the quantitative enumeration of fungi because of their tendency to form clumps. On the other hand, the histopathology of the fungal lesions in the experimental model is considerably different from that of bacterial vegetations. *Candida* and *Aspergillus* appear to proliferate in well-demarcated zones of an abscesslike lesion, whereas staphylococci and streptococci form collections of compact colonies extending from the surface of the vegetation to its base.(77,79,81,82) These morphological differences might also play a role in diminishing the rate of shedding of fungi into the bloodstream as compared with bacteria.

6.2.1.3. Adequate Culture Techniques

Adequate culture techniques are of obvious importance in the success of any effort to culture microorganisms from the bloodstream. The problem is that of suiting the culture techniques to the microorganisms to be cultured. The standard blood-culture techniques (trypticase soy or brain–heart infusion broth plus thioglycollate broth) are appropriate for at least 90% of the bacteria commonly implicated in intravascular infection. In most series of patients with IE, there are a certain number of patients (about 10%) in whom clinical or postmortem examination makes it highly probable that a microbial infection of the heart valves was present without its having been possible to culture the responsible organisms from the bloodstream. These patients are often referred to as having *blood-culture-negative endocarditis*. It is evident that the inability to culture microorganisms from the bloodstream in IE may be due to the influence of any one or more of the factors responsible for variation in the number of microorganisms detected in the circulation. The point to be made is that negative blood cultures in the presence of intravascular infection may be a consequence of either the biology of the infection or the appropriateness of the culture techniques employed. This subject is discussed in detail in Section 8.1.

6.2.1.4. Prior Administration of Antibiotics

The prior administration of antibiotics is an obvious explanation, and the most common one, for the inability to culture bacteria in patients with intravascular infection. There are two ways by which antibiotic administration can induce negative blood cultures in the presence of active valve infection:

1. Inhibition of growth in cultural media despite the presence of microorganisms in the bloodstream. This is the likely explanation for negative blood cultures taken shortly after the administration of antibiotics. It is theoretically possible to nullify the effect of circulating antibiotic by adequate dilution of the blood sample in culture medium, thereby reducing the concentration of antibiotic below that necessary to inhibit microbial growth. The effect of penicillin can be nullified by the addition of penicillinase to the cultures.

2. Diminution of the number of microorganisms in the intravascular vegetation, thereby producing a truly negative blood culture. This effect is seen when effective treatment is given for too short a period of time, or when treatment is given for what would be adequate periods of time, but with bacteriostatic rather than bactericidal antibiotics. This effect has been produced experimentally by treatment of sensitive α-streptococcal endocarditis in rabbits with 7 days of tetracycline. Therapy resulted in "sterilization" of vegetations in 2 animals and diminution of the number of streptococci in 2 additional rabbits, when bacteriological studies were carried out immediately after the last injection of tetracycline. When bacteriological studies were delayed until 48 hr after the last tetracycline injection, 13 of 14 rabbits had vegetations from which much greater numbers of streptococci could be recovered.[83]

It is sometimes surprising how long an antibacterial effect may persist in causing negative blood cultures. A patient with mitral insufficiency due to rheumatic heart disease was given 3 capsules of vibramycin 24 hr before coming to the hospital. She was febrile and had peripheral vascular lesions (petechiae, conjunctival hemorrhages) consistent with IE. Daily blood cultures, taken while the patient remained febrile, were sterile for 12 days. From the 13th day, blood cultures were regularly positive for *Str. viridans*. The patient had an uneventful recovery after therapy with penicillin and streptomycin.

The prolonged suppression of shedding of bacteria into the bloodstream is easily understood by reference to the experimental work of Durack,[82] in which he was able to show covering of an infected vegetation with elongated mononuclear cells 6 hr after a single injection of penicillin. The vegetation was not sterilized, but the decrease in the number of viable bacteria or the influence of their metabolic activity evidently permitted "endothelialization" of what was previously an open lesion, freely able to shed bacteria into the circulation.

The disappearance of fever in a patient with IE after the administration of antibiotics does not necessarily indicate that blood cultures have become negative. A patient with a clinical picture typical of endocarditis was given tetracycline for several days prior to coming to the hospital. While he was in the hospital for 3 days, his rectal temperatures were normal. Six of six blood cultures taken during this afebrile period were positive for *Str. viridans*. It is evident that the absence of fever does not rule out the possibility of a positive blood culture.

This patient makes one wonder what it is that is responsible for fever in patients with endocarditis; it is obviously not necessarily or solely the presence of circulating viable bacteria.[84]

6.2.1.5. Uremia

Uremia is traditionally cited as a stage in the evolution of IE when the blood culture is often sterile.[68,85] These observations date from the preantibiotic era, when cultural techniques were not as sophisticated as they are today. Furthermore, in order to implicate uremia as a cause of negative cultures, it would be necessary to have blood cultures during life and careful autopsy bacteriological studies establishing the presence of IE. These conditions are rarely fulfilled. In a study frequently referred to as providing evidence for the finding of negative blood cultures in uremic patients, only six patients were presented, two with uremia associated with aortic insufficiency. In no instance were criteria given for the diagnosis of IE.[86] The need for care in the interpretation of qualitative autopsy bacteriology is illustrated by the cultivation of streptococci from 40% of normal valves in 1929.[1] Furthermore, renal insufficiency is, if anything, a condition which increases susceptibility to infection,[87] and hemodialysis increases susceptibility to IE.[37,88]

Although I do not doubt the theoretical capacity of the blood to become sterile in the long-term evolution of IE and the likelihood that the frequency of glomerulonephritis in IE is related to the duration of the illness, I am not convinced that uremia has any effect on the ability to recover bacteria from the blood of patients with infected cardiac vegetations. Moreover, recent studies of patients with glomerulonephritis and uremia due to IE do not report the inability to culture microorganisms from the bloodstream.[89–93]

6.2.1.6. "Bacteria-Free" Stage of Infective Endocarditis

Libman and Friedberg[1] were convinced that a significant number of their patients were in a stage of evolution of IE wherein the vegetations (on the left side of the heart) sterilized themselves. The essential criterion for the diagnosis of this stage was the inability to find bacteria in valvular vegetations. Thus, although bacteria were not demonstrated in valvular vegetations with the techniques available at the time (see Section 8.2), they did not provide evidence that these vegetations had at one time been infected except for the sentence, "Occasionally patients have been observed in the active stage of the disease who, while under observation, pass into the bacteria-free stage."

Nevertheless, the illustrations provided by Libman and Friedberg make it difficult to discard completely the idea that a certain percentage of patients with even left-sided endocarditis heal spontaneously. They put the figure in the preantibiotic era between 3 and 4%.[1] In animals with IE, a capacity for spontaneous healing has been noted with intravascular infections, this capacity varying according to the location of the infection within the vascular system.[67,94] It is felt today that continued renal disease in patients with healed endocarditis can be explained by the prolonged circulation of immune complexes formed in antibody excess.[89] This, of course, raises the therapeutic possibility of plasmapheresis in these patients as treatment for the renal disease.[95]

6.2.2. Fever and Constitutional Symptoms

Fever in intravascular infection represents one of the hallmarks of the disease and was discussed in Section 6.1.1.7. The major point to be emphasized is that fever is frequently absent (perhaps in 25–30% of patients) in the presence of positive blood cultures and does not constitute an important argument against the diagnosis of intravascular infection, even when absent throughout the course of the illness.[84] This phenomenon suggests that bacteremia is not necessarily the factor of major importance in the production of fever in these patients. Fever might also result from hypersensitivity to bacterial products or from the presence of circulating immune complexes (CICs). Variations in the febrile state might thus occur according to the degree to which CICs are phagocytized by monocytes and the reticuloendothelial system (RES), that is, whether they are in the zone of antigen excess (less likely to be taken up) or in the zone of antibody excess (more likely to be taken up).[89]

Constitutional symptoms are very common, but the extent to which they are bothersome varies considerably from one patient to another.

6.2.3. Hematological Findings

Patients with intravascular infection often have changes in their peripheral blood count indicating the presence of infection, mild leukocytosis, and elevation of the sedimentation rate. However, both determinations may be normal. Anemia may be present and is usually of the nonregenerative type. The development of reticulocytosis can be a useful indication of the effectiveness of antibiotic therapy. IE in rabbits produces a hemolytic anemia improved by splenectomy.[96]

DIC may exist in the presence of infection with virtually any microorganism. It may be a prominent clinical feature of the illness, and hemorrhagic manifestations may be responsible for bringing the patient to the physician. Although thrombocytopenia is often seen in untreated intravascular infections, a systematic study of the occurrence of DIC in intravascular infection has not been carried out, but thrombocytopenia, activation, and coagulation abnormalities are common. The importance of hypercoagulability for the initiation and maintenance of NBTV, was discussed in Section 3.2.

6.2.4. Splenomegaly

A palpable spleen is found irregularly in patients with intravascular infection today (20–30% of subjects), whereas it was the rule (50–100% of subjects) in the preantibiotic era.[4,5,27,28] Splenic enlargement is undoubtedly due to the chronic stimulation of the phagocytic properties of the RES secondary to prolonged bacteremia and the presence of CICs. In rabbits, the splenomegaly associated with IE has been associated with increased red-cell destruction.[96]

6.2.5. Metastatic Infection

Metastatic infection can occur in the kidney, bone, spleen, lung, CNS, and skin. In most of these sites, it is probably associated with embolization in addition to bacteremia, and it is discussed in Section 5. The impressive finding is how infrequently bacteremia seems to be responsible for clinically evident metastatic infection in patients with intravascular infection. This may be attributed to the relative avirulence of some *viridans* streptococci, but group D streptococci, *Str. milleri,* and staphylococci are notorious for their capacity to produce metastatic infection in experimental animals (see Section 8.5). It is likely that the application of more sophisticated techniques, e.g., bone scanning, will demonstrate that metastatic infection is not at all uncommon. The presence of circulating antibody simultaneous with the presence of bacteria in the bloodstream may render the continual bacterial implants relatively innocuous. The presence of well-established antibody coating of bacteria would facilitate the action of polymorphonuclear leukocytes (PMN), which, in contrast to their role in intravascular sites of infection, play a most important role in the defenses against infection in peripheral tissues.

6.3. HOST RESPONSES TO BACTEREMIA

6.3.1. Intravascular Coagulation

Among the various host responses to bacteremia, intravascular coagulation is probably one of the most important, yet it is poorly understood. As mentioned in Sections 6.1.1.12 and 6.1.1.13, some patients with IE present the fully developed picture of DIC or thrombotic thrombocytopenic purpura.[42–52] Infecting organisms associated with these coagulation abnormalities include *Str. viridans,* group B streptococci, *Staph. aureus,* and *Aspergillus* species. In addition, pneumococci as well as a wide variety of other microorganisms have been identified as capable of provoking DIC even when not associated with IE.[97]

It is believed that bacteria can activate the clotting mechanism either directly or by activating complement or by causing release of clotting factors from damaged platelets or endothelium. Alternatively, the hypoperfusion and anoxemia resulting from severe infection may encourage the release of clotting factors from damaged tissues.[97,98] In addition, inhibition of fibrinolysis may result in secondary hypercoagulability.[99] Whatever the precise mechanism, there is no doubt concerning the importance of bacteria circulating in the bloodstream as one of the most important causes of intravascular coagulation. The combination of DIC, CICs, and hypercomplementemia is probably the mechanism by which diffuse glomerular damage is produced in patients with IE.[47,98,100]

In addition to serving as a stimulus for disseminated blood clotting, the presence of bacteremia in an intravascular vegetation is a powerful local stimulus to blood coagulation. There is rapid growth of intracardiac vegetations after challenge with microorganisms.[101] This local stimulus to blood clotting cannot be prevented in animals by aspirin, heparin, or thrombocytopenia.[102–104] On the other hand, fibrinolytic agents seem to be effective in altering the nature of infected vegetations in rabbits and dogs.[104,105]

It is of some interest to consider the consequences of local fibrin deposition around bacteria deposited on intravascular vegetations. The most visually impressive effect is that of packaging the bacteria so as to isolate them from phagocytic host defenses, thus favoring survival of the bacteria [see Figure 12 (Chapter 4)]. On the other hand, this packaging effect may also serve to limit the growth capacities of the bacterial colonies. This aspect is discussed in more detail in Chapter 7.

6.3.2. Anticoagulants

Anticoagulants have long been looked at with interest as a means of treating IE. Their use in the absence of effective antibiotic therapy is very dangerous, resulting in frequent fatal hemorrhagic complications.[53,106] After prosthetic-valve surgery, bleeding (in these anticoagulated patients) may be the first sign of the development of IE.[53] These observations have been reproduced in rabbits with experimental endocarditis. Left-heart infection plus anticoagulation leads to severe hemorrhage.[63,107] That this is not due to emboli is shown by experiments wherein the same hemorrhagic phenomena were seen as a consequence of right-sided infection.[63]

Thus, bacteremia seems to potentiate the anticoagulant effect of Dicumarol (and probably heparin also) in the presence of infective endocarditis. It is not clear, however, what effect anticoagulation has on the initiation and natural history of the infectious process. Curiously, the simple intravenous inoculation of bacteria in anticoagulated rabbits is not associated with decreased RE clearance of bacteria or hemorrhagic phenomena, and Dicumarol treatment of rabbits with intracardiac catheters in place does not increase their susceptibility to infection.[63] Heparin does not increase susceptibility to skin infection.[108] In a model of rapidly fatal *Pseudomonas* or pneumococcus infection with uniform DIC production, heparin was able to prevent DIC, but did not influence the mortality rate of the overwhelming infection.[109,110] Heparin treatment of *E. coli* bacteremia in rats may prolong survival, but only with quantities of heparin far in excess of those required to inhibit blood clotting.[111] Thus, although there can be no question of the importance of local and disseminated coagulation in IE, the role of blood clotting is much less clear in other types of infections.

One of the practical questions that derive from these studies is the role of anticoagulation after prosthetic-valve surgery in the susceptibility to, and evolution of, IE. Reference has already been made to the potentiation of the effect of Dicumarol in IE. In one series, anticoagulant treatment of patients with prosthetic heart valves was associated with an increased risk of intracranial hemorrhage.[22] On the other hand, another report speaks of the dangers of discontinuing anticoagulant therapy in patients with prosthetic heart valves and IE.[112] In my opinion, it must be accepted that anticoagulant therapy is hazardous in patients suspected of having IE; thus, particular attention must be directed to its regulation. On the other hand, if good control is possible, it would seem advisable to continue anticoagulants in patients with prosthetic heart valves who develop IE.[112] To continue anticoagulants without instituting effective antibiotic therapy is catastrophic. Therefore, every effort should be made to institute effective antibiotic therapy as soon as possible in such patients. For patients with IE receiving correct antibiotic treatment, I see no objection to the use of anticoagulants where there is a clear indication to do so. IE alone is not such an indication.

6.3.3. Specific Circulating Antibody

It has long been recognized that patients with IE have specific circulating antibody to their infecting organisms present simultaneously in the circulation.[104] This has been used as a diagnostic tool in patients with pneumococcal endocarditis[57] and has recently been proposed as a method for distinguishing between coagulase-positive *Staph. aureus* sepsis with and without endocarditis or metastatic infection.[113] In those patients with endocarditis, all but one had antibodies detected by counterimmunoelectrophoresis in the first serum sample (mean 7 days from onset of symptoms). Quantitation of the antibody by gel diffusion permitted good separation of the two groups of patients. This test may be useful in helping to determine the length of antibiotic therapy necessary for patients with staphylococcal sepsis and may also be useful in gauging the effectiveness of therapy.[113]

Similar techniques for the detection of antibodies are useful in patients suspected of having *Candida* infection, particularly since blood cultures may be negative with this infection.[114] On the other hand, precipitins and agglutinins to *Candida* have also been shown to develop nonspecifically in patients with IE of bacterial origin.[115] The detection of antibodies against streptococci could be useful in diagnosis in patients with negative blood cultures[116] (see Section 8.2).

Although heart antibody has been detected in a variety of heart diseases (myocardial infarction, myxoma), there is high frequency of such antibodies in patients with IE, usually associated with congestive heart failure.[117] Elevated titers in IE patients were not thought to be due to myocardial infarction and heart failure *per se*. Their persistence seems to be associated with a poor prognosis. Although the pathogenesis of these antibodies is not understood, it is interesting to speculate that they might be related to the myocardial-cell damage seen by electron-microscopic techniques in experimental endocarditis.[118,119]

There are references in the older literature to the action of preimmunization in facilitating the development of IE in animals inoculated with viable bacteria.[120-122] In the oft-quoted study by Wadsworth[121] of horses used for the production of antipneumococcal serum, it is not at all clear to me that IE was produced, since the horses had negative blood cultures. These studies are more likely a demonstration of the ability of immune complexes to produce NBTV, than they are of the role of antibody in inducing IE.

Because of the importance of early diagnosis of IE and because 10 days to 2 weeks may be necessary to develop a detectable antibody response, attention has recently been directed to the search for *circulating antigen* in IE. Techniques for the detection of *Staph. aureus* antigen by solid-phase radioimmunoassay look promising, although antigen is more difficult to detect in the presence of preformed antibody or right-sided IE.[222]

6.3.4. Circulating Immune Complexes

One of the most fascinating aspects of the biology of intravascular infection has been the documentation of the development of rheumatoid factor (anti-γ-globulin), cryoglobulins, and circulating immune complexes (CICs) in the serum of patients with IE. It is quite likely that it is by virtue of these immune reactions that many of the manifestations of IE, previously believed due to bacteremia or emboli, are brought about. These will be discussed under the general heading of CICs.

Earlier in Section 3.5, consideration was given to the role of CICs in the formation of lesions of NBTV. Our concern at that time was the pathogenesis of the underlying valve lesion susceptible to infection.

Whereas much of the earlier discussion was speculative, there is mounting evidence attesting to the importance of CICs in the pathogenesis of many of the consequences of IE formerly attributed to either bacteremia or embolization.

6.3.4.1. Formation

The formation of antigen–antibody (Ag-Ab) complexes in intravascular infection is not difficult to envision. A conventional Ab response coupled with prolonged and constant bacteremia puts Ag and Ab inescapably together simultaneously in the circulation.[89,123–124,223] The half-life of Ag-Ab is short, but that of Ag_2-Ab or Ag_2-Ab_2 is longer and may be prolonged still further by the saturation of the clearance mechanism (the RES), thus leaving CICs available for deposition in various tissues with the consequent production of tissue (endothelial-cell) injury.[126] Although unusual, in some patients, CIC-mediated disease continues even after sterilization of infected cardiac vegetations with antibiotics. It has been suggested that this is today's counterpart of Libman's "bacteria-free stage" of IE.[89,127,224]

It is important to bear in mind that most methods used for the detection of "immune complexes" are nonspecific, the serum reacting positively also with aggregated immunoglobulins. Nevertheless, detection of CICs combined with the identification of Ab, Ag, and complement in target tissues (e.g., kidney), lend support to the importance of CICs in the pathogenesis of tissue injury in IE.[100,125,126,128–131]

6.3.4.2. Pathogenesis of Tissue Damage

The deposition of CICs and complement in endothelial cells results in the release of chemotactic factors which attract PMN, which subsequently release digestive enzymes producing tissue injury. In rabbits, platelets are lysed by a similar mechanism. Immune complexes and complement activation are probably also capable of activating the events leading to DIC. In the renal injury (and perhaps in other tissues) produced by CICs, it is likely that both direct tissue damage and hypercoagulability contribute to the production of the final pathological lesion.[126,128] These mechanisms are believed to play a role in various infectious diseases, e.g., IE, leprosy, viral hepatitis, malaria, dengue fever, acute poststreptococcal glomerulonephritis, and perhaps gonococcal sepsis and schistosomiasis.[126,128]

The morphological consequences of tissue injury by CICs include arteritis, glomerulonephritis, synovial joint inflammation (arthritis), cardiac valvular lesions in lupus erythematosus, and probably arterial aneurysms.[126,128,132,225]. It is of particular interest that in rabbits with IE, it is possible to detect deposition of immunoglobulins, fibrinogen, and C3 on the aortic valve, suggesting that perpetuation of the disease might be related to continued valve injury by CICs.[133]

Diffuse glomerulonephritis has been produced in rabbits with streptococcal endocarditis when they were preimmunized against the infecting organism.[134,226] CICs and cryoglobulins have been detected in rabbits with experimental streptococcal endocarditis.[124,133,223]

6.3.4.3. Cryoglobulins

Cryoglobulins are cold-precipitable immune complexes (monoclonal or mixed IgA, IgG, IgM) which are found in many disease states such as multiple myeloma, Sjögren's syndrome, lupus erythematosus, acute poststreptococcal glomerulonephritis, and rheumatoid arthritis. They are frequently overlooked in routine laboratory studies because their capacity to precipitate at room temperature or in the cold traps them on the walls of the syringe in which blood was collected from the patient unless special precautions are taken.

Cryoglobulins have been found in 80–90% of patients with IE.[(129)] Although Ab in the complexes has been shown on a few occasions to be specific for the infecting organism, the majority of the time such specific antibody cannot be found. Thus, it is believed that the antibodies are to the patient's own IgG, altered in some way by its interaction with the Ag responsible for its formation, circulating bacteria.[(129,135–137)]

Patients with cryoglobulinemia, without IE, suffer from arthritis, purpuric skin lesions, Raynaud's phenomenon, arteritis, and glomerulonephritis. Thus, there is good reason to suspect a pathogenic role for these complexes in IE.

6.3.4.4. Rheumatoid Factor

Rheumatoid factor (RF) is an antiglobulin believed to be an antibody to altered native γ-globulin. In IE, the alteration of native γ-globulin is thought to be accomplished by an effect of the constant formation of Ag-Ab complexes on the unfolding of antigenic sites of γ-globulin.[(126)] Recent evidence supports the view that both IgG and IgM RF may be part of the Ab response to elevated levels of CICs which, in themselves, do not contain RF.[(138)]

Finding RF in the serum of patients with IE was the first clue to the probable presence of CICs in these patients. RF blocks the phagocytosis-promoting action of opsonin found in patients with IE.[(139)] It is possible, therefore, that RF interferes with one of the most important host defense mechanisms in infection. On the other hand, RF can perhaps prevent glomerulonephritis produced by soluble immune complexes in rats.[(140)] For the moment, one must conclude that its role in the pathogenesis of disease is unknown.

RF may be missed in routine determinations if it is part of a cold-precipitable immune complex, for the same reasons that cryoprecipitates themselves may be overlooked.

The usefulness of RF determinations in IE is both as an element perhaps favoring the diagnosis and, more frequently, as a means of evaluating the effectiveness of therapy. RF titers may descend to normal 2–3 weeks after the institution of effective antibiotic therapy.

RF is found frequently in addicts with IE, even at an early stage of disease.[(141)] Addicts without IE also have rates of positive RF higher than would be expected in the general population.[141] This evidence favors the hypothesis presented earlier (see Section 3.5) that CICs in addicts may produce NBTVs, thus predisposing the addicts to IE.

6.3.4.5. Hypercoagulability

The occurrence of DIC and hypercoagulability with bacteremia has already been discussed both from the standpoint of the pathogenesis of NBTVs and as a consequence of IE (see Section 3.2). It merely bears emphasizing here that from the point of view of tissue damage, the contributions of bacteremia, CICs, cryoprecipitates, hypocomplementemia, and hypercoagulability are difficult to separate. It is quite likely that with more sophisticated indices of intravascular coagulation such as the disappearance rate of radioactive fibrinogen, hypercoagulability will be found in most patients with IE.[47]

6.3.4.6. NBTV Formation

Although the role of CICs in the formation of NBTVs was considered in Section 3.5, it is important to recall here that the immune complexes formed as a consequence of intravascular infection have, theoretically at least, the same capacity to produce NBTVs as those which play a role in the original formation of NBTVs, thus contributing to the perpetuation of the infected vegetation.[133]

6.3.4.7. Clinical Consequences

a. Arthritis and Arteritis. The frequency with which arthritic and arteritic syndromes represent the symptomatic onset of IE is being recognized more and more frequently (see Section 6.1.1.11). Disabling polyarthritis and clinical syndromes typical of temporal arteritis with positive biopsy and polymyalgia rheumatica have recently been reported.[29,34] Of particular interest is that patients may respond well to 40–60 mg prednisone per day. One such patient was thus treated for 3 months before a reappearance of symptoms suggested the diagnosis of IE.[34] Joint fluid in such patients is sterile, and cellular responses reported are between 1200 and 16,500 leukocytes/mm^3, with one third to one fourth of the cells PMN. In two instances, latex fixation and complement studies of joint fluid were not suggestive of immune-complex disease, despite the finding of IC deposits in the synovial biopsy of one of these patients.[142] A similar syndrome of biopsy-positive vasculitis and multiple aneurysm formation has been documented in a patient with atrial myxomas.[143]

The role of CICs in the formation of mycotic aneurysms is unproven, but the finding of periarteritis with aneurysm formation in addicts and in patients with viral hepatitis lends support to their possible role in intravascular infection.[126-144]

Most investigators believe that petechiae, splinter hemorrhages, and Osler and Janeway lesions are probably also manifestations of CICs when they are seen in patients with IE.[126] It is curious that such lesions, once considered to be the hallmark of IE, are seen infrequently today. This may be due to the shorter duration of disease and the earlier administration of antibiotics. Indeed, splinter hemorrhages, in today's hospital population, occur so frequently under a wide variety of circumstances that they can no longer be considered pathognomonic, or even of significance for the diagnosis of IE.[145]

Recently, considerable attention has been directed to the skin manifestations of IE. Petechial hemorrhages are frequently seen and, rarely, in addition to the bleeding associated with DIC, raised purpuric nodules typical of leukocytoclastic angiitis have been reported.[146] There has long been confusion and controversy concerning lesions the description of which is attributed to Janeway and Osler. There is disagreement among authorities over the description and location of these lesions—macular, raised, erythematous, hemorrhagic. Most authors concede that they are found on the palms and the soles, with Osler lesions located principally in the pads of the fingers or toes. Everyone agrees that Osler lesions are tender and Janeway lesions are not. In cases where IE is due to *Staph. aureus* or *C. albicans,* microorganisms have been cultured from the lesions, whereas in streptococcal infections, bacteria are generally not isolated. Since the pathology of the lesions is consistent with either septic embolization or vascular damage due to CICs, it is not possible to say with certainty whether one or both of these mechanisms are operative. The finding of positive cultures of skin lesions in patients with positive blood cultures cannot be taken as evidence that the lesions are bacterial in origin. Furthermore, since immunoglobulins and complement may be found deposited in the perivascular regions of normal skin in patients with IE, this finding in skin lesions does not necessarily point to a pathogenetic mechanism. In addition, it has been pointed out that the absence of immunoglobulins in skin lesions does not mean that the lesions were not provoked by immune complexes.[147–149]

Thus, the pathogenesis of these skin lesions in IE remains ambiguous and the lesions themselves are rare; curiosity about them, however, continues unabated.[227]

b. Glomerulonephritis. Renal failure in IE is usually due to congestive heart failure (CHF). Despite the common finding of urinary abnormalities and microscopic glomerulonephritis, renal failure due to glomerulonephritis is a rarity. In four recent reviews describing 273 patients with IE, none developed renal insufficiency that could be attributed to glomerulonephritis.[5,23,27,28] Clinically important renal findings are more frequent in patients with infected cerebrospinal fluid (CSF) shunts (2–4%), probably due to the more insidious nature of the infection and the consequent longer duration of infection before the start of effective therapy.[150]

Nevertheless, there is considerable interest in the glomerulonephritis that develops in association with intravascular infection. This interest is due principally to the insight that can be gained from the study of diffuse renal disease provoked by immunological phenomena. Intravascular infection is one of the rare circumstances in man wherein the antigen responsible for glomerulonephritis is identifiable and the pathogenesis of the lesion susceptible to laboratory study in experimental animals.[134,226]

Glomerulonephritis is probably a universal histological finding in patients with IE. Of nine patients studied by Morel-Maroger *et al.*,[151] BUN and urinalyses were normal in eight, yet all were considered to have histological evidence of glomerulonephritis by renal biopsy. This finding is similar to the high frequency of glomerular changes in asymptomatic family members (even those with no or with minimal laboratory evidence of renal disease) of patients with overt poststreptococcal glomerulonephritis.[152]

At the other end of the clinical spectrum, patients with IE or infected A-V shunts may develop acute renal failure, requiring long-term hemodialysis, or the nephrotic syndrome.[81,89,92,153,154] The histological lesions may be indistinguishable from those of acute poststreptococcal glomerulonephritis or may be typical of membranoproliferative glomerulonephritis.[89,90,155,156] Extensive interstitial inflammatory reactions are common.[90,91,92,157] Although these may be due to immunological reactions in the interstitium of the kidney, it must be kept in mind that interstitial renal inflammation may result from antibiotics or other drugs administered for the various problems encountered in patients with IE, e.g., CHF, digestive disturbances, and musculoskeletal complaints.[158]

Inflammatory lesions of the renal arteries (arteritis) as well as renal artery aneurysms have also been observed as part of the spectrum of renal abnormalities in IE.[151,157]

It is important to distinguish the focal embolic lesions seen in the glomeruli of patients with IE from those lesions due to immune diffuse glomerulonephritis. Focal embolic lesions are seen commonly in the glomeruli of kidneys of rabbits with sterile aortic-valve vegetations or in rabbits with IE or recent onset (Figure 15).[134]

Various microorganisms have been implicated in the pathogenesis of immune glomerulonephritis in patients with IE: *Staph. aureus*,[90,159] *Coxiella burnetii*,[156,160,161] *Actinobacillus actinomycetemcomitans*,[35] psittacosis/lymphogranuloma venereum,[89] *Staph. albus*,[89] *Hemophilus parainfluenzae*,[127] and by far the most common, various species of α-hemolytic streptococci.[91–93,151] Glomerulonephritis in patients with infected CSF shunts is usually associated with *Staph. epidermidis* (type II A), or less often with *Staph. aureus* infection, the microorganisms most commonly responsible for infections of the shunt. It

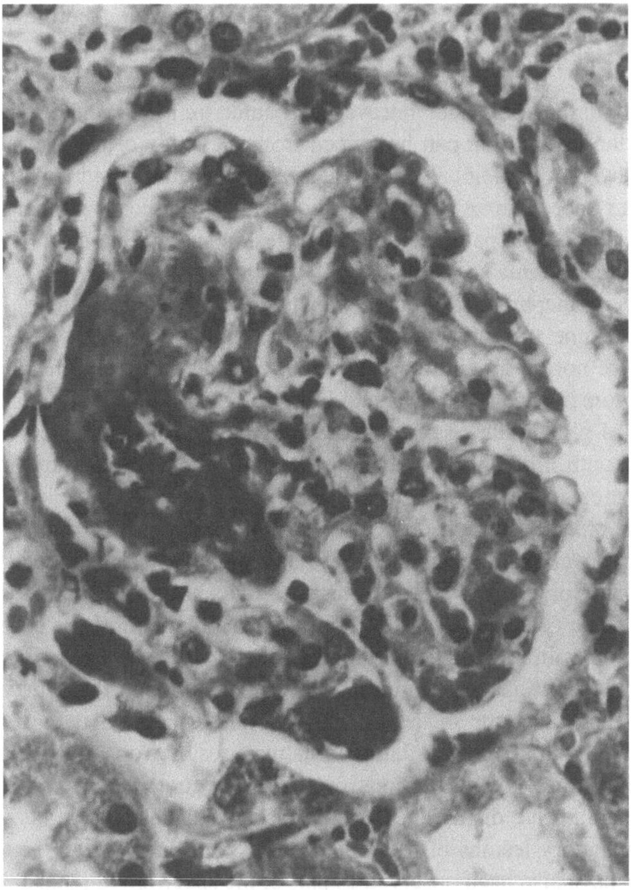

Figure 15. Photomicrograph of a glomerulus from a rabbit with aortic-valve IE due to *Str. sanguis* without preimmunization. Microembolic changes with fibrinoid and exudative necrosis involve several glomerular loops. The univolved capillary loops do not show proliferative changes. ×400. The same embolic lesions are seen in animals with NBTVs of the aortic valve. Reproduced from Arnold *et al*,[134] with permission.

is of particular interest that although diptheroid microorganisms *(Propionibacterium acnes, Corynebacterium bovis)* are rarely responsible for infection of shunts, when present, they are *usually* associated with the development of glomerulonephritis.[154,162,163] This raises the possibility that these microorganisms are particularly nephritogenic.

Studies of the pathogenesis of diffuse glomerular lesions in intravascular infection have, on the whole, supported the view that glomerulonephritis is produced by the deposition of immune complexes along the glomerular basement membrane with subsequent activation of the classic complement pathway.[89,92,135,137,153,155,159] The findings are similar to those in patients with lupus nephritis and acute poststreptococcal glomerular nepthitis. Similar immunofluorescent staining patterns have been demonstrated in rabbits with *Str. viridans* endocarditis which were preimmunized with the infecting microorganism. To date, it has not been possible to produce diffuse glomerulonephritis in the experimental animal without preimmunization, probably because there is not sufficient time for Ab development during the course of the infection (Figures 15 and 16).[134,226] In one patient with *Staph. aureus* endocarditis, the finding of antigen and C3 and the absence of immunoglobulin, C4, and C3 activator sug-

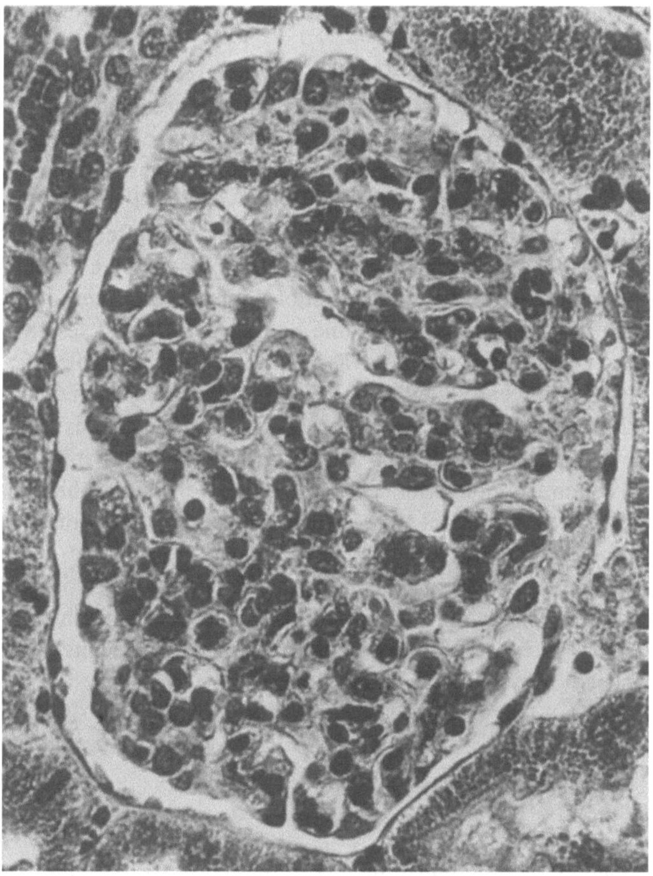

Figure 16. Glomerulus from a rabbit with *Str. sanguis* IE of the aortic valve preimmunized with *Str. sanguis*. There is hypercellularity, endothelial and mesangial-cell proliferation, capillary occlusion, and infiltration of PMN. ×400. Compare with normal portion of the glomerulus in Figure 15. Reproduced from Arnold *et al.*[134] with permission.

gested that *Staph. aureus* antigens could directly activate the complement system and that immune-complex deposition was not essential for the production of glomerular injury.[100,159,164] In some cases, the pathogenetic mechanism of glomerulonephritis in IE remained undetermined when it was not possible to detect immunoglobulin or C3 in the glomerular lesions.[89]

Serum levels of C3 are usually low in patients with intravascular infections and glomerulonephritis, and C4 levels may be depressed.[27,89,100,164] These levels return to normal with proper antibiotic treatment. Properdin, C3b inactivator, and factor B, components of the alternate complement pathway, may also be depressed in these patients.[100,137] Mixed cryoglobulins have been noted in a number of patients.[135,137] In some instances, Ag and bacterial Ab have been detected in cryoprecipitates which have been shown to be able to activate the classic complement pathway *in vitro*.[135,137]

The evolution of glomerulonephritis with intravascular infection is variable and has not yet been correlated with any particular immunological profile. Some patients have died of complications during the acute stage of their renal disease, whereas others have had a prompt and impressive improvement in renal function with the treatment of the infection.[89,92] Patients with evidence for CICs may continue to have evidence of active renal disease even after sterilization of infection.[127,165] In one instance, it was possible to discontinue chronic hemodialysis only 6 months after the completion of antibiotic treatment.[157]

Despite the uncertainty regarding the pathogenesis of all lesions of glomerulonephritis in patients with intravascular infections, the role of immune complexes seems sufficiently well established to suggest that removal of complexes (if indeed that is the principal effect) by plasmapheresis would be a reasonable therapeutic maneuver in any patient with intravascular infection whose renal function continued to deteriorate despite effective antimicrobial treatment. Plasmapheresis has been thought to be effective in the treatment of other forms of immune-complex nephritis.[166–169]

It is important to point out that immune-complex glomerulonephritis has been observed in patients with a variety of other microbial infections. Presumably, intravascular infections did not play a role in these patients.[170–172] One can only wonder how vigorously it was looked for (see discussion of size in Section 4.3.1).

6.4. LOCAL INVASION

Despite the general biological interest of intravascular infections, from the standpoint of mortality, the most important consequence of IE is to be found in the damage produced in the heart by the destructive effects of the infectious process on the local tissue. It is this local invasive process in IE which is responsible for valve destruction, valve-ring and other types of myocardial abscesses, and cardiac conduction defects, as well as the development of aneurysms of the sinus of Valsalva and major arteries. Valve-ring abscesses are the rule in prosthetic-valve endocarditis (PVE) and, rarely, growth of vegetations is so extensive as to produce valvular obstruction.

Of all the phenomena that accompany IE, local extension of infection is probably the easiest to visualize. There is virtually nothing known about the factors which influence this local destructive process.

6.4.1. Valve Destruction

Valve destruction is without question the most important and most frequent local phenomenon in IE. It is this lesion which is the principal cause of the appearance of CHF, and it is the complication most often responsible for the death of the patient.(173) Clinical evidence of valve destruction usually becomes apparent suddenly and may be noted for the first time perhaps as long as 7–10 days after the start of "effective" antibiotics.

The frequency of valve destruction is difficult to establish, but it has become apparent in recent reviews that the problem is common. In one series, regurgitant aortic-valve murmurs developed in an average of 62% of patients with left-sided infection, the range being 45–100% depending upon the responsible microorganism.(27) In another series, the overall percentage was similar, 43%, with no obvious difference according to the infecting microorganism.(5) Even if it should be found that some microorganisms are more prone to cause valve destruction than others, it is evident that this difference is small and is of no comfort to the physician, who should begin effective antibiotic therapy as soon as possible, irrespective of the infecting microorganism, in the effort to prevent this potentially lethal complication of IE.

6.4.2. Congestive Heart Failure

CHF resulting from valve destruction is the most common cause of death in patients with IE. Although reference is occasionally made to the development of CHF due to other causes,(27) I have not seen new CHF develop in the absence of valve perforation. In a large autopsy series of patients with IE, all the patients dying of CHF had severe valve destruction.(26) *Papillary muscle necrosis*, commonly seen at autopsy, is probably due to relative anoxemia as a result of the sudden development of CHF.(26) In two other large series, CHF was present in 90% of the patients who died.(5,27)

Although destruction of any cardiac valve is theoretically a potential cause of CHF, the rarity of right-sided IE and the relatively benign outcome of *destruction of the tricuspid valve* account for the negligible contribution of these lesions to the clinical problem. Although patients may appear to tolerate complete surgical removal of the tricuspid valve for weeks or months, it is likely that in the long run, prosthetic valve replacement will be necessary.[173,174] The ability to tolerate the absence of the tricuspid valve for varying lengths of time has led some surgeons to propose a two-stage procedure in cases where tricuspid-valve surgery is necessary: first, to remove infected valve tissue serving as the source of pulmonary emboli; second, at a later time, to insert a prosthetic valve in an operative field which has been properly sterilized with antibiotics.[175–177]

Destruction of the mitral valve has important hemodynamic consequences, but these may be difficult to distinguish from those of simultaneously occurring lesions of the aortic valve. Mitral-valve destruction alone appears to be relatively well tolerated,[5] whereas severe CHF with a fatal outcome is frequently seen when both aortic and mitral valves are involved.[27] Aortic- and mitral-valve vegetations commonly occur together (about 30–50% of the time at autopsy), and in the majority of instances in some series, mitral-valve infection may be secondary to infection of the aortic valve.[26]

Destruction of the aortic valve is the major cause of severe CHF in IE, and replacement of the damaged valve by a prosthesis represents the major approach to diminishing the mortality due to IE.[26,173,178] The clinical picture may be typical of that of aortic insufficiency with the sudden appearance of an aortic diastolic murmur and widened pulse pressure. The decisions as to the need for aortic-valve replacement and the timing of the operation are of the greatest importance. Ideally, one would like to wait for complete sterilization of the infection and operate when the congestive failure was well controlled medically. Unfortunately, the early and sudden appearance of severe intractable cardiac failure often forces a decision in favor of surgical intervention when the patient is in less than optimal condition.

Since the immediate risk of death is related to the development of CHF, it is the hemodynamic state of the patient which is decisive in determining the moment of operative intervention. Clearly, the earlier in the course of treatment that surgery is undertaken, the greater is the likelihood that viable bacteria remaining in the vegetation will bring about infection of the prosthesis. Fortunately, infection is frequently limited to the free edge of the valve cusps, and in these cases, surgical removal of the cusps is sufficient to remove all viable bacteria. So it is that successful valve replacement has been accomplished even in the presence of active infection of vegetations and in the presence of positive blood cultures.[179–182] Indeed, the immediate operative mortality of about 30% in these patients was dependent not on the bacteriological status of the infection, but rather on the overall cardiovascular condition of the patients.[179–182]

In some instances, the severity of CHF is such that hemodialysis is the only means of preparing the patient for operation. Hemodialysis has been employed simultaneously with the establishment of extracorporeal circulation in one patient on chronic hemodialysis requiring aortic-valve replacement as an emergency measure.[183]

It is important to emphasize that patients with acute aortic insufficiency due to valve destruction frequently pass through a phase of severe hemodynamic disturbance without manifesting the classic signs of aortic insufficiency (water-hammer pulse and widened pulse pressure). It is quite likely that it is the ability to recognize this early presymptomatic stage after acute aortic-valve perforation which will permit operative intervention under circumstances which are much more favorable for survival than if operation were carried out during the stage of intractable heart failure.

The primary compensatory mechanisms of the left ventricle have not had time to develop in patients with acute aortic insufficiency due to valve destruction by infection. Thus, radiographic and electrocardiographic evidence of left ventricular hypertrophy may be absent. Under these circumstances, the small left ventricle (relative to that found in chronic aortic insufficiency) prevents the exaggerated fall of diastolic arterial pressure and, with it, the clinical signs associated with a widened pulse pressure. Left ventricular pressure may exceed left atrial pressure in diastole, leading to premature closure of the mitral valve. This phenomenon is believed to be beneficial to the patient in that the pulmonary venous system is to a degree protected from the high diastolic pressures. These pressure changes result in a diminution or disappearance of the first heart sound and the appearance of the Austen–Flint murmur.

Thus, it has been proposed that patients with early mitral-valve closure (before the Q wave of the electrocardiogram) demonstrated by echocardiography should undergo early aortic-valve surgery.[(184)] Patients with these hemodynamic changes have sufficient valve damage to lead inevitably to the development of severe and ultimately intractable CHF. Operation at the stage before the appearance of overt congestive failure will undoubtedly improve their survival.[(185)]It is important to bear in mind that a diastolic murmur, easily confused with that of the murmur of aortic insufficiency, may be present in patients with chronic renal insufficiency (on hemodialysis) without any of the hemodynamic findings of aortic insufficiency. This murmur may be due to severe proximal stenosis of a large anterior descending coronary artery with good distal flow.[(186)]

6.4.3. Valve-Ring Abscess

Valve-ring abscess occurs in about 30% of patients with nonprosthetic IE and in almost 100% of patients with infection of prosthetic valves.[(187,188)] In patients without prosthetic valves, the abscesses are usually located in the region of the aortic valve, and are frequently associated with pericarditis and a high degree of A-V block. Aortic-valve involvement with aortic regurgitation is the rule. Valve-ring abscess is the most common cause of pericarditis in IE. Whereas most abscesses have been thought to be due to infection with bacteria other than α-hemolytic streptococci,[(189)] in a recent series there was no difference between the distribution of types of bacteria in those patients with and without such abscesses.[187] In PVE, about one third of valve-ring abscesses are associated with mitral-valve infection, whereas involvement of the mitral valve was rare in non-PVE.[188] Obviously, the regular occurrence of valve-ring abscess presents formidable problems to the surgeon in his effort to replace an infected prosthetic valve with a new one.[188] In some instances, antibiotic treatment seems to have sterilized the abscesses, but was not able to prevent dehiscence of the valve.[188]

Conduction abnormalities are common in IE. In a recent series of patients, A-V block and right bundle branch block were noted in 14 of 17 patients. An additional 21 patients had ventricular[13] or auricular[8] extrasystoles.[5] Of particular interest was the observation that mortality was highly associated with the infecting microorganism and not with the type of conduction abnormality. Conduction abnormalities were detected in 17 of 25 patients with infection due to staphylococci, group D streptococci, *E. coli,* and *Klebsiella,* and 12 of these 17 patients died. Similar disturbances of cardiac rhythm were found in 18 of 46 patients with infections due almost exclusively to various streptococci (not group D), and only 1 of these patients died.[5] The lethal nature of conduction abnormalities in patients with infections due to staphylococci, *E. coli,* β-hemolytic streptococcus, and *Klebsiella* has been confirmed in other reports.[190]

Left bundle branch block (LBBB) is uncommon in IE, but has been reported in a patient with fatal IE due to *Staph. aureus* infection.[191] Other cases of LBBB have been recorded.[26,178,192]

The pathogenesis of conduction abnormalities is related to the extension of ring abscesses or *septal perforations* involving the conduction system.[26,178,190,192,193] In several large series of patients with IE, A-V conduction defects were noted on the average in about 8% of patients. In the presence of septal perforation, A-V block is found about 60% of the time.[192] It is remarkable that such perforations may occur in the absence of electrocardiographic abnormalities.[194,195]

Other destructive lesions resulting from local tissue invasion include: *rupture of chordae tendinae,*[196] *thrombophlebitis of the coronary sinus,*[197] *abscess and aneurysm of the sinus of Valsalva,*[198] and *purulent pericarditis.*[26,199,200] Purulent pericarditis is usually the result of extension of an aortic-valve-ring abscess to the pericardium and is considered an indication for surgical intervention.[200] An occasional patient with purulent pericarditis probably develops the infection on the basis of septic emboli.[178]

6.4.4. Valve Obstruction

Rarely, valvular vegetations may grow to such a size that they produce acute obstruction of the involved valves.[178,201–203,228] Diagnosis is possible with the aid of echocardiography and is an indication for prompt surgical treatment.

Fungal infections may reach very large proportions, particularly on prosthetic valves, causing serious valve dysfunction.[80] Rarely, vegetations may be so large as to *occlude a coronary ostium*.[204]

6.5. PERIPHERAL EMBOLI

Emboli from sites of intravascular infection are undoubtedly more common than is clinically recognized. Their frequency depends on the definition of embolization, and detailed pathological study, when carried out, is possible only at autopsy. Judging from the frequency of emboli in rabbits with IE, they occur in all patients (see Figure 15). This is also the impression one gets from reading the description by Libman and Friedberg[1] and the data collected by Kerr.[60] The organs most commonly affected are the brain, spleen, kidneys, and myocardium. In these target organs, large emboli are easily identified grossly and

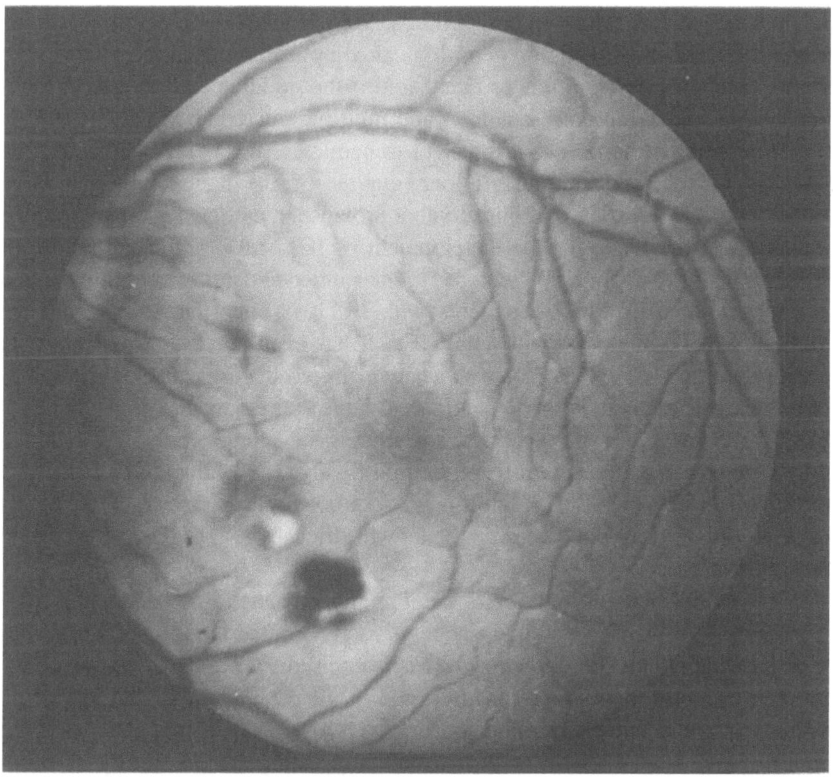

Figure 17. Photograph of the optic fundus of a patient with *Str. viridans* IE showing large white-centered hemorrhages. This patient experienced obstruction of his brachial artery with an embolus as well perforation of his aortic valve.

produce infarcts which are often infected. Emboli are frequently the factor which brings the patient to the hospital (20%) and may occur as long as 2–5 weeks after antibiotic therapy is completed.[28] The clinical consequences or the expression of such emboli depends upon their size and location. Pulmonary emboli are common in addicts with right-sided endocarditis.[28] Patients with prosthetic-valve infections are particularly prone to develop peripheral arterial emboli.[28] Embolic lesions are often seen by examination of the optic fundus (Figure 17). Other ocular complications of IE include cytoid bodies or soft exudates described by Roth, choroiditis, papillitis, neuritis, and metastatic endophthalmitis.[205]

6.5.1. Nervous System

A wide variety of neurological signs and symptoms may occur in IE (30–50% of patients), this being the reason 10–15% of patients with IE are initially referred to neurologists. The mortality rate of patients with neurological manifestations of IE is much higher than in the general group of patients with IE: 50% in patients with cerebral infarcts, 90% in those with cerebral hemorrhage.[18,21] The most common neurological complications seen in patients with IE are: cerebral infarction due to occlusion of the middle cerebral artery, meningeal signs and symptoms, seizures, and multiple microemboli.

It is important to note that transient ischemic episodes (TIEs) preceded the onset of neurological findings in one quarter of the patients in one large series.[21] It is interesting that mitral-valve prolapse, a cardiac lesion susceptible to serving as the focus for the development of IE, is also a frequent cause of TIEs, particularly in young patients.[206] Since anticoagulants are contraindicated for the treatment of TIEs in patients with IE, it is important to consider the possibility of IE in any patient with TIEs. It has been noted that patients with atherosclerotic TIEs return to normal between episodes of neurological symptoms, whereas patients with IE continue to have symptoms and signs of infection.[21] Curiously, in one analysis, the finding of cerebral emboli was much more common in patients with IE of the mitral valve (52%) than in patients with aortic-valve infections (28%), but this was not noted in other series.[22,26] Major cerebral emboli were not seen in patients with tricuspid-valve IE, as one would have anticipated.

It is estimated that symptomatic cerebral mycotic aneurysm occurs in 2–10% of patients with IE.[22] Since these aneurysms are located in peripheral branches of major cerebral arteries, they may be easily excised.[20] Ziment[20] has proposed that ". . . carotid angiography is indicated in all patients under the age of 50 with a neuropsychiatric syndrome accompanied by any significant changes in the cerebrospinal fluid when there is evidence suggesting the possibility of endocarditis." Others propose angiography for " . . . those patients with an abnormal CSF and or computerized axial tomography, or unexplained neurological deterioration."[22]

Studies of the effects of septic cerebral embolism in dogs show, interestingly, that mycotic aneurysm with hemorrhage was the complication of emboli infected with staphylococci and *E. coli,* while *Str. viridans* and enterococcus contamination of emboli resulted in the insidious development of brain abscess in infarcted areas.[207]

Other major neurological syndromes seen in IE include toxic encephalopathy, brain abscess (usually multiple), meningitis (with normal CSF sugar despite positive cultures and pleocytosis), organic headache, mononeuritis, convulsions, and visual impairment.[21,22] It is not clear that all these clinical pictures are due to embolic phenomena; it is entirely possible that vasculitis due to CICs makes a significant contribution to the spectrum of neurological illness in IE.

Neurological complications of IE are seen less often with infection due to *viridans* streptococci (28%) than with infection due to other microorganisms (*Staph. aureus:* 53%; enterobacteriaceae: 90%).[22] CSF findings vary more in relation to the infecting organism than to the nature of the neurological complication. *Viridans* streptococci are associated with a normal or sterile CSF, whereas other organisms are usually associated with CSF infection in the presence of clinical neurological findings.[22]

6.5.2. Spleen, Gallbladder, and Liver

Although emboli to the spleen are common at autopsy (about 50% of patients), they are usually not evident clinically.[178] If they are of sufficient size, they may produce infarcts which are painful. In contrast, renal infarcts are usually not painful, probably because the renal capsule has its own arterial blood supply. Splenic infarcts are important, since they may develop in abscesses and serve as a source of reinfection of the cardiac vegetations.[7,8] Splenectomy has been carried out in such cases.

Recently, I saw a patient with IE admitted to the hospital with an acute abdomen who, at surgery, proved to have a ruptured splenic abscess. Splenic rupture as the presenting sign of IE is rare,[9] as is infarction of the liver or gallbladder.[6]

6.5.3. Kidney

Emboli to the kidney are common and may result in the formation of septic or bland infarcts or focal embolic lesions to portions of the glomerular capillaries of variable numbers of glomeruli. Both these lesions are very common, but give rise to very few clinical symptoms. They are probably responsible for the hematuria which is commonly seen in IE. Although it is sometimes possible and sometimes very important to be able to culture the responsible bacteria from the urine, in my experience this is unusual, except in patients with staphylococcal IE.

Embolic renal lesions rarely, if ever, are responsible for the development of significant proteinuria or renal failure. Embolic lesions are commonly seen in experimental endocarditis of the aortic valve in rabbits (see Figure 15). In fact, the presence of renal infarcts can be used as a gross indication of the presence of infection of the vegetations, since there is a good correlation between the two.

From a clinical point of view, the renal lesions of greatest significance in IE are immune-complex glomerulonephritis and interstitial nephritis due to drug toxicity. These subjects are discussed in Section 6.3.4.

6.5.4. Bone

Abcess formation in bone, of embolic origin, is probably very common in IE. With the use of radioactive bone scanning, it is possible to identify zones of hyperfixation in many patients, perhaps in the majority. Most of the time, these lesions are asymptomatic and disappear with antibiotic treatment of the IE, not to give rise subsequently to any conventional radiological signs of osteomyelitis. Occasionally, however, these bone lesions are symptomatic and may even be the patient's initial complaint. In a patient who recently presented with back pain, typical radiological evidence of vertebral osteomyelitis developed at the time he completed 6 weeks of antibiotic treatment for enterococcal endocarditis.

Musculoskeletal complaints, including polyarthritis, are occasionally seen in IE, but are most likely secondary to inflammatory changes brought about by the deposition of CICs.

Osteomyelitis and septic arthritis are being reported more frequently in IE.[37,39-41] Septic polyarthritis was the presenting finding in two dogs which presented with chronic shifting lameness and who were later found to have IE.[208] It is likely that the finding of osteomyelitis due to *viridans* streptococci is always an indication of the presence of IE.[39,40] In addicts with staphylococcal endocarditis, examination of joint fluid may offer a rapid means of establishing the presence and the nature of the infection.[209]

6.5.5. Major Arteries

Sudden occlusion of a major artery is rare in IE due to infection with α-hemolytic streptococci. When this complication occurs, one should think particularly of infection with large, friable vegetations, such as are seen with *Bacteroides* or fungal endocarditis.[80,210,211] Indeed, the recovery of fungi from surgically removed infected emboli is at times the method by which the etiological diagnosis of IE is made. Patients with PVE are at special risk of embolization.(80) Obviously, emboli may occlude arteries anywhere in the body. In one case, there was infarction of zones of the liver and of the entire gallbladder.(6) Emboli removed from major arteries should be cultured and examined histologically.

6.5.6. Mycotic Aneurysms

With the exception of the nervous system, mycotic aneurysms resulting from IE are rare. This is interesting, since IE was the principal cause of mycotic-aneurysm formation in the preantibiotic era. When extracerebral mycotic aneurysms occur in IE, the arteries most commonly affected are the mesenteric and splenic as well as the coronary, pulmonary, and abdominal aorta. Although there is still speculation as to the pathogenesis of mycotic aneurysms, e.g., the arrival of bacteria in the arterial wall by way of the vasa vasorum, the tendency today is to believe that these infections begin on the intimal surface of the vessel. Intimal deposition of CICs may also play a role. The peculiar localization of these lesions remains unexplained.(178) Mycotic aneurysms sometimes form in the root of the aorta and the heart, but the mechanism here is most likely that of local extension of infection.

6.5.7. Heart

Myocardial infarction is unusual clinically (about 10% of patients), but it is a common autopsy finding (about 50% of cases).(27,28,178) Although it would seem reasonable to expect that such damage would contribute to congestive failure, there is little clinical evidence to support this view. In patients in whom myocardial infarction and congestive failure are diagnosed clinically, this is almost always associated with major valvular damage. Replacement of the damaged valve is associated with improvement of cardiac function.(182) In one instance, heart-valve replacement and removal of an embolus to the coronary artery were carried out simultaneously.(212)

In a recent review of *myocardial abscesses* at autopsy, about 20% were due to IE.(213) There was about one such finding per year at autopsy in a university hospital. All the abscesses were hematogenous, since in no instance was there any evidence of direct extension from an infected vegetation. In one series of autopsied patients with IE, 20% had myocardial abscesses, but it was not clear whether valve-ring abscesses were included in these cases.(214)

A variety of *myocardial inflammatory lesions* are regularly found at autopsy in patients dying of IE, perhaps in as many as 100% of cases.(26) The pathogenesis of these lesions is unknown, and although it is not possible to attribute the presence of CHF to these lesions alone, it is not unlikely that they contribute to myocardial dysfunction. Diffuse myocardial-cell damage is a regular finding in rabbits with experimental endocarditis.[118,119]

6.6. MORTALITY AND FACTORS AFFECTING PROGNOSIS

As stated in Section 6.1, so much depends on the population under study that it is difficult to speak globally about the prevalence of this disorder. The same arguments hold in discussing the mortality of these infections. Age, underlying heart disease, site of infection, infecting microorganism, delay in starting effective treatment, prior cardiovascular surgery, alcoholism, hemodialysis, drug addiction, any underlying disease, e.g., cancer, will all obviously influence outcome.[28,215] To evaluate the lethal consequences of infection with a particular microorganism, one would have to control all the aforementioned variables. In addition, one would have to take into consideration prior medical treatment received, since inadequate antibiotic treatment is a factor in obscuring the diagnosis, prolonging the illness, and increasing the likelihood of the development of serious complications.

The predominant cause of death in IE is CHF secondary to valve perforation.[173] Additional deaths are due to myocardial infarction (abscess) or, rarely, dysrhythmia. A small percentage of deaths is due to the complications of septic emboli to the CNS, cerebral infarct, rupture of a mycotic aneurysm, or cerebral infection (abscess or meningitis). Renal insufficiency is a rare cause of death. Interest in the pathogenesis of the renal lesions gives the impression that it is a more important cause of death than it in fact is.

Addicts with right-sided staphylococcal infection usually do very well. Probably anyone with right-heart infection will do well. Even *Pseudomonas* and *Serratia* infections have a relatively good prognosis if located on the right side of the heart.[216–218]

Rupture of a mycotic aneurysm is usually lethal. Therefore, any patient suspected of this complication should be under very careful surveillance during the period of diagnosis, with an eye toward surgical treatment whenever possible.

Infections caused by streptococci, formerly 100% lethal, are now sterilized by antibiotics in the great majority of instances, and immediate mortality is generally low (10%).[215,219] On the other hand, staphylococci, gram-negative bacilli, and fungi are associated with high rates of mortality (50–80%), but these infections also occur in different populations.[215]

Interestingly, a recent analysis of 125 patients by Pelletier and Petersdorf[27] does not show any important difference in mortality in relation to infecting organism, save for infections due to gram-negative bacilli, in which case mortality was also correlated with prior surgery or uncontrollable infection. Aside from infection with antibiotic-resistant organisms such as occurs after cardiac prosthetic-valve placement in the presence of "prophylactic" antibiotics or in immuno-depressed patients, the inability to sterilize infection is an unusual cause of death.

In considering nonenterococcal streptococcal infections in patients with natural heart valves (all ages), despite bacteriological cure rates of about 90%, immediate mortality remains about 10–25%.[27,28] Survival at follow-up 2–5 years later (all natural valve infections) is only 50–60%, the major causes of death being CHF and cerebral emboli.[28,215]

Thus, it is evident, leaving aside infections after cardiac surgery, drug addicts, and patients on chronic hemodialysis, that valve destruction accounts for 70–90% of deaths in IE. Valve destruction may take place despite "appropriate" antibiotic treatment. However, the majority of the time, perforation has occurred before the patient comes to the hospital or very shortly thereafter. Evidently, reducing the mortality of this disease will depend to a major degree on being able to establish the diagnosis at an early stage and being able to institute correct antibiotic treatment as rapidly as possible. It will also be important to determine the optimal antibiotic treatment, not only to achieve eventual sterilization of the infected vegetations, but also to limit to a minimum the local destructive capacities of the infection.

Now that experience with echocardiography in patients with IE has increased, it has been possible to correlate the finding of vegetations with risk of valve perforation and major embolic events (see Section 8.2). More experience is necessary to be certain of this correlation, but it appears that echocardiography will be of considerable help in identifying patients at high risk of potentially fatal complications of IE. In the future, evaluations of the efficacy of treatment programs designed to limit the local destructive capacities of IE will benefit greatly from the identification of these patients at high risk.

REFERENCES

1. Libman, E., Friedberg, C. K.: *Subacute Bacterial Endocarditis*. Oxford University Press, New York, 1941, 108 pages.
2. Hunter, T. H.: Bacterial endocarditis. *Am. Heart J.* **42**(3):472–482, 1951.
3. Watanakunakorn, C.: Changing epidemiology and new aspects of infective endocarditis, in: *Advances in Internal Medicine*, Stollerman, G. H., ed. Year Book Medical Publishers, Chicago, pp. 21–47, 1977.
4. Weinstein, L., Rubin, R. H.: Infective Endocarditis—1973. *Prog. Cardiovas. Dis.* **16**:239–274, 1973.
5. Crittin, J., Waldvogel, F. A.: Endocardites bactériennes: Aspects cliniques, bactériologiques et facteurs de pronostic. *Schweiz. Med. Wochenschr.* **107**(21)(Suppl. 5):1–26, 1977.
6. Henrich, W. L., Huehnergarth, R. J., Rösch, J., Melnyk, C. S.: Gallbladder and liver infarction occurring as a complication of acute bacterial endocarditis. *Gastroenterology* **68**(6):1602–1607, 1975.

7. Lingeman, C. J., Smith, E. B., Battersby, J. S., Behnke, R. H.: Subacute bacterial endocarditis—Splenectomy in cases refractory to antibiotic therapy. *Arch. Intern. Med.* **97**:309–314, 1956.
8. Gallavardin, P., Coiffier, B., Tissot, E., Brun, F.: Abcès de la rate revelant une endocardite infectieuse—À propos d'un cas. *Lyon Med.* **242**(16):297–300, 1979.
9. Gonin, A., Berthou, J. D., Simonin, C., Delaye, J., Roques, J. C., Dufoix, V.: Ruptures spontanées de rate au cours de l'endocardite infectieuse—A propose de 3 nouvelles observation. *Lyon Med.* **229**(12):1269–1271, 1973.
10. Godeau, P., Wechsler, B., Herreman, G., Balafrej, M., Bletry, O., Squalli, S.: Rupture de rate au cours des endocardites bactériennes: 2 observations. *Nouv. Presse Med.* **8**:2811–2814, 1979.
11 Klein, R. S., Recco, R. A., Catalano, M. T., Edberg, S. C., Casey, J. I., Steigbigel, N. H.: Association of *Streptococcus bovis* with carcinoma of the colon. *N. Engl. J. Med.* **297**(15):800–802, 1977.
12. Noble, C. J., Uttley, A. H. C., Falk, R. H., Richardson, P. J.: *Streptococcus bovis* endocarditis and colonic cancer (letter). *Lancet* **1**(8067):766, 1978.
13. Brooks, R. J., Ravreby, W. D., Keusch, G., Bottone, E.: More on *Streptococcus bovis* endocarditis and bowel carcinoma (letter). *N. Engl. J. Med.* **298**(10):572, 1978.
14. Levy, B. S., von Reyn, C. F., Arbeit, R. D., Friedland, J., Crumpacker, C.: More on *Streptococcus bovis* endocarditis and bowel carcinoma (letter). *N. Engl. J. Med.* **298**(10):572–573, 1978.
15. Snyder, N., Atterbury, C. E., Correia, J. P., Conn, H. O.: Increased concurrence of cirrhosis and bacterial endocarditis—A clinical and postmortem study. *Gastroenterology* **73**(5):1107–1113, 1977.
16. Buchbinder, N. A., Roberts, W. C.: Alcoholism—An important but unemphasized factor predisposing to infective endocarditis. *Arch. Intern. Med.* **132**:689–692, 1973.
17. Smith, F. E., Palmer, D. L.: Alcoholism, infection and altered host defenses: A review of clinical and experimental observations. *J. Chron. Dis.* **29**:35–49, 1976.
18. Greenlee, J. E., Mandell. G. L.: Neurological manifestations of infective endocarditis: A review. *Stroke* **4**:958–963, 1973.
19. Hickie, J. B.: Bacterial endocarditis in Sydney 1950–1959. *Med. J. Austr.* **1**:929–934, 1961.
20. Ziment, I.: Nervous system complications in bacterial endocarditis. *Am. J. Med.* **47**:593–607, 1969.
21. Jones, H. R., Jr., Siekert, R. G., Gerac Geraci, J. E.: Neurological manifestations of bacterial endocarditis. *Ann. Intern. Med.* **71**(1):21–28, 1969.
22. Pruitt, A. A., Rubin, R. H., Karchmer, A. W., Duncan, G. W.: Neurological complications of bacterial endocarditis. *Medicine* **57**(4):329–343, 1978.
23. Schnurr, L. P., Ball, A. P., Geddes, A. M., Gray, J., McGhie, D.: Bacterial endocarditis in England in the 1970's: Review of 70 patients. *Q. J. Med. N. Ser.* **46**(184):499–512, 1977.
24. Thell, R., Martin, F. H., Edwards, J. E.: Bacterial endocarditis in subjects 60 years of age and older. *Circulation* **51**(1):174–182, 1975.
25. Tan, J. S., Watanakunakorn, C., Terhune, C. A., Jr.: *Streptococcus viridans* endocarditis: Favorable prognosis in geriatric patients. *Geriatrics* **28**:68–73, 1973.
26. Roberts W. C.: Characteristics and consequences of infective endocarditis (active or healed or both) learned from morphologic studies, in: *Infective Endocarditis*, Rahimtoola, S. H., ed. Grune & Stratton, New York, pp. 55–123, 1978.
27. Pelletier, L. L., Petersdorf, R. G.: Infective endocarditis: A review of 125 cases from the University of Washington hospitals, 1963–72. *Medicine* **56**(4):287–313, 1977.
28. Garvey, G. J., Neu, H. C.: Infective endocarditis—an evolving disease. *Medicine* **57**(2):105–127, 1978.

29. Gretillat, F., Debievre, J., Lubetzki, J.: Endocardite d'Osler révélée par un tableau de pseudopolyarthrite rhizomélique. *Nouv. Presse. Med.* **5**(24):1534, 1976.
30. Churchill, M. A., Jr., Geraci, J. E., Hunder, G. G.: Musculoskeletal manifestations of bacterial endocarditis. *Ann. Intern. Med.* **87**:754–759, 1977.
31. Bayer, A. S., Brenner, R. J., Galpin, J. E., Guze, L. B.: Severe disabling polyarthritis associated with bacterial endocarditis. *West. J. Med.* **123**(5):404–406, 1975.
32. Meyers, O. L., Commerford, P. J.: Muscoloskeletal manifestations of bacterial endocarditis. *Ann. Rheum. Dis.* **36**:517–519, 1977.
33. Holler, J. W., Pecora, J. S.: Backache in bacterial endocarditis. *N. Y. State J. Med.* **3**:1903–1905, 1970.
34. Lawrence, E. C., Mills, J.: Bacterial endocarditis mimicking vasculitis with steroid-induced remission. *West. J. Med.* **124**(4):333–334, 1976.
35. Geraci, J. E., Griepp, P. R., Wilkowske, C. J., Wilson, W. R., Washington, J. A., II: *Cardiobacterium hominis* endocarditis—Four cases with clinical and laboratory observations. *Mayo Clin. Proc.* **53**:49–53, 1978.
36. Dzindzio, B. S., Meyer, L. R., Osterholm, R., Hopeman, A., Woltjen, J., Forker, A. D.: Isolated gonococcal pulmonary valve endocarditis: Diagnosis by echocardiography. *Circulation* **59**(6):1319–1324, 1979.
37. Leonard A., Raij, L., Shapiro, F. L.: Bacterial endocarditis in regularly dialyzed patients. *Kidney Int.* **4**:407–422, 1973.
38. Storck, D., Jeanmaire, H., Geitner, S., Kuntz, J. L., Hermann, P.: Endocardites bactériennes revelées par des manifestations rhumatismales. *J. Med. Strasbourg* **8**:537–540, 1977.
39. Choubrac, P., Mathé, G., Haas, C., Crickx, B., Robin, P.-M., Dyan, A., Dubois, G.: Spondylodiscites révélatrices d'endocardites bactériennes. *Ann. Med. Interne* **127**(2):117–121, 1976.
40. Acar, J.-F., Durin, R., Deloux, G., Barthalo, M., Guibert, J.: A propos de deux cas de spondylodiscites révélatrices d'une endocardite a *Streptocoque viridans. Gas. Med. Fr.* **81**:2351–2356, 1974.
41. Good, A. E., Hague, J. M., Kauffmann, C. A.: Streptococcal endocarditis initially seen as septic arthritis. *Arch. Intern. Med.* **138**:805–806, 1978.
42. Powell, E. B.: Non-suppurative lesions in staphylococcal septicaemia. *Pathol. Bacteriol.* **82**:141–149, 1961.
43. McKeel, D.: Pemphigus vulgaris, large dose glucocorticoid therapy and staphylococcal bacteremia. *Am. J. Med.* **63**:152–160, 1977.
44. Murray, H. W., Tuazon, C. U., Sheagren, J. N.: Staphylococcal septecemia and disseminated intravascular coagulation. *Arch. Intern. Med.* **137**:844–847, 1977.
45. Case records of the Massachusetts General Hospital. Castleman, B., ed. Case 26—1971: Rapidly fatal sepsis with consumption coagulopathy in heroin addict. *N. Engl. J. Med.* **285**(1):40–48, 1971.
46. Beylot, C., Castaing, R., Poisot, D., Bioulac, P., Cazaugade, M.: "Acral cyanosis": Manifestation d'une coagulation intravasculaire disséminée au cours d'une endocardite bactérienne aiguë. *Ann. Dermatol. Syphiligr.* **101**(4):375–382, 1974.
47. Wardle, E. N., Floyd, M.: Fibrinogen catabolism study of three patients with bacterial endocarditis and renal disease. *Br. Med. J.* **3**:255–257, 1973.
48. Stimmel, B., Dack, S.: Infective endocarditis, in narcotic addicts, in: *Infective Endocarditis,* Rahimtoola, S. H., ed. Grune and Stratton, New York, pp. 195–209, 1978.
49. Glumeck, N., Dereume, J. P., Hubrechts, J. M., Parmentier, R., Sternon, J.: Bacterial endocarditis, intravascular coagulation and aortic bifurcation embolism. *Acta Clin. Belg.* **31**(5):292–294, 1976.
50. Doughten, R. M., Pearson, H. A.: Disseminated intravascular coagulation associated with Aspergillus endocarditis. *J. Pediatr.* **73**:576–582, 1968.

51. Robboy, S. J., Salisbury, K., Ragsdale, B., Bobroff, L. M., Jacobson, P. M., Colman, R. W.: Mechanism of Aspergillus induced microangiopathic hemolytic anemia. *Arch. Intern. Med.* **128**:790–793, 1971.
52. Bayer, A. S., Theofilopoulos, A. N., Eisenberg, R., Friedman, S. G., Guze, L. B.: Thrombotic thrombocytopenic purpuralike syndrome associated with infective endocarditis—A possible immune complex disorder. *J. Am. Med. Assoc.* **238**(5):408–410, 1977.
53. Bailey, I. K., Richards, J. G.: Infective endocarditis in a Sydney teaching hospital—1962–1971. *Aust. N. Z. J. Med.* **5**:413–420, 1975.
54. Beeson, P. B., Brannon, E. S., Warren, J. V.: Observations on the sites of removal of bacteria from the blood in patients with bacterial endocarditis. *J. Exp. Med.* **81**:9–23, 1945.
55. Werner, A. S., Cobbs, C. G., Kaye, D., Hook, E. W.: Studies on the bacteremia of bacterial endocarditis. *J. Am. Med. Assoc.* **202**(3):199–203, 1967.
56. Hook, E. W.: Annotation. *Yale J. Biol. Med.* **38**:521–526, 1966.
57. Bennett, I. L., Jr., Beeson, P. B.: Bacteremia: A consideration of some experimental and clinical aspects. *Yale J. Biol. Med.* **26**:241–262, 1954.
58. Kaye, D.: Infecting microorganisms, in: *Infective Endocarditis,* Kaye, D., ed. University Park Press, Baltimore, pp. 43–54, 1976.
59. O'Keefe, J. P., Gorbach, S. L.: Laboratory diagnosis of infective endocarditis, in: *Infective Endocarditis,* Rahimtoola, S. H., ed. Grune and Stratton, New York, pp. 307–325, 1978.
60. Kerr, A.: *Subacute Bacterial Endocarditis.* Charles C. Thomas, Springfield, Illinois, 1955.
61. Keefer, C. S.: Subacute bacterial endocarditis: Active cases without bacteremia. *Ann. Intern. Med.* **11**:714–734, 1937–1938.
62. Freedman, L. R., Arnold, S., Valone, J.: Experimental endocarditis. *Ann. N. Y. Acad. Sci.* **236**:456–465, 1974.
63. Freedman, L. R., Valone, J.: Experimental endocarditis. *Prog. Cardiovasc. Dis.* **22**:169–180, 1979.
64. Durack, D. T., Beeson, P. B., Petersdorf, R. G.: Experimental bacterial endocarditis. III. Production and progress of the disease in rabbits. *Br. J. Exp. Pathol.* **54**:142–151, 1973.
65. Carrizosa, J., Tanphaichitra, D., Levison, M. E.: Experimental *Bacteroides fragilis* endocarditis in rabbits. *Infect. Immun.* **15**(3):871–873, 1977.
66. Liekweg, W. G., Jr., Levinson, S. A., and Greenfield, L. J.: Infections of vascular grafts: Incidence, anatomic location, etiologic agents, morbidity, and mortality, in: *Infections of Prosthetic Heart Valves and Vascular Grafts,* Duma, R. J., ed. University Park Press, Baltimore, pp. 239–251, 1977.
67. Francioli, P., Freedman, L. R.: Streptococcal infection of endocardial and other intravascular vegetations in rabbits: Natural history and effect of dexamethasone. *Infect. Immun.* **24**:483–491, 1979.
68. Cannady, P. B., Sanford, J. P.: Negative blood cultures in infective endocarditis: A review. *South. Med. J.* **69**(11):1420–1424, 1976.
69. Editorial: Culture-negative endocarditis. *Lancet* **2**:1164–1165, 1977.
70. Hampton, J. R., Harrison, M. J. G.: Sterile blood cultures in bacterial endocarditis. *Q. J. Med.* **36**(142):167–174, 1967.
71. Gleckman, R.: Culture negative bacterial endocarditis confirming the diagnosis. *Am. Heart J.* **94**(1):125–126, 1977.
72. Petit, J.-C., Sicard, D.: Endocardite à streptocoque deficient cultivant en satellitisme. *Med. Mal. Infect.* **7**(11):506–508, 1977.
73. Carey, R. B.: Culture-negative endocarditis. *Lancet* **1**:278, 1978.
74. Sonnenwirth, A. C. (ed.): *Bacteremia: Laboratory and Clinical Aspects.* Charles C. Thomas, Springfield, Illinois, 1973.

75. Washington, J. A., II: Blood culture techniques: Techniques in the diagnosis of infective endocarditis, in: *Infective Endocarditis*, Kaplan, E. L., Taranta, A. V., eds. American Heart Association Monograph No. 52, Dallas, pp. 44–45, 1977.
76. Piepkorn, M. W., Reichenbach, D. D.: Infective endocarditis associated with cell wall-deficient bacteria. *Human Pathol.* **9**(2):163–173, 1978.
77. Freedman, L. R., Johnson, M. L.: Experimental endocarditis. IV. Tricuspid and aortic valve infection with *Candida albicans* in rabbits. *Yale J. Biol. Med.* **45**:163–175, 1972.
78. Sande, M. A., Bowman, C. R., Calderone, R. A.: Experimental *Candida albicans* endocarditis: Characterization of the disease and response to therapy. *Infect. Immun.* **17**(1):140–147, 1977.
79. Carrizosa, J., Kohn, C., Levison, M. E.: Experimental Aspergillus endocarditis in rabbits. *J. Lab. Clin. Med.* **86**(5):740–753, 1975.
80. McLeod, R., Remington, J. S.: Fungal endocarditis, in: *Infective Endocarditis,* Rahimtoola, S. H., ed. Grune and Stratton, New York, pp. 211–290, 1978.
81. Garrison, P., Freedman, L. R.: Experimental endocarditis. I. Staphylococcal endocarditis in rabbits resulting from placement of a polythelene catheter in the right side of the heart. *Yale J. Biol. Med.* **42**:394–410, 1970.
82. Durack, D. T.: Experimental bacterial endocarditis. IV. Structure and evolution of very early lesions. *J. Pathol.* **115**:81–89, 1975.
83. Southwick, F. S., Durack, D. T.: Chemotherapy of experimental streptococcal endocarditis. III. Failure of a bacteriostatic agent (tetracycline) in prophylaxis. *J. Clin. Patho.* **27**:261–264, 1974.
84. Teich, E. M.: Afebrile bacterial endocarditis. *J. Mount Sinai Hosp.* **35**:566–577, 1968.
85. Kerr, A.: *Subacute Bacterial Endocarditis*. Charles C. Thomas, Springfield, Illinois, 1955.
86. Villarcal, H., Sokoloff, L.: The occurrence of renal insufficiency in subacute bacterial endocarditis. *Am. J. Med. Sci.* **220**:655–661, 1950.
87. Montgomerie, J. Z., Kalmanson, G. M., Guze, L. B.: Renal failure and infection. *Medicine* **47**(1):1–32, 1968.
88. Goodman, J. S., Crews, H. D., Ginn, H. E., Koenig, M. G.: Bacterial endocarditis as a possible complication of chronic hemodialysis. *N. Engl. J. Med.* **280**(16):876–877, 1969.
89. Boulton-Jones, J. M., Sissons, J. G. P., Evans, D. J., Peters, D. K.: Renal lesions of subacute infective endocarditis. *Br. Med. J.* **2**:11–14, 1974.
90. Freeman, B. C., Kreps, E. M., Ronsheim, N. J., Lejano, R. F., Sommers, S. C.: Post-staphylococcal glomerulonephritis in heroin addicts. *N. Y. State J. Med.* **74**(12):2241–2243, 1974.
91. Levy, R. L., Hong, R.: The immune nature of subacute bacterial endocarditis (SBE) nephritis. *Am. J. Med.* **54**:645–652, 1973.
92. Perez, G. O., Rothfield, N., Williams, R. C. Jr.: Immune-complex nephritis in bacterial endocarditis. *Arch. Intern. Med.* **136**:334–336, 1976.
93. Keslin, M. H., Messner, R. P., Williams, R. C., Jr.: Glomerulonephritis with subacute bacterial endocarditis. *Arch. Intern. Med.* **132**:578–581, 1973.
94. Perlman, B. B., Freedman, L. R.: Experimental endocarditis. III. Natural history of catheter induced endocarditis after catheter removal. *Yale J. Biol. Med.* **44**:214–223, 1971.
95. Landewehr, D. M., Evans, P. S., Fischer, L. M., Ruddy, S.: Removal of immune complexes by plasmapheresis in glomerulonephritis with subacute bacterial endocarditis. *Clin. Res.* **25**:507A, 1977.
96. Joyce, R. A., Sande, M. A.: Mechanism of anaemia in experimental bacterial endocarditis. *Scand. J. Haematol.* **15**:306–311, 1975.
97. Yoshikawa, T., Tanaka, K. R., Guze, L. B.: Infection and disseminated intravascular coagulation. *Medicine* **50**(4):237–258, 1971.

98. Zimmerman, T. S., Fierer, J., Rothenberger, H.: Blood coagulation and the inflammatory response. *Semin. Hematol.* **14**:391–408, 1977.
99. Lipinski, B., Cybulska, J., Worowski, K., Jeljaszewicz, J.: Blood clotting and fibrinolysis in experimental staphylococcal infection. *Pathol. Microbiol.* **34**:295–304, 1969.
100. O'Connor, D. T., Weisman, M. H., Fierer, J.: Activation of the alternate complement pathway in *Staph. aureus* infective endocarditis and its relationship to thrombocytopenia, coagulation abnormalities and acute glomerulonephritis. *Clin. Exp. Immunol.* **34**:179–187, 1978.
101. Carrizosa, J., Kaye, D.: Development of the vegetation in experimental streptococcal endocarditis. *Clin. Res.* **25**:373A, 1977.
102. Levison, M. E., Carrizosa, J., Tanphaichitra, D., Schick, P. K., Rubin, W.: Effect of aspirin on thrombogenesis and on production of experimental aortic valvular *Streptococcus viridans* endocarditis in rabbits. *Blood* **49**(4):645–650, 1977.
103. Thompson, J., Eulderink, F., Lemkes, H., van Furth, R.: Effect of warfarin on the induction and course of experimental endocarditis. *Infect. Immun.* **14**(6):1284–1289, 1976.
104. Durack, D. T., Beeson, P. B.: Pathogenesis of infective endocarditis, in: *Infective Endocarditis,* Rahimtoola, S. H., ed. Grune and Stratton, New York, pp. 1–53, 1978.
105. Parker, B. M., Andrésen, D. C., Thomas, W. A., Smith, J. R.: Effect of intravenous fibrinolytic enzymes on the vegetation of experimental bacterial endocarditis. *J. Lab. Clin. Med.* **52**:588–595, 1958.
106. Petch, C. P.: Anticoagulants in bacterial endocarditis (letter). *Br. Med. J.* **3**:502, 1973.
107. Hook, E. W. III, Sande, M. A.: Role of the vegetation in experimental *Streptococcus viridans* endocarditis. *Infect. Immun.* **10**(6):1433–1438, 1974.
108. Miles, A. A., Miles, E. M., Burke, J.: The value and duration of defence reactions of the skin to the primary lodgement of bacteria. *Br. J. Exp. Pathol.* **38**:79–96, 1957.
109. Guckian, J. C.: Coagulopathy in experimental sepsis with *Streptococcus pneumoniae* in rabbits: Effect of drug therapy and splenectomy. *J. Infect. Dis.* **134**(2):150–157, 1976.
110. Corrigan, J. J., Kiernat, J. F.: Effect of heparin in experimental gram-negative septicemia. *J. Infect. Dis.* **131**(2):138–143, 1975.
111. Horwitz, D. L., Ballantine, T. V. N., Coran, A. G., Herman, C. M.: Heparin treatment of live *Escherichia coli* bacteremia in rats. *J. Surg. Res.* **13**(3):120–125, 1972.
112. Wilson, W. R., Geraci, J. E., Danielson, G. K., Thompson, R. L., Spittell, J. A., Jr., Washington, J. A., II, Giuliani, E. R.: Anticoagulant therapy and central nervous system complications in patients with prosthetic valve endocarditis. *Circulation* **57**:1004–1007, 1978.
113. Nagel, J. G., Tuazon, C. U., Cardella, T. A., Sheagren, J.N.: Teichoic acid serologic diagnosis of staphylococcal endocarditis—Use of gel diffusion and counterimmunoelectrophoretic methods. *Ann. Intern. Med.* **82**(1):13–17, 1975.
114. Iannini, P. B., Everett, E. D., Pappas, G., LaForce, F. M.: Candida precipitins as a diagnostic aid in Candida endocarditis. *J. Am. Med. Assoc.* **236**(22):2518–2520, 1976.
115. Bacon, P.A., Davidson, C., Smith, B.: Antibodies to Candida and autoantibodies in subacute bacterial endocarditis. *Q. J. Med. N. Ser.* **43**(172):537–550, 1974.
116. Shanson, D. C., Hince, C.: An immunofluorescent method for detecting antibodies against viridans streptococci in *Streptococcus viridans* endocarditis. *J. Clin. Pathol.* **31**(3):292–293, 1978.
117. Das, S. K., Cassidy, J. T.: Importance of heart antibody in infective endocarditis. *Arch. Intern. Med.* **137**:591–593, 1977.
118. Dhalla, N. S., Ziegelhoffer, A., Singal, P. K., Panagia, V., Dhillon, K. S.: Subcellular changes during cardiac hypertrophy and heart failure due to bacterial endocarditis. *Basic Res. Cardiol.* **75**:81–91, 1980.
119. Tomlinson, C. W., Dhalla, N.S.: Myocardial cell damage during experimental infective endocarditis. *Lab. Invest.* **33**(3):316–323, 1975.
120. Swift, H. F.: The heart in infection. *Am. Heart J.* **3**(6):629–648, 1928.

121. Wadsworth, A. B.: A study of the endocardial lesions developing during Pneumococcus infection in horses. *J. Med. Res.* **39**:279–291, 1919.
122. Wright, H. D.: The production of experimental endocarditis with pneumococci and streptococci in immunised animals. *J. Pathol. Bacteriol.* **29**:5–11, 1926.
123. Bayer, A. S., Theofilopoulos, A. N., Eisenberg, R., Dixon, F. J., Guze, L. B.: Circulating immune complexes in infective endocarditis. *N. Engl. J. Med.* **295**:1500–1505, 1976.
124. Bayer, A. S., Theofilopoulos, A. N., Dixon, F. J., Guze, L. B.: Circulating immune complexes in experimental *Streptoccus viridans* endocarditis: A monitor of therapeutic efficacy. *J. Infect. Dis.* **139**:1–8, 1979.
125. Mohammed, I., Ansell, B. M., Holborow, E. J., Bryceson, A. D. M.: Circulating immune complexes in subacute infective endocarditis and poststreptococcal glomerulonephritis. *J. Clin. Pathol.* **30**:308–311, 1977.
126. Reed, P., Williams, R. C., Jr.: Immune complexes in infectious diseases, in: *Advances in Internal Medicine,* Stollerman, G. H., ed. Year Book Medical Publishers, Chicago, Vol. 22, pp. 49–72, 1977.
127. Nomeir, A. M. Watts, E., Philp, J. R.: Bacterial endocarditis: Echocardiographic and clinical evaluation during therapy. *J. Clin. Ultrasound* **4**(1):23–37, 1975.
128. Zubler, R. H., Lambert, O. H.: Immune complexes in clinical investigation, in: *Recent Advances in Clinical Immunology, I,* Thompson, R. A., ed. Churchill, Livingston, Edinburgh, London, and New York, Chapt. 6, pp. 125–147, 1977.
129. Hurwitz, D., Quismorio, F. P., Friou, G. J.: Cyroglobulinaemia in patients with infectious endocarditis. *Clin. Exp. Immunol.* **19**:131–141, 1975.
130. Woodroffe, A. J., Border, W. A., Theofilopoulos, A. N., Götze, O., Glassock, R. J., Dixon, F. J., Wilson, C. B .: Detection of circulating immune complexes in patients with glomerulonephritis. *Kidney Int.* **12**:268–278, 1977.
131. Tung, K. S. K., Kim, B., Bjorvatn, B., Kronvall, G., McLaren, L. C., Williams, R. C. Jr.: Discrepancy between C1q deviation and Raji cell tests in detection of circulating immune complexes in patients with leprosy. *J. Infect. Dis.* **136**(2):216–221, 1977.
132. Shapiro, R. F., Gamble, C. N., Wiesner, K. B., Castles, J. J., Wolf, A. W., Hurley, E. J., Salel, A. F.: Immunopathogenesis of Libman–Sacks endocarditis. *Ann. Rheum. Dis.* **36**:508–516, 1977.
133. Allen, J. E., McIntosh, R. M.: Experimental streptococcal endocarditis—Immunological aspects. *Clin. Res.* **26**:389A, 1978.
134. Arnold, S. B., Valone, J. A., Askenase, P. W., Kashgarian, M., Freedman, L. R.: Diffuse glomerulonephritis in rabbits with *Streptococcus viridans* endocarditis. *Lab. Invest.* **32**(6):681–689, 1975.
135. Kaufman, D. B., McIntosh, R.: The pathogenesis of the renal lesion in a patient with streptococcal disease infected ventriculoatrial shunt cryoglobulinemia and nephritis. *Am. J. Med.* **50**:262–268, 1971.
136. Hardin, J. A., McCluskey, R. T.: Mixed cryoglobulinemia with impaired renal function. *N. Engl. J. Med.* **292**(24):1285–1290, 1975.
137. Strife, C. F., McDonald, B. M., Ruley, E. J., McAdams, A. J., West, C. D.: Shunt nephritis: The nature of the serum cryoglobulins and their relation to the complement profile. *J. Pediatr.* **88**(3):403–413, 1976.
138. Carson, D. A., Bayer, A. S., Eisenberg, R. A., Lawrence, S., Theofilopoulos, A.: IgG rheumatoid factor in subacute bacterial endocarditis: Relationship to IgM rheumatoid factor and circulating immune complexes. *Clin. Exp. Immunol.* **31**:100–103, 1978.
139. Messner, R. P., Laxdal, T., Quie, P. G., Williams, R. C. Jr.: Serum opsonin, bacteria, and polymorphonuclear leukocyte interactions in subacute bacterial endocarditis. *J. Clin. Invest.* **47**:1109–1120, 1968.

140. Marnikov, M., Loshuma, A., Marson, P. L., Heremans, J. I.: Prevention by rheumatoid-factor of glomerulonephritis caused in rats by soluble Ag–Ab complexes (abstract). *Eur. J. Clin. Invest.* **4**(5):326, 1974.
141. Sheagren, J. N., Tuazon, C. U., Griffin, C., Padmore, N.: Rheumatoid factor in acute bacterial endocarditis. *Arthritis Rheum.* **19**(5):887–890, 1976.
142. Myers, A. R., Schumacher, H. R.: Arthritis of subacute bacterial endocarditis (SBE). *Arthritis Rheum.* **19**(4):813–814, 1976.
143. Leonhardt, E. T. G., Kullenberg, K. P. G.: Bilateral atrial myxomas with multiple arterial aneurysm: A syndrome mimicking polyarteritis nodosa. *Am. J. Med.* **62**:792–794, 1977.
144. Gilroy, J., Andaya, L., Thomas, V. J.: Intracranial mycotic aneurysms and subacute bacterial endocarditis in heroin addiction. *Neurology* **23**(11):1193–1198, 1973.
145. Kilpatrick, Z. M., Greenberg, P. A., Sanford, J. P.: Splinter hemorrhages—Their clinical significance. *Arch. Intern. Med.* **115**:730–735, 1965.
146. Rubenfeld, S., Min, K. W.: Leukocytoclastic angiitis in subacute bacterial endocarditis. *Arch. Dermatol.* **113**:1073–1074, 1977.
147. Alpert, J. S., Krous, H. F., Dalen, J. E., O'Rourke, R. A., Bloor, C. M.: Pathogenesis of Osler's nodes. *Ann. Intern. Med.* **85**:471–473, 1976.
148. Farrior, J. B., Silverman, M. E.: A consideration of the differences between a Janeway's lesion and an Osler's node in infectious endocarditis. *Chest* **70**(2):239–243, 1976.
149. Lowenstein, M. B., Urman, J. D., Abeles, M., Weinstein, A.: Skin immunofluorescence in infective endocarditis. *J. Am. Med. Assoc.* **238**(11):1163–1165, 1977.
150. Schoenbaum, S. C., Gardner, P., Shillito, J.: Infections of cerebrospinal fluid shunts: Epidemiology, clinical manifestations and therapy. *J. Infect. Dis.* **131**(5):543–552, 1975.
151. Morel-Maroger, L., Sraer, J. D., Herreman, G., Godeau, P.: Kidney in subacute endocarditis. *Arch. Pathol.* **94**:205–213, 1972.
152. Dodge, W. R., Spargo, B. H., Travis, L.B .: Occurrence of acute glomerulonephritis in sibling contacts of children with sporadic acute glomerulonephritis. *Pediatrics* **40**:1029–1030, 1967.
153. Labrune, B., Levy, M., Bauby, C., Gubler, M. C., Maller, R.: Les glomerulonephrites secondaires aux dérivations ventriculoatriales ("shunt nephritis"). *Arch. Fr. Pediatr.* **30**:793–808, 1973.
154. Bolton, W. K., Sande, M. A., Normansell, D. E., Sturgill, B. C., Westervelt, F. B.: Ventriculojugular shunt nephritis with *Corynebacterium bovis*. *Am. J. Med.* **59**:417–423, 1975.
155. Spitzer, R. E., Stitzel, A. E., Urmson, J. R.: Is glomerulonephritis after bacterial sepsis always benign? (letter). *Lancet* **1**:871, 1978.
156. Uff, J. S., Evans, D. J.: 11. Glomerular disease in infective endocarditis, in: Proceedings of the Pathological Society of Great Britain and Ireland. *J. Med. Microbiol.* **10**:Pi, 1977.
157. Baglin, A., Normand, J. P., Tancrède, C., Callard, P., Brunet, A., Fritel, D.: Anurie prolongée au cours d'une endocardite bactérienne. *Ann. Med. Interne* **126**(4):241–250, 1975.
158. Freedman, L. R.: Interstitial renal inflammation, including pyelonephritis and urinary tract infection, in : *Stauss and Welt's Diseases of the Kidney,* 3rd ed., Early, L. E., Gottschalk, C. W., eds. Little, Brown, Boston, pp. 817–876, 1979.
159. Pertschuk, L. P., Vuletin, J. C., Sutton, A. L., Velazquez, L. A.: Demonstration of antigen and immune complex in glomerulonephritis due to *Staphylococcus aureus*. *Am. J. Clin. Pathol.* **66**(6):1027, 1976.
160. Hall, G. H., Hart, R. J. C., Davis, S. W., George, M., Head, A. C.: Glomerulonephritis associated with *Coxiella burnetii* endocarditis (letter). *Br. Med. J.* **2**:275, 1975.
161. Rosman, M. S., Lubbe, W. F., Hayden, M., Basson, N., Uys, C. J.: Q fever endocarditis: A report of 2 cases. *S. Afr. Med. J.* **53**:296–300, 1978.
162. Beeler, B. A., Growder, J. G., Smith, J. W., White, A.: Propionibacterium acnes: Pathogen in central nervous system shunt infection—Report of 3 cases including immune complex glomerulonephritis. *Am. J. Med.* **61**:935–938, 1976.

163. Moss, S. W., Gary, N. E., Eisinger, R. P.: Nephritis associated with a diptheroid-infected cerebrospinal fluid shunt. *Am. J. Med.* **63:**318–319, 1977.
164. Sheagren, J. N., Tuazon, C. V., Quie, P. G.: Alternate complement pathway activation by strains of *S. aureus* isolated from patients with disseminated intravascular coagulation. *Clin. Res.* **26:**526A, 1978.
165. Spitzer, R. E., Stitzel, A. E., Urmson, J. R.: Evidence that immune complex glomerulonephritis associated with indolent bacterial sepsis may lead to progressive renal disease. *Pediatr. Res.* **12:**548, 1978.
166. Chan, Y. L., Long, B., To, B. L., Kwitko, A., Seymour, A. E., Thompson, A., Taylor, H., Clarkson, A. R.: Plasmapheresis in the management of glomerulonephritis. *Aust. N. Z. Med. J.* **7:**225, 1977.
167. D'Apice, A. J. F.: Plasmapheresis in the treatment of glomerulonephritis. *Aust. N. Z. J. Med.* **7:**441, 1977.
168. Rossen, R. D., Hersh, E. M., Sharp, J. T., McCredie, K. B., Gyorkey, F., Suki, W. N., Eknoyan, G., Reisberg, M. A.: Effect of plasma exchange on circulating immune complexes and antibody formation in patients treated with cyclophosphamide and prednisone. *Am. J. Med.* **63:**674–682, 1977.
169. Becker, G. J., d'Apice, A. J. F., Walker, R. G., Kincaid-Smith, P.: Plasmapheresis in the treatment of glomerulonephritis. *Med. J. Aust.* **2:**693–696, 1977.
170. Beaufils, M., Morel-Maroger, L., Sraer, J. D., Kanfer, A., Kourilsky, O., Richet, G.: Acute renal failure of glomerular origin during visceral suppurations. *N. Engl. J. Med.* **295:**185–189, 1976.
171. Chesney, R. W., O'Regan, S., Drummond, K. N.: Candida endocrinopathy syndrome with membranoproliferative glomerulonephritis—Demonstration of glomerular candida antigen. *Clin. Nephrol.* **5**(5)**:**232–238, 1976.
172. Forrest, J. W., Jr., John, F., Mills, L. R., Buxton, T. B., Moore, W. L., Jr., Hudson, J. B. H., Ozawa, T.: Immune complex glomerulonephritis associated with *Klebsiella pneumoniae* infection. *Clin. Nephrol.* **7**(2)**:**76–80, 1977.
173. Cohen, L., Freedman, L. R.: Damage to the aortic valve as a cause of death in bacterial endocarditis. *Ann. Intern. Med.* **55:**562–564, 1961.
174. Sethia, B., Williams, B. T.: Tricuspid valve excision without replacement in a case of endocarditis secondary to drug abuse. *Br. Heart J.* **40**(5)**:**579–580, 1978.
175. Simberkoff, M. S., Isom, W., Smithivas, T., Noriega, E. R., Raha, J. J.: Two-stage tricuspid valve replacement for mixed bacterial endocarditis. *Arch. Intern. Med.* **133:**212–216, 1974.
176. Wright, J. S., Glennie, J. S.: Excision of tricuspid valve with later replacement in endocarditis of drug addiction. *Thorax* **33**(4)**:**518–519, 1978.
177. Arneborn, P., Björk, V. O., Rodriguez, L., Svanbom, M.: Two-stage replacement of tricuspid valve in active endocarditis. *Br. Heart J.* **39**(11)**:**1276–1278, 1977.
178. Weinstein, L., Schlesinger, J. J.: Pathoanatomic, pathophysiologic and clinical correlations in endocarditis. *N. Engl. J. Med.* **291:**832–837, 1122–1126, 1974.
179. Bastin, R., Vilde, J. L., Frottier, J., Lejeune, A.: La chirurgie cardiaque dans les endocardites à la période infectiuse. Coeur—No. spécial: Journées internationales de cardiologie consacrées aux remplacements valvulaires, Oct. 1974, Deauville.
180. Stinson, E. B., Griepp, R. B., Vosti, K., Copeland, J. G., Shumway, N. E.: Operative treatment of active endocarditis. *J. Thorac. Cardiovasc. Surg.* **71**(5)**:**659–665, 1976.
181. Boyd, A. D., Spencer, F. C., Isom, O. W., Cunningham, J. N., Reed, G. E., Acinapura, A. J., Tice, D. A.: Infective endocarditis—An analysis of 54 surgically treated patients. *J. Thorac. Cardiovasc. Surg.* **73**(1)**:**23–30, 1977.
182. Gonin, A., Cressens, J. P., Beaune, J., Delaye, J.: Aspects actuels de l'endocardite bactérienne—L'évolution vers l'insuffisance cardiaque précoce. *Lyon Med.* **237**(11)**:**875–883, 1977.

183. Amouroux, C., Willems, P., Clerget-Gurnaud, J. M., Ducret, J., Leoni, F., Mikaeloff, P. H.: Circulation extra-rénale pour insuffisance aortique par endocardite infectieuse. *Lyon Med.* **239**(4):195–198, 1978.
184. Mann, T., McLaurin, L., Grossman, W., Craige, E.: Assessing the hemodynamic severity of acute aortic regurgitation due to infective endocarditis. *N. Engl. J. Med.* **293**(3):108–113, 1975.
185. Dorschner, F., Steinbrunn, W., Turina, J., Krayenbühl, H. P.: Schwierigkeit der Diagnosestellung und Beurteilung des Schweregrades der akuten Aorteninsuffizienz bei bakterieller Endokarditis. *Schweiz. Med. Wochenschr.* **106**:1816–1819, 1976.
186. Falicov, R. E., Behara, S., Oyama, J. H.: Diastolic murmur in uremia (letter). *N. Engl. J. Med.* **300**(23):1333, 1979.
187. Arnett, E. M., Roberts, W. C.: Valve ring abscess in active infective endocarditis—Frequency, location and clues to clinical diagnosis from the study of 95 necropsy patients. *Circulation* **54**(1):140–145, 1976.
188. Arnett, E. N., Roberts, W. C.: Clinicopathology of prosthetic valve endocarditis, in: *Infection of Prosthetic Heart Valves and Vascular Grafts*. Duma, R. J., ed. University Park Press, Baltimore, pp. 17–41, 1977.
189. Sheldon, W. H., Golden, A.: Abscesses of the valve rings of the heart, a frequent but not well recognized complication of acute bacterial endocarditis. *Circulation* **4**:1–12, 1951.
190. Théry, C., Folliot, J. P., Gosselin, B., Lekieffre, J., Warembourg, H.: Les blocs auriculo-ventriculaires des endocardites bactériennes. *Arch. Mal. Coeur* **70**(1):15–23, 1977.
191. Fenichel, N. M., Jiminez, F. A., Polachek, A. A.: 2:1 Left bundle branch block in acute bacterial endocarditis with septal abscess. *J. Electrocardiol.* **10**(3):287–290, 1977.
192. Chestier, Y., Duval, A., Luxereau, P., Chabrol, C., Acar, J.: Les communications interventriculaires acquises au cours des endocardites bactériennes. *Arch. Mal. Coeur* **71**(1):23–32, 1977.
193. De Cock, K. M., Rees, J. R.: Staphylococcal aortic valve endocarditis with aortic root to right atrial fistula. *Postgrad. Med. J.* **54**:413, 1978.
194. Jouven, J. C., Rapuzzi, A., Escogido, H., Baille, Y., Malmejac, C., Houel, J.: Communications interventriculaires par perforations septales au cours del endocardites évolutives. *Ann. Chir. Thorac. Cardio-vasc.* **16**(3):227–233, 1977.
195. Godeau, P., Herreman, G., Dechy, H., Bletry, O., Cahen, C., Guiraudon, G., Gailly, J., Veyssier, J.: Perforations auriculo-ventriculaires au cours d'une endocardite bactérienne: Guérison chirirgicale. *Sem. Hop. Paris* **53**(10):621–626, 1977.
196. Roberts, W. C., Buchbinder, N.A.: Healed left-sided infective endocarditis: A clinicopathologic study of 59 patients. *Am. J. Cardiol.* **40**(6):876–888, 1977.
197. Dryer, R., Goldman, D., Nelson, R.: Septic thrombophlebitis of the coronary sinus in acute bacterial endocarditis. *Lancet* **2**:369, 1976.
198. Wennevold, A., Rygg, I. H., Jacobsen, J.R.: Acute aortic regurgitation and abscess of sinus of Valsalva due to fulminating ulcerative endocarditis—Report of three fatal cases in children. *Scand. J. Thorac. Cardiovasc. Surg.* **10**:7–10, 1976.
199. Mildvan, D., Goldberg, E., Berger, M., Altchek, M. R., Lubkan, S. B.: Diagnosis and successful management of septal myocardial abscess: A complication of bacterial endocarditis. *Am. J. Med. Sci.* **274**(3):311–316, 1977.
200. Klacsmann, P. G., Bulkley, B. H., Hutchins, G. M.: The changed spectrum of purulent pericarditis—An 86 year autopsy experience in 200 patients. *Am. J. Med.* **63**:666–673, 1977.
201. Prasquier, R., Gibert, C., Witchitz, S., Valere, P., Beaufils, P., Vachon, F.: Acute mitral valve obstruction during infective endocarditis. *Br. Med. J.* **50**:9–11, 1978.
202. Copeland, J. G., Salomon, N. W., Stinson, E. B., Popp, R. L., Shumway, N. E.: Acute mitral valvular obstruction from infective endocarditis. *J. Thorac. Cardiovasc. Surg.* **78**(1):128–130, 1979.

203. Pease, H. F., Matsumoto, S., Cacchione, R. J., Richards, K. L., Leach, J. K.: Lethal obstruction by aortic valve vegetation. *Chest* **73**(5):658–660, 1978.
204. Greenberg, B.H., Hoffman, O., Schiller, N. B., Miller, M., Chatterjee, K.: Sudden death in infective endocarditis (letter). *Chest* **71**:794–795, 1977.
205. McCue, J. D., Dreher, R. J.: Bilateral endophthalmitis with *Streptococcus viridans* endocarditis. *J. Maine Med. Assoc.* **70**:463–465, 1979.
206. Barnett, H. J. M., Boughner, D. R., Taylor, D. W., Cooper, P. E., Kostuk, W. J., Nichol, P. M.: Further evidence relating mitral-valve prolapse to cerebral ischemic events. *N. Engl. J. Med.* **302**:139–144, 1980.
207. Molinari, G. F.: Experimental cerebral infection. I. Selective segmental occlusion of intracranial arteries in the Doc; II. Clinicopathological model of deep cerebral infarction. *Stroke* **1**:224–232, 1972.
208. Caywood, D. D., Wilson, J. W., O'Leary, T. P.: Septic polyarthritis associated with bacterial endocarditis in two dogs. *J. Am. Vet. Med. Assoc.* **171**(6):549–552, 1977.
209. Thadepalli, H., Francis, C. K.: Diagnostic clues in metastatic lesions of endocarditis in addicts. *West. J. Med.* **128**:1–5, 1978.
210. Nastro, L. J., Finegold, S. M.: Endocarditis due to anaerobic gram-negative bacilli. *Am. J. Med.* **54**:482–496, 1973.
211. Felner, J. M., Dowell, V. R., Jr.: Anaerobic bacterial endocarditis. *N. Engl. J. Med.* **283**(22):1188–1192, 1970.
212. Pfeifer, J. F., Lipton, M. J., Oury, J. H., Angell, W. W., Hultgren, H. N.: Acute coronary embolism complicating bacterial endocarditis: Operative treatment. *Am. J. Cardiol.* **37**:920–922, 1976.
213. Kim, H. S., Weibaecker, D. G., Lie, J. T.: Myocardial abscesses without and with coexisting infectious endocarditis. *Circulation* **55**:11–21, 1976.
214. Lerner, P. I., Weinstein, L.: Infective endocarditis in the antibiotic era. *N. Engl. J. Med.* **274**:199–206, 259–266, 323–331, 388–393, 1966.
215. Kaye, D.: Cure rates and long-term prognosis, in: *Infective Endocarditis,* Kaye, D., ed. University Park Press, Baltimore, pp. 201–211, 1976.
216. Mills, J., Drew, D.: *Serratia marcescens* endocarditis: A regional illness associated with intravenous drug abuse. *Ann. Intern. Med.* **84**(1):29–35, 1976.
217. Riad El-Khatib, M., Wilson, F. M., Lerner, A. M.: Characteristics of bacterial endocarditis in heroin addicts in Detroit. *Am. J. Med. Sci.* **271**(2):197–201, 1976.
218. Sklaver, A. R., Hoffman, T. A., Greenman, R. L.: Staphylococcal endocarditis in addicts. *South. Med. J.* **71**(6),638–643, 1978.
219. Relson, S. R., White, P. D.: Notes on 250 cases of subacute bacterial (streptococcal) endocarditis studied and treated between 1927 and 1939. *Ann. Intern. Med.* **22**:40–60, 1945.
220. Baglin, J. Y., Poinseau, J., Dechy, H., Dorra, M., Poisson, M.: Movements choréiques révélateurs d'endocardites bactériennes à streptocoques. *Nouv. Presse Med.* **9**:1383–1384, 1980.
221. Govindan, S., Itani, A. L., Garcia, J. H.: Inflammation of the temporal artery associated with subacute bacterial endocarditis and hepatitis B antigen. *Arch. Neurol.* **37**:318, 1980.
222. Wheat, L. J., Kohler, R. B., White, A.: Solid-phase radioimmunoassay for detection of staphylococcal antigen in serum of rabbits with endocarditis due to *Staphylococcus aureus*. *J. Infect. Dis.* **138**:174–180, 1978.
223. Burton-Kee, J., Morgan-Capner, P., Mowbray, J. F.: Nature of circulating immune complexes in infective endocarditis. *J. Clin. Pathol.* **33**:653–659, 1980.
224. Harkiss, G. D., Brown, D. L., Evans, D. B.: Longitudinal study of circulating immune complexes in a patient with *Staphylococcus albus*-induced shunt nephritis. *Clin. Exp. Immunol.* **37**:228–238, 1979.

225. Bidani, A., Roberts, J., Schwartz, M., Lewis, E.: Immunopathology of cardiac lesions in fatal systemic lupus erythematosus. *Am. J. Med.* **69**:849–858, 1980.
226. Thörig, L., Daha, M. R., Eulderink, F., Kooy-Bauer, W. C., Thompson, J.: Experimental *Streptococcus sanguis* endocarditis: Immune complexes and renal involvement. *Clin. Exp. Immunol.* **40**:469–477, 1980.
227. Kerr, A., Jr., Tan, T. S.: Biopsies of the Janeway lesions of infective endocarditis. *J. Cutaneous Pathol.* **6**:124–129, 1979.
228. Neimann, J. L., Godenir, J. P., Roche, G., Voirot, P.: Végétations mitrales obstructives aucours d'une endocardite bactérienne. *Arch. Mal. Coeur Vaiss.* **73**:1217–1222, 1980.
229. Kauffmann, R. H., Thompson, J., Valentijn, R. M., Daha, M. R., Van Es, L. A.: The clinical implications and the pathogenetic significance of circulating immune complexes in infective endocarditis. *Am. J. Med.* **71**:17–25, 1981.

7

Host Defense Mechanisms

Very little is known about the mechanisms of host defense in intravascular infections. Considerable emphasis is put on the ineffectiveness of conventional mechanisms: the lack of a lytic effect of antibody and complement on the gram-positive cocci responsible for the vast majority of infections and the inability of polymorphonuclear leukocytes (PMN) to penetrate the fibrin barrier surrounding developing bacterial colonies. These two factors, in addition to the diminished metabolic activity of colonies located deep in the vegetations (with the consequence that they would be theoretically less susceptible to the action of antibiotics, such as penicillin), serve as the theoretical basis for the empirical clinical reality that it takes long-term treatment with bactericidal antibiotics to cure intravascular infections.

Yet there is good reason to believe that host defense mechanisms do exist—we just don't know much about them. One of the principal reasons to suspect the presence of host defense mechanisms is the relative rarity of the establishment of intravascular infection despite the known frequency of bacteremia theoretically capable of inducing infection and the known frequency of intravascular abnormalities capable of serving as a nidus for the development of infection.

It is the juxtaposition of these two arguments, the ineffectiveness of conventional mechanisms and the likelihood that mechanisms do exist, that lend particular interest and importance to the subject. It is the purpose of this chapter to consider what we know about these mechanisms with an eye toward formulating future studies in the hope that such information might provide clues which will help to improve our ability to prevent the development of infection and to treat patients with this disease. Furthermore, there is the possibility that the study of bacterial infections in which conventional host defense mechanisms do not operate will lead to the discovery of hitherto unrecognized factors in the body's defense.

7.1. LOCATION WITHIN THE VASCULAR SYSTEM

As was pointed out in Section 4.3, there are considerable differences in the ease with which it is possible to infect vegetations located in different parts of the vascular system. There are clinical indications that this is the case; after all, infection is rare in patients with interauricular septal defects, on the right side of the heart, and in the commonplace vegetations covering ulcerated arteriosclerotic plaques in the aorta.

Not until it was possible to experimentally produce comparable lesions in these various locations, however, was it possible to speak of differing susceptibilities to infection. In rabbits with nonbacterial thrombotic vegetations (NBTVs) provoked by the placement of indwelling plastic catheters in different parts of the vascular system, the intravenous inoculation of bacteria has regularly resulted in infection when the lesions were in the heart or the aortic arch, the abdominal aorta, and the inferior vena cava (IVC).

There were important differences, however, in the evolution of infection in these parts of the vascular system which varied according to the location of the vegetations. In the left heart, infection persisted and usually resulted in the death of the animal. On the right side of the heart, infection evolved toward spontaneous sterilization over a period of weeks to months. In the aortic arch, infections also became sterile spontaneously and more rapidly than in the right side of the heart. In the abdominal aorta and IVC, infections resolved spontaneously in a very short time (Figures 18 and 19).[(1)]

Thus, there can be no doubt that the nature of the vegetation formed, or the effectiveness of cellular host defense mechanisms, is different in different intravascular locations and that these factors are important in determining the evolution of the infection.

Even in left-heart infections in rabbits due to *Staphylococcus aureus,* when the catheter which provoked the initial NBTV was removed, a certain percentage of infections were sterilized spontaneously.[(2)] This probably occurs in man also, albeit rarely, judging by the cases in the "bacteria-free" stage of infective endocarditis (IE) presented by Libman and Friedberg.[(3)]

The reasons for these variations in microbiological differences with the location of infection within the vascular system are not known. Nevertheless, they point to the presence of host defense factors which play an important role in determining the outcome of infection.

Oxygen tension and intravascular pressure cannot explain these findings, since remarkable differences exist between infections on the same side of the circulation. On the other hand, anaerobic infections in the rabbit have a different short-term evolution on the right side of the heart than aerobic infection. Anaerobic bacteria reach higher densities in the right side of the heart as compared to aerobic bacteria.[(4)]

It is possible that turbulence is an important factor in increasing the tendency

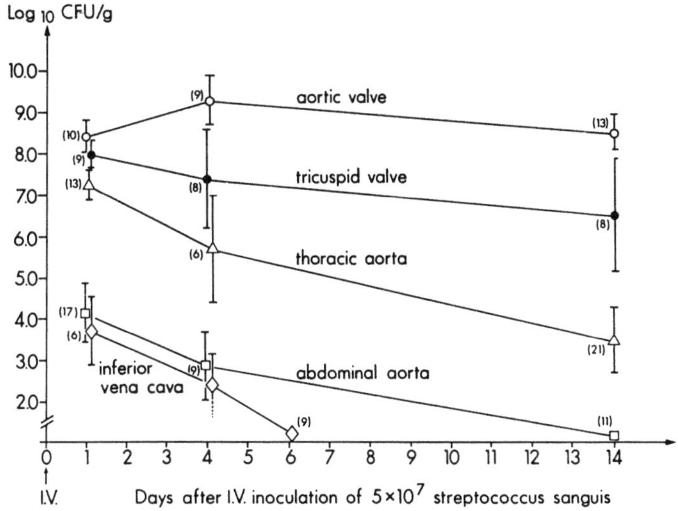

Figure 18. Quantitative cultures of vegetations at different intravascular sites after intravenous injection of 5 × 10^7 *Streptococcus sanguis*. Each point represents the mean ± 95% confidence limits. The numbers of rabbits are shown in parentheses. "Sterile" vegetations were considered to contain 10^2 bacterial colony-forming units (CFU)/g vegetation for purposes of calculating the mean. Reproduced from Francioli and Freedman[1] with permission.

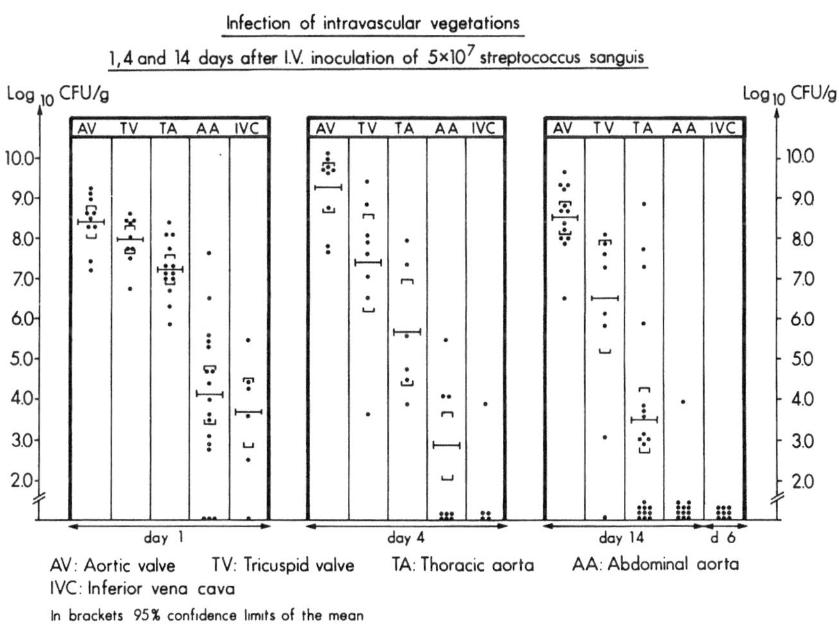

Figure 19. Data from individual rabbits used in the construction of curves in Figure 18. Notice the complete progressive spontaneous sterilization of intravascular vegetations depending upon their location within the vascular system.[1]

to deposit platelets and fibrin over infected vegetations (the Venturi effect).[5] It is thus conceivable that turbulence plays a role equivalent to that of the polythelene catheter in preparing the terrain for infection and in maintaining it.[1] However, the fact that infections sterilize themselves everywhere except in the left heart in rabbits, despite the continued presence of the agent (catheter) responsible for the development of the platelet–fibrin thrombus, argues against turbulence, or the lack of it, as the sole or determining factor influencing the course of infection.[1] Furthermore, the ability to block sterilization of IE with dexamethasone even in the absence of the catheter, at the time when the blood culture was sterile, is a strong argument pointing to a host mechanism, probably cellular, operating within the infected vegetation, independent of factors responsible for the turbulence-producing contribution to the infected vegetation.[1]

7.2. POLYMORPHONUCLEAR LEUKOCYTES

Attention has long been directed to the paucity of PMN in histological studies of the infected vegetations in man and animals with IE, and it was long ago recognized that the relative absence of PMN might be important in facilitating the development and persistence of infection.

On the other hand, PMN are often seen heavily infiltrating the base of an infected vegetation and probably play an important role in limiting the extension of the lesion. This role of PMN may be limited, however, by the presence of rheumatoid factor in the serum of patients with IE, which has been shown to interfere with the phagocytic capacity of PMN *in vitro*,[6] as well as by a reversible defective bactericidal activity of PMN recovered from patients with untreated IE.[7]

Since adrenal corticosteroids are known to inhibit the accumulation of PMN at a site of inflammation, it was thought that one way to biologically test the importance of PMN in IE was to administer dexamethasone to rabbits with IE.

Experiments in rabbits with IE due to *Candida albicans* and simultaneous *Candida* pyelonephritis showed that dexamethasone, in a quantity sufficient to promote infection in the kidney, had no effect on the density of infection in the cardiac vegetation.[8] Dexamethasone did not influence the size of the vegetation or the susceptibility of the NBTV to hematogenous infection. Similar experiments in rabbits with left-sided α-hemolytic streptococcal endocarditis also failed to show any effect due to dexamethasone on the density of bacteria in the vegetation. There was no difference in mortality between control and dexamethasone-treated rabbits.[1,8]

Thus, in quantities sufficient to promote acute fungal infection in the kidney, dexamethasone had no effect on an infected vegetation in the left side of the heart. If it is interference with the activity of PMN in acute candidal infection of the kidney that accounts for the effect of dexamethasone, this interference does not affect the early events in experimental IE. In addition, the electron-microscopic photographs of Durack[9] show how difficult it would be for PMN to approach bacterial colonies which seem almost "protectively" bundled up in layers of fibrin. Thus, in the rabbit, there are good reasons for believing that PMN do not play a role in host defenses in early infection (with the microorganisms studied) when that infection is located in the left heart.

In infected vegetations in the aortic arch or right heart, the response to dexamethasone was different. Carrying out the same experiments with dexamethasone and α-hemolytic streptococci, we were able to show within a period of 2 weeks after the initiation of infection that whereas in control animals aortic-arch or right-heart (catheter removed) vegetations were either sterile or contained very few bacteria, aortic-arch and right-heart vegetations in animals treated with dexamethasone were not sterilized and contained about as many colony-forming units of bacteria as vegetations on the aortic valve or in the right heart with the catheter left in place.[1] Sterilization of right-sided vegetations is also blocked by nitrogen-mustard-induced agranulocytosis and leukopenia.[10]

The distance between the aortic valve and the vegetations on the interior of the aortic arch is a few millimeters, yet this distance was sufficient to alter the biology of infection in a fundamental way. It would seem from these experiments that there is a dexamethasone-sensitive cellular defense mechanism which operates in the aortic arch—as well as in the right side of the heart and probably elsewhere in the arterial and venous system—which is not as effective on the aortic valve. This mechanism could be the availability of host phagocytes. If PMN were found to be important in intravascular infections, we would have to revise the widely held conclusions derived from histological studies in man and animals. If, on the other hand, PMN do not play a role in intravascular infections and dexamethasone and leukocytes were to exert their effect by some other mechanism, this model offers a means of studying a hitherto-unrecognized host defense mechanism. Whatever the mechanism, it operates with much greater effectiveness in the aorta, the IVC, and the right side of the heart than on the aortic valve.

Recent experiments concerning the possible role of PMN as a host defense mechanism in IE are of particular interest. Indium-111-labeled platelets, *but not PMN*, accumulate in aortic-valve vegetations tested 3–5 days after the induction of infection.[11] In addition, there appears to be a reversible defect in the bactericidal function of PMN in patients with untreated IE.[7] The pathogenesis of this defect is unknown. Both these studies argue against a role for PMN in IE.

On the other hand, encapsulation of *Staph. aureus*, generally accepted as a factor diminishing the effectiveness of phagocytic antibacterial defenses, appears to render test bacteria more resistant to host defense mechanisms within vegetations.[32]

The role of PMN in the initial stages of infection of NBTVs was considered in Section 5.1. The probable absence of an effective role for PMN in the biology of IE transforms the therapeutic problem from that of treating a patient with PMN which are available to that of treating patients without an effective PMN response. This is most commonly seen in clinical medicine in patients with agranulocytosis. Patients with IE should probably be considered, therefore, to have *"localized agranulocytosis."* It is likely, incidentally, that what we are learning about the antibiotic treatment of IE in man and animals is applicable to patients with generalized agranulocytosis.

7.3. HEALING–ENDOTHELIALIZATION

An infected vegetation is a virtual whirlpool of activity. At the base, there is the tendency of infection to spread inward, with the conventional host defense mechanisms opposing this spread. At the edge of the vegetation, there is the constant deposition of bacteria and platelet–fibrin thrombi. Durack[9] has illustrated the rapidity (6 hr) with which elongated mononuclear phagocytes cover the vegetation after the beginning of penicillin therapy. Clearly, these monocytes are prevented from covering infected vegetation prior to the administration of antibiotics, but can do so once either the number or the metabolic activity of the bacteria in the vegetations is diminished. The fact that infected right-heart vegetations (and some left-sided ones after catheter removal) become endothelialized and sterilized spontaneously without therapy suggests that this is a powerful mechanism which fails to succeed in the rabbit on the left side of the heart. Perhaps a role of the catheter in perpetuating infection is exactly that of creating conditions which prevent this "endothelialization."

Although covering the vegetation would seem logically to be an effective way of preventing infection, the clinical reality is that even well-endothelialized cardiac abnormalities promote the development of fresh lesions of NBTV, probably continually. Thus, the patient with a prosthetic valve or vascular graft is continually and probably forever at risk of developing intravascular infection. The conditions of risk are so different in the immediate postoperative period and later, however, that it is not possible to evaluate the risk of infection according to the length of time the prosthesis has been in place.

In animals, vascular grafts infected after intravenous inoculation of staphylococci were found not to be completely endothelialized, whereas those which did not become infected were endothelialized.[12] The question remains unanswered as to whether this relation is causative and in which direction. In rabbits, there is rapid diminution in susceptibility to infection with time after removal of the catheter from both sides of the heart.[8]

In summary, there is an obvious logic to the importance of covering the infected vegetation with monocytes or endothelium in order to break the vicious circle of infection and reseeding of the vegetation. Similarly, it would seem reasonable to assume that endothelialization of a sterile vegetation would diminish its susceptibility to infection. These questions are just beginning to be studied in the laboratory and for the moment remain interesting hypotheses.

7.4. ROLE OF FOREIGN BODY

The role of a foreign body in increasing susceptibility to bacterial infection is well known. In intravascular infection, foreign bodies are particularly important in infections associated with indwelling intravenous catheters and prosthetic heart valves. The animal model for the production of intravascular infection using an indwelling plastic catheter is of particular interest in that it provides a means of studying this phenomenon in the laboratory.

As was discussed in Chapter 2, the principal role of a foreign body in producing conditions suitable for the development of infection is its capacity to induce the formation of NBTVs. It is interesting that removal of the catheter after induction of infection results in more rapid spontaneous sterilization of infection on the right side of the heart in rabbits than on the left.[1,2] The effect of catheter removal from the left side of the heart differs according to the bacteria responsible for infection: streptococcal infections persist, whereas staphylococcal infections heal after catheter removal.[1,2] Evidently, the presence of the catheter produces an environment favorable to the persistence of infection. It is likely that one of the effects of the catheter is the continued production of fresh platelet–fibrin vegetations which are highly susceptible to infection by bacteria emanating from the already infected vegetation. Alternatively, the mechanical agitation produced by the catheter might favor the discharge of free bacteria, thus favoring the reseeding of fresh zones of vegetation.

Histological studies of right-heart infections have shown that there is a preferential localization of bacterial colonies in zones of the vegetation adjacent to the plastic catheter.[1] Thus, the presence of the catheter seems to alter the microenvironment in such a way as to favor the survival and growth of bacteria. That dexamethasone produces the same result on bacterial content of the vegetation raises the interesting possibility that they both exercise their effects by altering the *acellular* microenvironment in which bacteria find themselves in IE. Vegetations infected with streptococci in the aortic arch and right side of the heart behave similarly, whereas those on the aortic valve seem to be much less dependent on this "environmental factor" and are less affected by either removal of the catheter or administration of dexamethasone.[1] Removal of the catheter also facilitates the antibiotic treatment and antibiotic prophylaxis of IE.[13,14]

Thus, the catheter (and presumably the prosthetic heart valve) have been shown to have the effects on the production and maintenance of intravascular infection listed in Table 7.

The fascinating aspect of the study of the role of the catheter in promoting

TABLE 7
Role of Foreign Body (Catheter or Prosthetic Valve) in the Production and Maintenance of Intravascular Infection

Effect	Mechanisms
1. Production of NBTV.	Trauma—endothelial injury. Hypercoagulability. ?Activation of complement leading to: Endothelial damage Hypercoagulability
2. Susceptibility of NBTV to infection (?).	Not tested.
3. Retards sterilization of infected vegetations by host defense mechanisms.	?Impairs endothelialization of vegetations. ?Interferes with cellular host defenses. ?Interferes with undefined host defense mechanisms.
4. Interferes with action of antibiotics; prophylaxis and treatment.	?Inactivates antibiotics. ?Inactivates host defenses which influence antibiotic activity: Cellular Humoral

intravascular infection is that it offers some prospect of identifying the mechanisms by which foreign bodies influence infections in general. Of special pertinence to general problems of infection is the role of the catheter in interfering with the action of antibiotics. If one considers, for example, the inhibition of the activity of vancomycin in the prophylaxis of streptococcal IE, it is evident that the catheter must make the newly arrived bacteria inaccessible to the already present antibiotic, or it must inactivate the antibiotic, or it must inhibit a cellular or humoral mechanism which enhances the activity of the antibiotic.(14) In this regard, it is pertinent to recall that careful studies of the early vegetation did not reveal any significant accumulation of leukocytes or any evidence of phagocytosis during the 20 hr following colonization of an experimental NBTV in rabbits.(33) Since it is difficult to imagine how bacteria, newly arrived on the surface of a vegetation, could be rendered inaccessible to the antibiotic, we are left with two possibilities which heretofore have not been recognized as playing a role in the biology of intravascular infection. There is little information concerning the direct effect of polythelene catheters on the action of antibiotics. Preliminary *in vitro* studies suggest that there is no effect.(10) On the other hand, there is evidence demonstrating an effect of leukocyte granules on antibiotic-damaged bacteria.(34) These experiments raise the interesting possibility that phagocytes might influence bacterial infections by means other than direct contact with bacteria resulting in phagocytosis. Such a mechanism has not yet been demonstrated.(35)

7.5. AGING OF BACTERIA

The role of aging of bacteria in their viability is an intriguing area of study. Occasionally, one sees patients with staphylococcal osteomyelitis with recurrences after an interval of 20 years with the same phage-type bacterium. Patients thought to have been "cured" of *Candida* sepsis or *Candida* endocarditis are now being seen years later with what is undoubtedly a reawakening of what was a dormant infection.[15,16]

In view of the ability of unusual microorganisms to survive for prolonged periods of time, sometimes in an unrecognizable form, it is interesting to speculate on the pathogenesis of the "aging" apparent in bacterial colonies at the base of a vegetation after only a few days and the possibility that this represents a "host defense mechanism" in IE.[17] It seems to me that these microorganisms were too young to die a "natural" death in such a short time. I am impressed by the dense packing of bacteria in a tight fibrin wrapping as a possible mechanism of bacterial killing.[9] In view of the rapid multiplication going on within the colony, there must be considerable competition for nutrients. The fact that it is the bacteria in the center of the colony which seem to die first suggests that the center of the colony runs out of nutrients. Although this might result in the death of many bacteria, I would be surprised if a colony could sterilize itself this way.

How, then, do certain vegetations in rabbits, and probably some in man as well, sterilize themselves? Why only certain vegetations and not others? The answers to these questions will undoubtedly provide us with insight into phenomena of general interest in the area of host defense mechanisms.

7.6. SERUM BACTERICIDAL ACTIVITY

The only host defense mechanism which has been characterized and which is probably effective in intravascular infections is the bactericidal property of the serum. Bacteria susceptible to the bactericidal activity (antibody and complement) of normal rabbit serum have the capacity to initiate infection (aortic valve IE) in prepared rabbits, but within 24–48 hr, the vegetations are sterilized.[18-20] The ability of serum bactericidal to the test organism to diffuse into infected vegetations and kill the microorganisms in the vegetations is the principal antimicrobial defense in these infections. It is of interest that rifampin has the capacity to render *Escherichia coli* sensitive to the serum bactericidal system in rabbits, thus decreasing their capacity to induce IE[21] (see Section 4.1 for further discussion of this subject).

Although early studies of streptococci recovered from IE in man were said to demonstrate a bactericidal effect of immune serum on the test organisms, it is highly unlikely that this is an effective bactericidal mechanism.[22,23] Indeed, paradoxically, it was originally believed that the presence of antibody to the test organism was a factor favoring infection.[22–24] Recent studies have reexamined this question, and it appears that preexisting circulating antibody to streptococci tends to protect against the development of IE after intravenous inoculation of bacteria in rabbits with NBTVs on the aortic valve.[24,25] In one study, it was possible to show that the effect of preformed antibody might be to diminish the initial sticking of streptococci to the NBTV.[25] On the other hand, the effect of preimmunization was not always demonstrable with streptococci, sometimes, but not always, depending upon the amount of circulating antibody.[24,26,27] Immunization of rabbits against a strain of serum-resistant *Pseudomonas aeruginosa* had a tendency to increase susceptibility to infection.[28]

Thus, although immunization may protect animals against the development of IE after intravenous inoculation of certain test bacteria, perhaps by diminishing sticking of bacteria to NBTVs, there is no evidence at hand to show that preimmunization is capable of promoting the sterilization of gram-positive infections. The evolution of aortic-valve IE with streptococcal infection was in no way influenced by prior immunization, except that preimmunization permitted the development of diffuse glomerulonephritis.[26,29,30]

Serum bactericidal activity is one of the indices used in judging the adequacy of antibiotic treatment of IE. In most instances, the natural serum bactericidal effect has been additive or synergistic to the effect produced by antibiotics *in vitro*.[31] The therapeutic consequences of this *in vitro* additive (or syngeristic) effect of serum are not known.

REFERENCES

1. Francioli, P., Freedman, L. R.: Streptococcal infection of endocardial and other intravascular vegetations in rabbits: Natural history and effect of dexamethasone. *Infect. Immun.* **24**:483–491, 1979.
2. Perlman, B. B., Freedman, L. R.: Experimental endocarditis. III. Natural history of catheter induced endocarditis after catheter removal. *Yale J. Biol. Med.* **44**:214–223, 1971.
3. Libman, E., Friedberg, C. K.: *Subacute Bacterial Endocarditis*. Oxford University Press, New York, 1971, 108 pages.
4. Carrizosa, J., Tanphaichitra, D., Levison, M. E.: Experimental *Bacteroides fragilis* endocarditis in rabbits. *Infect. Immun.* **15**(3):871–873, 1977.
5. Rodbard, S.: Blood velocity and endocarditis. *Circulation* **27**:18–28, 1963.
6. Messner, R. P., Laxdal, T., Quie, P. G., Williams, R. C., Jr.: Serum opsonin, bacteria, and polymorphonuclear leukocyte interactions in subacute bacterial endocarditis. *J. Clin. Invest.* **47**:1109–1120, 1968.
7. Repine, J. E., Clawson, C. C., Burchell, H. B., White, J. G.: Reversible neutrophil defect in patients with bacterial endocarditis. *J. Lab. Clin. Med.* **88**(5):780–787, 1976.
8. Freedman, L. R., Valone, J.: Experimental endocarditis. *Prog. Cardiovasc. Diseases* **22**:169–180, 1979.

9. Durack, D. T.: Experimental bacterial endocarditis. IV. Structure and evolution of very early lesions. *J. Pathol.* **115:**81–89, 1975.
10. Yersin, B., Glauser, M., Freedman, L. R.: Unpublished observations.
11. Riba, A. L., Thakur, M. T., Gottschalk, A., Andriole, V. T., Zaret, B. L.: Imaging experimental infective endocarditis with indium-111-labeled blood cellular components. *Circulation* **59**(2)**:**336–343, 1979.
12. Moore, W. S.: Experimental studies relating to sepsis in prosthetic vascular grafting, in: *Infections of Prosthetic Heart Valves and Vascular Grafts*. Duma, R. J., ed. University Park Press, Baltimore, pp. 267–285, 1977.
13. Pelletier, L. L., Petersdorf, R. G., Nielson, K.: Chemotherapy or experimental streptococcal endocarditis. V. Effect of duration of infection and retained intracardiac catheter on response to treatment. *J. Lab. Clin. Med.* **87**(4)**:**692–702, 1976.
14. Heraief, E., Glauser, M., Freedman, L. R.: Vancomycin prophylaxis of streptococcal endocarditis in rats, in: *Current Chemotherapy and Infectious Disease* (Proceedings of the 11th International Congress of Chemotherapy and 19th Interscience Conference on Antimicrobial Agents and Chemotherapy), American Society for Microbiology, Washington, D. C., pp. 911–913, 1980.
15. Galgiani, J. N., Stevens, D. A.: Fungal endocarditis: Need for guidelines in evaluating therapy-experience with two patients previously reported. *J. Thorac. Cardiovasc. Surg.* **73**(2)**:**293–296, 1977.
16. McDermott, W.: Inapparent infection—Relation of latent and dormant infections to microbial persistence. *Public Health Rep.* **74**(6)**:**485–499, 1959.
17. Durack, D. T., Beeson, P. B.: Experimental bacterial endocarditis. II. Survival of bacteria in endocardial vegetations. *Br. J. Exp. Pathol.* **53:**50–53, 1972.
18. Durack, D. T., Beeson, P. B.: Protective role of complement in experimental *Escherichia coli* endocarditis. *Infect. Immun.* **16**(1)**:**213–217, 1977.
19. Archer, G., Fekety, F. R., Jr.: Experimental endocarditis due to *Pseudomones aeruginosa*. I. Description of a model. *J. Infect. Dis.* **134:**1–7, 1976.
20. Kaspar, R. L., Drutz, D. J.: Perihepatitis and hepatitis as complications of experimental endocarditis due to *Neisseria gonorrhoeae* in the rabbit. *J. Infect. Dis.* **136**(1)**:**37–42, 1977.
21. Alexander, W. J., Curtiss, R., III, Bradac, J. A., Cobbs, C. G.: Rifampin modifies serum susceptibility of *E. coli* and its virulence in rabbit endocarditis model (abstract). *Clin. Res.* **26**(1)**:**26A, 1978.
22. Swift, H. F.: The heart in infection. *Am. Heart J.* **3**(6)**:**629–648, 1928.
23. Wright, H. D.: The production of experimental endocarditis with pneumococci and streptococci in immunised animals. *J. Pathol. Bacteriol.* **29:**5–11, 1926.
24. Durack, D. T., Gilliland, B. C., Petersdorf, R. G.: Effect of immunization on susceptibility to experimental *Streptococcus mutans* and *Streptococcus sanguis endocarditis*. *Infect. Immun.* **22:**52–56, 1978.
25. Scheld, W. M., Thomas, J. H., Sande, M. A.: Influence of preformed antibody on experimental *Streptococcus sanguis endocarditis*. *Infect. Immun.* **25:**781–785, 1979.
26. Thorig, L., Thompson, J., Eulderink, F., van Furth, R.: The role of host factors in the pathogenesis of bacterial endocarditis. *Neth. J. Med.* **22**(5)**:**174–175, 1979.
27. Hinthorn, D. R., Mitchell, G. W., Liu, C.: Importance of preformed antibody in pathogenesis of experimental endocarditis. 18th Interscience Conference on Antimicrobial Agents and Chemotherapy. Abstract 279, 1978.
28. Archer, G. L., Johnston, J. L.: Effect of type-specific active immunization on the development and progression of experimental *Pseudomonas aeruginosa* endocarditis. *Infect. Immun.* **24**(1)**:**167–173, 1979.
29. Arnold, S. B., Valone, J. A., Askenase, P. W., Kashgarian, M., Freedman, L. R.: Diffuse glomerulonephritis in rabbits with *Streptococcus viridans* endocarditis. *Lab. Invest.* **32**(6)**:**681–689, 1975.

30. Thörig, L., Daha, M. R., Eulderink, F., Kooy-Bauer, W. C., Thompson, J.: Experimental *Streptococcus sanguis* endocarditis: Immune complexes and renal involvement. *Clin. Exp. Immunol.* **40**:469–477, 1980.
31. Bryan, C. S., Marney, S. R., Alford, R. H., Bryant, R. E.: Gram negative bacillary endocarditis. *Am. J. Med.* **58**:209–215, 1975.
32. West, T., Cantey, J. R., West, M., Yoakum, S., Burdash, N.: Encapsulation as a virulence factor in experimental coagulase-negative staphylococcal endocarditis. *Clin. Res.* **28**:382A, 1980.
33. McGowan, D. A., Gillett, R.: Scanning electron microscopic observations of the surface of the initial lesion in experimental streptococcal endocarditis in the rabbit. *Br. J. Exp. Pathol.* **61**:164–171, 1980.
34. Pruul, H., Wetherall, B. L., McDonald, P. J.: Activity of human leucocyte granule extract on antibiotic-damaged bacteria. 20th Interscience Conference on Antimicrobial Agents and Chemotherapy, Sept. 1980, Abstract 732.
35. Gerding, D. M., Peterson, L. R., Moore, B. M., Bean, B.: Effect of local polymorphonuclear leucocytes (PMN) on resolution of *S. aureus* abscesses treated with cephalothin (K). 20th Interscience Conference on Antimicrobial Agents and Chemotherapy, Sept. 1980, Abstract 685.

8

Treatment

8.1. DECISION TO TREAT

Throughout this discussion, considerable emphasis has been placed on establishing a bacteriological diagnosis because of the obvious importance of instituting effective antibiotic therapy for intravascular infection at the earliest possible moment. In most analyses of series of patients with infective endocarditis (IE), those patients treated for the presumption of IE in the absence of a positive blood culture had higher mortality rates than those patients in whom microorganisms responsible for infection had been identified.[1,2]

The importance of identifying the infecting microorganism must, however, be weighed against the devastating risks of untreated infection; the patient with IE is "sitting on a keg of dynamite" which can go off at any minute. The aortic valve of a young patient only mildly ill may suddenly perforate, or the patient may have a massive cerebrovascular occlusion resulting in either death or prolonged incapacity. The physician is under pressure, therefore, to start antibiotic therapy as soon as possible, the underlying assumption being that the earlier correct antibiotic therapy is begun, the lower is the risk that the patient will develop the complications of IE.

Fortunately, in practice, the problem is not as difficult as it might appear. The great majority of patients present either with a mild illness or in a clinical state suggestive of severe infection. In the former case, the diagnosis is so uncertain that two or three pairs of blood cultures are obtained per day, and the diagnosis is established when the microbiology laboratory announces the presence of microorganisms in the blood cultures. In the latter case, the condition of the patient is such that antibiotic therapy is begun immediately after at least two or three pairs of blood cultures are obtained. Treatment is indicated under these circumstances whether the patient has endocarditis or not.

Nevertheless, there remains a significant number of patients in whom the presence of IE is suspected, but in whom the indications for antibiotic therapy are not clear and blood cultures remain negative. Unfortunately, there does not seem to be a satisfactory way to define a constellation of criteria sufficient to identify the clinical problem with greater precision.

8.2. NEGATIVE BLOOD CULTURES

The decision as to when to start treatment for suspected infective endocarditis (IE) in the face of negative blood cultures will be influenced by the evolution and gravity of the clinical state of the patient. Attention must be directed to those aspects of the biology of intravascular infection known to influence the appearance of microoganisms in the bloodstream as well as technical problems known to influence the ability to culture microorganisms *in vitro*.

In studies in which the frequency of culture-negative IE has been examined, about 20% of patients considered to have IE had negative blood cultures.[1–3] However, when blood cultures are carried out with careful techniques, a percentage as low as 3% culture-negative endocarditis has been reported.[2] It is difficult to be certain about the frequency of such cases because so much depends on the criteria utilized for establishing the diagnosis of IE in the absence of positive blood cultures. For example, valvular vegetations are not uncommon in patients with intracardiac catheters and pacemakers, cancer, and various immunological abnormalities and in association with disseminated intravascular coagulation (see Section 3.2). Thus, the finding of vegetations alone would not seem to be sufficient to establish the diagnosis.

The identification of microorganisms within vegetations would certainly add weight to the suspicion of IE. On the other hand, it is difficult to evaluate such studies without quantitative estimates of the number of bacteria detected and without information about the ability to detect microorganisms in "noninfected" intravascular vegetations. It is well known, for example, that in febrile patients *not* subsequently proven to have infections, it is common to find intraleukocytic bacteria in buffy-coat preparations.[4] Perhaps such "bacteria-laden" polymorphonuclear leukocytes (PMN) stick to any intravascular vegetations without their presence indicating infection of the vegetation. Furthermore, it has been demonstrated in rabbits with IE that it is sometimes necessary to employ conventional histological or immunofluorescent techniques to demonstrate microorganisms in vegetations which are negative by culture in animals with negative blood cultures.[5,6]

An example of these difficulties in interpretation is illustrated by a recent careful study of the problem.[1] Of 25 patients included as examples of culture-negative IE whose hearts were examined at surgery or at autopsy, 3 cases were included who had positive blood cultures, 4 were found not to have vegetations, and in an additional 6 patients with vegetations, microorganisms were neither seen nor cultured.

The fact that only 1 or 2 such patients were seen per year at a large university hospital is obviously another reason for the difficulty in applying consistent diagnostic criteria. The 52 cases analyzed in the aforementioned series occurred over a period of 30 years.[1]

It would seem to me that any study of this problem would demand: (1) a clinical definition of those patients to be included as cases of possible culture-negative endocarditis; (2) detailed evaluation of the vegetations seen at autopsy or at surgery, including conventional and perhaps immunofluorescent histological studies and a determination as to whether erosion or perforation of a valve had taken place; (3) quantitative bacteriological studies (histological and cultural) of vegetations—including stains and culture techniques capable of detecting newly discovered microorganisms such as *Legionella* species; (4) similar morphological and microbiological examinations of vegetations found at autopsy and at cardiac surgery in patients considered clinically *not* to have IE.

The most important cause of negative blood cultures in patients with IE is the *prior administration of antibiotics,* the frequency of which has varied considerably in different analyses of blood-culture-negative IE.[3] It is probably a more common cause of negative blood cultures than has been generally believed, accounting for perhaps as many as two thirds of cases.[1,7] Patients receiving single doses of penicillin or tetracycline before coming to the hospital may have negative blood cultures for weeks (despite the persistence of fever) before bacteria can be culured from the blood.[1,2] Conversely, I have seen a patient who became afebrile and asymptomatic after taking tetracycline, but whose blood cultures remained positive. A patient has also been recorded whose blood cultures became positive only after discontinuation of penicillin takin as prophylaxis for rheumatic fever.[1]

It is likely that antibiotics can act in the following several ways to clear the blood of bacteria: (1) Inhibit the *in vitro* growth of bacteria present in the blood. (2) Decrease the density of bacteria in the vegetation, thus decreasing the number of bacteria shed into the bloodstream. (3) Increase the efficiency of the phagocytosis and killing of bacteria in the bloodstream by the reticuloendothelial system. This mechanism is hypothetical, but its existence would be consistent with recent studies showing the increased killing of bacteria by PMN in the presence of subinhibitory concentrations of antibiotics.[8]

In subjects suspected of having intravascular infection who are known to have taken antibiotics, a certain number of measures should be taken to minimize the *in vitro* antimicrobial effectiveness of the antibiotics:

1. Assure ample dilution of the blood in the culture media (10 ml blood in 100–200 ml culture medium) so as to minimize the concentration of antibiotic.

2. If the patient is currently receiving antibiotics, obtain blood for culture just before the next administration of antibiotics in order to have blood containing the lowest concentration of antibiotic.

3. Add sodium polyanetholsulfonate (SPS) to the culture media to a maximum concentration of 0.025%.[9] This anticoagulant, which has several properties which decrease the antibacterial effect of whole blood, inactivates aminoglycosides, poylmixin, and colistin.

4. Add penicillinase to the culture media when appropriate, simultaneously making sure of the sterility of the penicillinase.

5. Supplement media with 15% sucrose in an effort to recover cell-wall-deficient bacterial forms.

6. Incubate the cultures for long periods of time—perhaps 1 month.

All the propositions listed above are directed against any antibiotic that might be present in the bloodstream at the time of blood culture. If, on the other hand, the effect of the antibiotic was either to decrease the shedding of bacteria into the peripheral blood or increase peripheral clearance of bacteria, it is evident that such laboratory devices would not be expected to improve the recovery of bacteria from the bloodstream. In the case where the effect of antibiotics was to decrease the number of circulating bacteria, this effect could be nullified either by neutralizing the *in vivo* action of the antibiotic or by waiting until its effect wore off. Since there is no known way to nullify the effect of any antibiotic *in vivo,* the essential question is: how long can one afford to wait for the dissipation of the antibiotic effect in the hope of obtaining the positive blood cultures? For the present, there is not a satisfactory way of answering this question.

The possibility of identifying bacterial antigens as a means of diagnosing "bacteremia" in patients with negative blood cultures is discussed at the end of this section.

The *location of intravascular infection* has been considered in detail as a factor of importance in determining the probability of finding a positive blood culture. Infections outside the heart or in the right side of the heart are associated with lower microbial densities (except for anaerobic infection) than the more frequent infections within the left side of the heart.[10,11] Mycotic aneurysms can be investigated by *arteriography,* and *forward angiography* may be helpful in identifying intracardiac vegetations.[12–14] *Cardiac catheterization,* despite its obvious risk of dislodging vegetations, has been employed successfully to document infection of the right heart when peripheral-blood cultures were sterile.[12,14,15] The principle here is a simple one— that the concentration of bacteria will be higher in the blood which has just been in contact with an infected vegetation than in blood that has been diluted or has passed through capillary beds capable of filtering bacteria, e.g., liver and lung. Similarly, blood leaving a peripheral atrioventricular shunt, established for purposes of hemodialysis, will contain a much higher density of bacteria than peripheral blood. It seems to me that this same principle should be utilized in patients with indwelling intravenous catheters who are suspected of having developed intravascular infection. Blood cultures taken through the suspicious catheter should be more often positive than those from the general pool of peripheral blood and should be easier to interpret than cultures of catheter tips withdrawn through the skin.

Echocardiography is a particularly interesting technique which, because of its ease of application, has been applied extensively to identify and localize intracardiac vegetations. This technique is useful to detect abnormal valve movements, such as mitral-valve preclosure, which seems particularly to be associated with the finding of aortic insufficiency in IE.[16] The disappearance of vegetations by echocardiography may be useful in evaluating treatment, or the persistence or sudden disappearance of vegetations may explain the source of continued embolic episodes.[17–19] A negative echocardiogram does not rule out the presence of vegetations on the heart valves. In a recent study comparing echocardiograms with autopsy confirmation of the presence of vegetations in 20 patients with IE, vegetations were found by echocardiography 11 times, 1 of which was considered to be a false-positive finding. On the other hand, vegetations found at autopsy in 8 patients were not detected by echocardiography.[20] Echocardiography is less sensitive in detecting lesions of the tricuspid than of the mitral valve.[21]

It must be borne in mind that even when vegetations are found by echocardiography, this does not establish the presence of infection, since this technique is also useful in detecting nonbacterial thrombotic vegetations.[22] In addition, findings compatible with atrial myxoma (diagnosis easily confused with IE) do not rule out the possibility of concomitant IE.[23–25] The use of two-dimensional echocardiography is a useful supplement to the conventional M-mode technique.[26] It is likely that diagnostic accuracy in IE will improve with technical advances.

Of particular interest is the relationship between the presence of vegetations by M-mode echocardiography and the frequency of severe complications and mortality in IE.[27–31] With combined data from five studies (left-sided IE in all but 3 patients) in which outcome was related to echocardiographic findings, the relations presented in Table 8 were evident.

TABLE 8
Outcome of Infective Endocarditis According to Presence of Vegetation by M-Mode Echocardiography[a]

Patients	Vegetation present	Normal
Deaths	13/63 (21%)	0/74 (0%)
Valve surgery	59/80 (74%)	4/88 (5%)
Cured with antibiotics only	8/63 (13%)	72/74 (97%)
Emboli	22/69 (32%)	3/80 (4%)

[a] Data from references 27–31.

Thus, echocardiography not only is useful in the detection of vegetations as a diagnostic aid in IE (about 50% of patients), but also is an important indication of the risk of serious valve damage, emboli, and mortality. In 74 patients with IE and normal echocardiograms, 72 were cured with antibiotics alone; there were no deaths and only 2 surgical valve replacements. Only 3 patients of 80 had peripheral emboli recognized. In patients with vegetations detected by echocardiography, 13 of 63 died, 42 of 80 required valve replacement, and only 8 of 63 were cured by antibiotics alone. Emboli were detected in 22 of 69 of these patients.

There was no relation between the infecting microorganism and the finding of vegetations by echocardiography in these series. Duration of symptoms of infection was an important determinant of positive echocardiograms in one series (<6 weeks, 1/9 echocardiograms positive; >6 weeks, 10/10 positive),[29] whereas such a correlation was not evident in the other study in which this relation was examined.[30]

Other noninvasive techniques are also useful in evaluating the status of patients with suspected IE. *Electrocardiography* is useful in the search for conduction abnormalities and evidence for myocardial infarction; phonocardiography is important for documenting changes in heart sounds. In patients with prosthetic heart valves, *cineradiography* may be useful to detect abnormalities or changes in valve movement.

A variety of *myocardial imaging* techniques have been utilized to try to identify endocardial vegetations: gallium-67technetium-99^{m}-pertechnetate-labeled antistaphylococcal antibody (staphylococcal endocarditis in rabbits), indium-111-labeled platelets, and technetium-99^{m} stannous pyrophosphate.[32–36] Although a few observations have been carried out in patients, the most satisfactory marker, technetium-99^{m} stannous pyrophosphate, is also taken up by nonbacterial endocardial vegetations and a variety of nonbacterial inflammatory myocardial lesions. The labeling of antibody would appear to have greater specificity, but for the present is limited by the need to label specific antibacterial antibody. The specificity of imaging with indium-111-labeled platelets for IE remains to be established. These techniques must be considered to be in the early stages of experimental development and evaluation.

A variety of *technical microbiological problems* known to influence the ability to culture microorganisms *in vitro* are pertinent to the identification of the infecting microorganism in patients suspected of having IE who have negative blood cultures.

Blood cultures should be repeated and consideration given to *arterial blood cultures* in the search for fungus infection. Biphasic *(Casteneda-type) media* are useful for culturing fungi and *Brucella* species.[9,35] Cultures of urine may be useful in the search for staphyloccocci, fungi, and enterococci. *Bone-marrow cultures* should be a routine part of the search for hematological or granulomatous disorders or fungal infections in this group of patients.[37]

Nutritional supplements may be essential for the *in vitro* cultivation of certain bacteria. Acar recently reported that 6 of 100 bacteria recovered from patients with IE required such supplements to establish the diagnosis.[38] At the New York Hospital, 3 of 55 streptococci recovered from patients with IE required pyridoxal supplements for laboratory cultivation.[39] Some streptococci grow only as satellite colonies adjacent to staphylococci.[7,9,40–42] Both pyridoxal and "satellite" streptococci will grow in the presence of L-cysteine supplements, but supplements of both pyridoxal and L-cysteine are not recommended, since excess concentrations of either will inhibit growth.[41]

Cell-wall-deficient bacteria should be searched for using hypertonic culture media. Electron microscopy has revealed cell-wall-deficient bacterial forms in vegetations which would have been considered nonbacterial by conventional light-microscopic techniques.[43] In one instance, cell-wall-deficient forms were detected in vegetations in the absence of prior antibiotic therapy.[43] However, in general, cell-wall-deficient bacteria have not been found to play an important role in IE.

Venting of blood-culture bottles has been recommended to accelerate growth of *Pseudomonas* and *Candida* species. However, venting may inhibit growth of anaerobic bacteria.[9]

In summary, there are a variety of bacteriological techniques which are important in isolating unusual microorganisms from the peripheral blood. It is of particular interest, as mentioned earlier, that at the New York Hospital, where there has been a long-standing interest in the bacteriology of IE, only 3% of 243 patients considered to have IE had negative blood cultures.[44] The technique for processing routine blood cultures at that hospital is as follows[44] :

5 ml of blood is inoculated into each of 3 bottles containing 70–90 ml of:

1. Trypticase soy broth (TSB)
2. Thioglycollate broth (TB) without indicator
3. Beef-heart infusion (BHI) broth (prepared weekly at the New York Hospital)

All blood cultures are then passed blindly to chocolate agar from TSB and BHI after incubation for 24 hr and from BHI after incubation for 4 days.

If growth is not apparent by the seventh day of incubation, the blood cultures are discarded.

If IE is suspected on clinical grounds, all blood cultures are passed blindly to TSB with pyridoxal and blood agar after 7 days; the initial BHI and TB cultures are discarded at 10 days, and TSB cultures are discarded at 14 days.

Of course, an effort should be made to culture fluid obtained from any peripheral skin lesions or inflamed joint cavities as well as emboli removed at the time of surgery. A careful *ophthalmological examination* should be carried out in the search for lesions due to *Candida* septicemia. Certain infections can be diagnosed *serologically,* e.g., *Candida, Aspergillus,* histoplasmosis, Q fever, and psittacosis. In addition, staphylococcal antigen and teichoic acid antibodies should be sought as an indication of infection with *Staphylococcus aureus* and antibodies to *Staph. albus S 11A,* particularly in children with ventriculoatrial shunts.[45–51] The detection of antibodies to streptococci, *Listeria*, and *Propionibacterium acnes* may also be helpful in patients with negative blood cultures.[49,52–54] A search should also be made for rheumatoid factor, circulating immune complexes, and heart antibody, and complement levels should be measured (see Section 6.3.4). None of the results of these serological studies are specific for IE, but they are useful in accumulating evidence favoring the diagnosis and some of them for evaluating the effect of antibiotic therapy. *Gas–liquid chromatography* may prove to be useful for the diagnosis of fungal and perhaps certain bacterial infections.[55,56]

8.3. POSITIVE BLOOD CULTURES

Whereas it is always difficult to know whether, or when, to treat for IE a patient who has negative blood cultures, it may also be difficult to know whether a positive blood culture indicates intravascular infection or just a transient bacteremia due to an extravascular infection.

If bacteremia is *prolonged* (hours to days), that can be taken as evidence favoring intravascular infection, but it is not specific (as discussed in Section 6.2). Besides, most of the time a decision to commence antibiotic therapy is too important to be delayed in order to determine the constancy of bacteremia.

If specific *antibodies* to the microorganism are identified in the same sample of blood from which bacteria were cultured, that would constitute strong evidence in favor of intravascular infection, but it is not usual to save serum samples at the time of taking blood cultures. This might be worth doing, however, even in the postoperative state. It is surprising how rapidly teichoic acid antibodies are useful in the diagnosis of staphylococcal endocarditis, even during the early phase of infection.[47] Although sepsis, particularly due to *Staph. aureus,* is less likely to represent intravascular infection when there is an identifiable focus of infection, this is a statistical judgment, since such a focus may serve as the portal of entry for infective endocarditis (IE) or may be a metastatic infection from previously unrecognized (or even asymptomatic) IE.[57] Of course, the total clinical picture must play a large role in evaluating the question of whether or not to treat a patient with positive blood cultures for IE. My tendency is to err on the side of long-term treatment, particularly in view of the potential hazards of inadequate treatment of IE.

In the *postoperative period after cardiac-valve surgery,* it has been shown that not all patients with bacteremia have infection of their prosthetic valves; however, this also is a statistical judgment, and for the moment, there is no way of being certain as to whether a freshly placed heart valve has become infected by, or is the source of, a particular episode of bacteremia postoperatively.[58,59] The findings which favor valvular infection include the development of conduction abnormalities by ECG, evidence of valvular dysfunction or dehiscence (phonocardiogram), echocardiographic evidence of vegetation formation, or cineradiographic evidence of abnormal motion of the valve. Emboli or other usual manifestations of IE would of course also favor the diagnosis of valvular infection. The problem is difficult and requires the judgment of experienced physicians. Ultimately, the question is whether the risks of prolonging antibiotic therapy (to 6 weeks) for a presumptive diagnosis of IE are greater than the risks of treating patients with postoperative bacteremia without evidence of valvular involvement for only 2–3 weeks. As mentioned earlier, I am inclined toward longer treatment for the great majority of patients in these circumstances.

The treatment of late prosthetic-valve endocarditis (PVE) is particularly difficult, since the bacteria recovered are often resistant to usual antibiotics. Treatment often requires a combination of medical and surgical-valve-replacement therapy. It is of interest that patients with late PVE due to *viridans* streptococci have a mortality of "only" 25–40%, and many have been cured without its being necessary to replace the prosthetic valve.[60–62] The indications for surgery in the management of IE and PVE are considered in Section 8.6.

It is often difficult to decide whether a patient with an *indwelling right-heart catheter* (total parenteral nutrition, central venous pressure, pacemaker) who develops bacteremia has IE. This issue is similar to that described for postoperative patients, but the risks of serious consequences from right-sided intracardiac infection are considerably less, as are the therapeutic problems (as discussed earlier). I would be more inclined, in these instances, to remove the intracardiac device and give short courses of antibiotic therapy (1–2 weeks) in the absence of signs of endocarditis. Patients with persistent staphylococcal bacteremia associated with a removable intravenous device or with a slow clinical response to appropriate antimicrobial therapy should be treated for 6 weeks.[63] In instances where it is too dangerous to consider removing an infected pacemaker, there is little alternative to treating the patient with antibiotics for 6 weeks.[64] The management of patients with isolated fungemia is also a complex and difficult problem (see Section 8.5.8).

8.4. ANTIBIOTICS

8.4.1. Principles

The principles of antibiotic therapy for infective endocarditis (IE) are well established: bactericidal drugs, administered parenterally, for long periods of time. The reasons for requiring long-term intensive therapy have been described earlier; they are due principally to the absence of effective polymorphonuclear-leukocyte activity and the dormant metabolic state of older bacteria in the vegetations, thus slowing the effectiveness of cell-wall-active antibiotics such as penicillin. The unreliability of oral absorption of antibiotics argues strongly for parenteral administration in the treatment of IE.

Beyond these principles, our knowledge of the outcome of treatment in man is based on clinical studies of antibiotic regimens arrived at empirically. In other words, we know about the effectiveness of certain regimens in infections with particular microorganisms. For example, 4–6 weeks of penicillin–streptomycin treatment of an infection due to penicillin-sensitive [minimal inhibitory concentration (MIC) < 0.1 μg/ml] α-hemolytic streptococci can be counted upon to sterilize all vegetations. However, there are important risks of embolization and valve perforation related to the presence of infection. We do not know whether a different antibiotic treatment program would diminish these risks. In infections with other microorganisms, there is less information, and the ability to achieve 100% sterilization of vegetations is even less well established.

Animal studies have been particularly helpful in this regard. Although they can be criticized, as can the effort to extrapolate all animal studies to man, they nevertheless provide us with a means of determining antibiotic activity in a valvular vegetation which is very close, if not identical, to that seen in man. There is no way of obtaining similar information from patients with IE. Of course, the pharmacodynamics of antibiotics are different in animals and in man, and there may also be important differences in protein binding. Nevertheless, the studies which have been carried out are considered of sufficient value to have already altered what were previously generally accepted practices of antibiotic usage in man.

There are many factors which stand in the way of unambiguous treatment recommendations in man. Some of the variables which influence patient outcome and thus have to be taken into consideration in the evaluation of antibiotic effect include: age, duration of symptoms, presence of underlying systemic disease, presence of underlying valvular disease, localization of infected vegetations (side of heart, valve), nature of infecting microorganism, and antibiotic sensitivity of the microorganism. Furthermore, since relatively few patients are seen in a single hospital, the changes in medical practice with the passage of time may outstrip the possibilities of evaluating a single management protocol. Collaborative studies are essential to make headway in this area, but the desirability of these studies exceeds, for the moment at least, our capacity to overcome the obstacles imposed by the size of the effort necessary to obtain an interpretable result.

The medical literature is replete with reports of 1 or 2 or even 5–10 patients with IE purporting to demonstrate usefulness of a particular antibiotic treatment program. These reports are useful to the extent that they demonstrate which antibiotic regimens may work or which may not work, but they are not helpful in determining the quantity and the nature of antibiotics (alone or in combination) which are optimal for the treatment of IE. Furthermore, since a wide variety of antibiotic treatment programs may be successful in some patients, the choice of optimal therapy is necessarily based on a statistical evaluation of therapeutic success.

Unfortunately, it is not easy to decide upon the criteria for evaluating antimicrobial agents in IE. In the preantibiotic era, the prompt cure of a single patient could be considered proof of the usefulness of a therapeutic agent, since the mortality rate of IE was 100%. Today, however, with many antibiotics available, all of which may be partially effective, yet which differ in effectiveness in relatively minor ways, the problem of determining the best mode of treatment is complicated. For example, although inability to eliminate bacteria from the bloodstream or relapse of infection after completion of treatment is an obvious index of bacteriological failure, it is not certain to what extent relapse, for example, is a consequence of inability to sterilize the valvular vegetations or whether it represents reseeding from sites of metastatic infection. Metastatic infection is the rule in animals with staphylococcal or *Candida* infection, and the interaction of infecting agent, host defenses, and antibiotic activity is quite different in an intracardiac vegetation and a renal abscess.[10,65] In addition, it may not be a simple matter to determine whether a second episode of IE is a treatment failure or a new infection. It is highly probable that some bacteria may remain dormant for years before provoking symptomatic illness.[66]

Mortality is obviously another endpoint for the evaluation of antibiotic therapy in IE. However, it has been known for some time that the principal cause of death in IE on natural valves is congestive heart failure resulting from valve destruction or perforation.[67] This potentially fatal complication of IE is seen despite effective sterilization of vegetations by antibiotics. It would seem to me, therefore, that any judgment of the effectiveness of treatment programs should include the effect on the frequency of valve destruction.

8.4.2. Recommended Treatment Programs

When a microorganism is identified as the cause of IE, antibiotics are chosen according to the statistical probability of their being effective. Studies are then carried out as rapidly as possible to determine the antibiotic sensitivities of the particular microorganism isolated. Disk sensitivity methods are not sufficiently accurate for the purposes of guiding antibiotic treatment in IE. At present, there is no substitute for determining the MIC and the minimal bactericidal concentration (MBC) of antibiotic effective against the test bacterium as an initial guide to the long-term therapy of the patient. Subsequent adjustments in the quality and quantity of antibiotic administered will depend on tests of serum bactericidal activity (SBA) of the patient's serum while receiving antibiotics. SBA has already been considered from the standpoint of a host defense mechanism in Section 7.6 and is discussed again in Chapter 9.

Until very recently, the major laboratory result guiding antibiotic therapy has been the MIC of the antibiotic. This is rather curious, since it has long been known that bacteriostatic antibiotics are not effective in the treatment of IE. Recent studies have called attention to the fact that for certain strains of bacteria, the MBC is sufficiently higher than the MIC to justify reference to these strains as being tolerant to the antibiotic tested.[403] In rabbits, penicillin treatment which would have been considered to be adequate according to the MIC and SBA was ineffective for tolerant *Streptococcus sanguis,* whereas a nontolerant strain was rapidly sterilized.[68] A study of the same phenomenon in rabbits infected with nontolerant and tolerant staphylococci and treated with methicillin did not reveal difference in antibiotic efficacy according to tolerance. However, it is known that tolerance to antibiotics exhibited by staphylococci may be extremely variable, depending upon the precise laboratory conditions chosen to demonstrate the phenomenon.[69,404] On the other hand, tolerance may be important in explaining the relatively slow response of IE due to *Lactobacilli* to penicillin in rabbits.[70]

Prior antibiotic therapy may select for antibiotic-tolerant mouth streptococci, thereby diminishing the effectiveness of antibiotics used for the treatment of IE.[405]

Having underlined the potential importance of determining the MIC and MBC of infecting microorganisms for guiding antibiotic therapy, I must emphasize that the lack of standardization of laboratory methods makes it essential to keep an open mind concerning the precision with which this information can be applied to clinical problems.[71,72] It has been said of the MIC that[72]

> the mysteries which keep the bacterial inoculum below the threshold of visibility at the particular time the test is read in the specific environment in which the test is performed might well test the skills of a clairvoyant. . . . Variability in the results of testing for bactericidal activity does not prompt much optimism for this test as a more uniform *in-vitro* method than the MIC.

Despite these reservations, MIC and MBC results will be used in the following discussion as a guide to the choice of antibiotics in the treatment of IE, since they are cited in the literature. Some authors, however, acknowledge their questionable usefulness and do not always predicate therapy based on such nonstandardized laboratory procedures.[71]

8.4.2.1. Streptococci

a. Streptococci Inhibited by 0.1 μg/ml of Penicillin G or Less. With bacteriological sterilization as the criterion of success, it is an easy matter to cure IE due to penicillin-sensitive streptococci. Antibiotics are extraordinarily successful, reducing the relapse rate to virtually zero and the overall mortality from 100 to about 15%. Despite uncertainties concerning the standardization of laboratory techniques, it has generally be found that the great majority of *viridans* streptococci are inhibited by 0.1 μg/ml of penicillin or less.[71,73]

To my knowledge, the following regimen has not been associated with any reports of bacteriological failure in patients with penicillin-sensitive streptococci[73,74]:

Penicillin G, 20 million units I.V. per day for 4 weeks

(or 1.2 million units I.M. every 4 hr)

plus

Streptomycin, 0.5 g I.M. or I.V. every 12 hr for 2 weeks

Although there are those who advocate 4 weeks of penicillin without streptomycin[75,76] and those who advocate 2 weeks of penicillin and streptomycin,[71] bacteriological relapses have been recorded with these treatment programs.[74] Other treatment programs which have been proposed advocate oral instead of parenteral penicillin.[77] The argument against streptomycin is based on the impression that penicillin alone is just as effective[75,76] and that streptomycin adds an unnecessary toxic risk. Obviously, the propositions are related; if 4 weeks of penicillin alone is just as effective as 4 weeks of penicillin with 2 weeks of streptomycin, then the risk of streptomycin toxicity is unnecessary. If, on the other hand, penicillin alone is not as good as combined therapy, the minimal risk of 1 g streptomycin per day for 14 days is fully justified. Although relapses have been recorded with the use of 4 weeks of penicillin alone, the quantity of penicillin used in these cases was small[78] or the duration of symptoms prior to the start of treatment was long.[76,79,406] I am not aware of relapses in patients treated with 4 weeks of penicillin and 2 weeks of streptomycin, as recommended above.

Toxicity associated with the recommended 2-week course of streptomycin consists of reversible vestibular symptoms in, at most, 2% of patients.[80] Obviously, in the presence of symptoms of toxicity, streptomycin should be discontinued. Attention must also be directed to adjusting the quantity of streptomycin given to patients with abnormal renal function, to the elderly, to patients with preeexisting vestibular disease, and to patients receiving other potentially ototoxic drugs.

It is also argued that 2 weeks of penicillin and streptomycin is sufficient and will decrease the length of hospitalization.[71] If the patient's clinical status is satisfactory and if his home circumstances permit, he can certainly receive his last 2 weeks of penicillin intramuscularly at home.

Obviously, there may not be a great difference among the recommendations of 4 weeks of penicillin plus 2 weeks of streptomycin, 2 weeks of penicillin and 2 weeks of streptomycin, and 4 weeks of penicillin alone, considered from the standpoint of bacteriological relapse alone. Nevertheless, my interpretation of the existing published data conforms with that of Hook and Guerrant[74] and Bryant and Kimbrough,[81] as well as of Resnick and Cohen,[80] Svanbom and Strandell,[82] and Sande and Scheld,[407] in recommending 4 weeks of penicillin and 2 weeks of streptomycin.

However, the issue of bacteriological cure is only one aspect of the problem ot treatment of IE. Although detailed attention has not been directed to the problem in published reports, valve destruction requiring cardiac surgery is an important consequence of IE, even with penicillin-sensitive streptococci. In recent series, about 20–28% of patients developed this complication.[71,75,83] If one assumes that valve perforation is related to bacterial growth in vegetations, it would seem reasonable to try to sterilize these vegetations as rapidly as possible in the hope of decreasing this and perhaps other complications such as cerebral emboli. Combined penicillin–streptomycin treatment of experimental IE has been shown to be unequivocally superior to penicillin alone in the *speed* with which vegetations infected with penicillin-sensitive streptococci are sterilized, thus adding another important reason for treating with combined therapy (Figure 20).[84–86]

It is evident that any future effort to evaluate the therapy of IE in man must consider not only bacteriological response and mortality but also the duration of the disease before the onset of treatment, the nature of the findings by echocardiography, and a detailed evaluation of the complications of the disease such as valve perforation and metastatic infectin (bone scan) as well as damage to other organ systems such as the brain and the kidneys. Taking into consideration the numbers of patients in different categories necessary to clarify these questions, it is unlikely that a practical study can be organized in the near future.[87] On

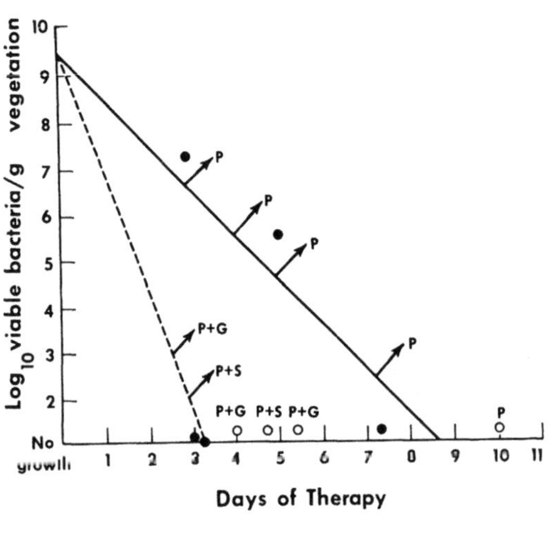

Figure 20. Approximate rate of bacterial eradication from the cardiac vegetations of rabbits with *Str. viridans* endocarditis during therapy with penicillin (P) alone (——) or P plus either streptomycin (S) or gentamicin (G) (-----). Rates were determined by titers of viable *Str. viridans* (●) per gram of vegetation removed from animals sacrificed during therapy and by the presence (↗) or absence (○) of bacteriological relapse after discontinuation of antibiotic therapy. Reproduced from Sande and Irwin[86] with permission.

the other hand, it has been estimated that the reduction of the length of hospitalization of patients treated for IE due to penicillin-sensitive streptococci from 4 weeks to 2 weeks could result in savings nationally in the United States of more than $40 million per year.[83] Perhaps, in view of the large sums of money involved, an effort to resolve this question would be economically feasible.

In case of penicillin allergy, I prefer to use vancomycin 0.5 g I.V. every 6 hr.[88] The cephalosporins have been used successfully under these circumstances, but the possibility of allergic cross-reactivity is not negligible.[79]

The treatment of pneumococcal, gonococcal, or meningococcal endocarditis is similar to that of streptococcal infection. In these infections, there is neither experimental nor clinical evidence to suggest that streptomycin is a useful adjunct to penicillin therapy.

b. Streptococci Resistant to 0.1 μg/ml of Penicillin G (including Enterococci). There is a great deal written about the importance of the correct classification of a streptococcus in order to determine the proper antibiotics to be administered to a patient with IE. It is evident today that one cannot rely on the name of the streptococcus to determine the choice of antibiotics. As discussed in Section 8.4.2, there are uncertainties associated with the determination of the MIC and MBC of a particular infecting microorganism; nevertheless, these uncertainties seem relatively minor compared with the difficulties of giving a name to a particular streptococcus. To quote Wannamaker and Parker[89]: "The streptococci associated with infective endocarditis are a heterogenous and individualistic lot . . . [which for years] . . . have resisted regimentation and the numerous efforts of taxonomists to place them in tidy groups."

In fact, the problem facing the physician is simpler than that facing the microbiologist. With the discovery (or the strong suspicion) of a streptococcus as the etiological agent in a patient with IE, therapy should be begun with penicillin intravenously and streptomycin as described above for penicillin-sensitive streptococci.

Once it is determined that the MIC of the streptococcus is more than 0.1 μg/ml of penicillin G, or more than 0.2 μg/ml according to some authors[71,90]—no matter what name seems appropriate according to classification schemes—the patient should be treated with:

Penicillin G, 20 million units I.V. per day for 6 weeks

plus

Streptomycin, 1.0 g I.M. every 12 hr for 2 weeks

then: 0.5 g I.M. every 12 hr for 4 additional weeks.

There is general agreement that the patient should *not* be treated with penicillin or ampicillin alone; clinical relapses are more frequent with a penicillin alone, and animal studies have clearly established the superiority of combined treatment.[91–93] In rabbit endocarditis, penicillin plus gentamicin was superior to a penicillinase-resistant penicillin plus gentamicin, suggesting that initial treatment of a patient with suspected IE due to "penicillin-resistant" streptococci should include penicillin G and an aminoglycoside.[94]

In case of penicillin allergy, vancomycin (0.5 g I.V. every 6 hr) can be substituted for penicillin; synergy is frequent with vancomycin and streptomycin,[95] but is more predictable (100%) with vancomycin and gentamicin.[96] There is agreement that the cephalosporins are not capable of substituting for penicillin despite evidence of effectiveness *in vitro*. Although cephalosporin is as effective in rabbit IE as penicillin, providing that the serum level of cephalosporin exceeds the MIC of the organism to the same degree as that of penicillin,[97] the quantity of cephalosporin necessary to achieve these *in vivo* concentrations in man is prohibitive.[98]

Although ampicillin is more effective than penicillin *in vitro*, the difference is small and more than compensated for by the achievable serum levels of penicillin *in vivo*.[99] In view of the extensive clinical experience with penicillin, this drug remains the penicillin of choice in the treatment of "penicillin-resistant" streptococci.

The administration of the recommended amount of streptomycin for 6 weeks produced vestibular toxicity in about 25% of patients.[74] Toxicity developing during therapy argues for discontinuation of streptomycin after 4 weeks. It is primarily the toxicity of streptomycin in the doses recommended which raises several questions in the treatment of this category of infection: Is 6 weeks of streptomycin better than 4 weeks? Is 6 weeks of streptomycin necessary for the treatment of nonenterococcal "penicillin-resistant" streptococci? There are no data which help in answering these questions. The question of whether there is a difference in antibiotic requirements of enterococcal and nonenterococcal "penicillin-resistant" streptococci could perhaps be examined experimentally.

Another question which has given rise to much discussion is how to treat patients in whom streptomycin–penicillin synergy is not demonstrable *in vitro*, i.e., patients in whom the streptococcus is resistant to 2000 μg/ml of streptomycin. There is growing evidence that streptomycin resistance is increasing in frequency, and in two recent series, it has been reported to be as high as 25–50%.[99–101] In the presence of resistance to streptomycin, synergy with penicillin is not demonstrable. On the other hand, synergy between penicillin and gentamicin is virtually always demonstrable and raises the question as to whether penicillin–gentamicin should not be recommended instead of penicillin–streptomycin.[99–102] There are several aspects of this question which deserve consideration.

Conventional disk antibiotic sensitivities are inadequate to judge the antibiotic sensitivities of streptococci so as to guide therapeutic decisions. Streptococci will always appear resistant to the concentration of streptomycin in disks, and resistance to a penicillin disk does not preclude a satisfactory synergistic effect between penicillin and streptomycin.[101] Thus, streptomycin resistance can be established only by tube-dilution sensitivities. The finding of high-level streptomycin resistance does not automatically mean that penicillin–streptomycin synergy is absent.[100]

The risk of toxicity with 6 weeks of gentamicin treatment is not well defined. Judging from the consequences of high-dose therapy (8 mg/kg per day) in 14 young patients with *Pseudomonas* endocarditis, the risk of conventional therapy (3–5 mg/kg per day) may not be greater than that seen with streptomycin.[100] In patients with high-dose therapy, 50% developed ototoxicity; however, in only one patient was diminished acuity to low and middle frequencies noted.[103] Swartz[90] is sufficiently convinced of the advantage of penicillin–gentamicin therapy in enterococcal endocarditis to recommend these antibiotics in preference to penicillin–streptomycin. On the other hand, the prevailing view is that penicillin–gentamicin treatment should be reserved for those patients who do not respond to, or who relapse after, treatment with penicillin–streptomycin.[74,81]

8.4.2.2. Staphylococci

The treatment of staphylococcal IE depends on the antibiotic sensitivities of the organism and perhaps the location of the infection. Staphylococci inhibited by 0.1 μg/ml of penicillin should be treated for 6 weeks with intravenous penicillin and streptomycin, as recommended for penicillin-sensitive streptococci (see Section 8.4.2.1a).

All other staphylococci should be treated with penicillinase-resistant penicillins, since even if the staphylococcus is relatively sensitive to penicillin, penicillinase production may be induced in the presence of penicillin.[74] Current recommendations are to give:

Nafcillin, methicillin, or oxacillin, 2.0 g I.V. every 4 hr for 6 weeks

On the basis of animal experiments demonstrating the more rapid sterilization of staphylococcal IE with combined therapy,[104–106] I recommend that gentamicin also be given in conventional doses, 3–5 mg/kg per day, the dosage being adjusted according to serum levels and renal function, for a period of 7–14 days.

The same kind of controversy exists concerning the indications for gentamicin in these circumstances as has been described for the combined treatment of penicillin-sensitive streptococci.[107–109] Clinical data are not convincing[110,111]; one prospective study in drug addicts did show more rapid development of negative blood cultures and more rapid fall in temperature in patients treated with combined therapy, but the differences were not significant.[112] It has long been known that the prognosis of staphylococcal IE in addicts (with predominantly right-heart infection) was far superior to that of left-sided IE[113,114]; however, the experimental studies showing the advantage of combined treatment have been carried out in rabbits with left-sided IE.[104–106] Thus, the existing clinical data do not negate the possible validity of the rabbit studies for man.

The increasing frequency with which staphylococci are found to be tolerant to various antibiotics and resistant to methicillin has stimulated the search for other combinations of antibiotics effective in treatment, particularly of left-sided staphylococcal IE.[115,116] Treatment programs which have been found effective in circumstances of poor clinical response, penicillin allergy, or methicillin resistance include:

Vancomycin, 0.5 g I.V. every 6 hr, alone or with gentamicin

or

Vancomycin plus rifampin, 18 mg/kg P.O. per day (children)[115]

300 mg P.O. every 8 hr (adults)[117]

For the present, there are insufficient data to do more than note the kinds of antibiotics that have been effective in selected cases.

Studies in rabbits have not been able to demonstrate a difference in the effectiveness of methicillin, nafcillin, or oxacillin in the treatment of staphylococcal IE, despite differences in *in vitro* activity, protein binding, and pharmacodynamics in the rabbit.[118] On the other hand, nafcillin and methicillin have been found to be significantly more effective than cephalothin and cephazolin in sterilizing left-heart vegetations.[119,120] There is controversy as to whether cefazolin has particular deficiencies as a therapeutic agent in man.[81,121–124]

Staphylococcus epidermidis is a frequent cause of IE after prosthetic-valve placement and is usually resistant to methicillin or nafcillin. All methicillin-resistant isolates in one study had subpopulations resistant to cephalosporins. Resistance to the aminoglycosides was also frequent, thus leaving vancomycin and rifampin the most consistently effective antibiotics.[125] Of course, antibiotic resistance in these instances is probably related to the prophylactic antibiotics administered at the time of valve surgery (see Section 8.5)

8.4.2.3 Negative Blood Cultures

In patients in whom there is a strong suspicion of IE and yet negative blood cultures, most authorities favor a trial of antibiotics as recommended for penicillin-resistant streptococcal endocarditis (see Section 8.4.2.1b) or staphylococcal endocarditis (see Section 8.4.2.2). Of course, it is necessary to take into consideration any epidemiological clues which may increase the probabilities of eventually finding a particular microorganism. For example, if the clinical illness began after dental surgery, one would think of mouth streptococci, whereas if symptoms began after transurethral resection, one would be more concerned about enterococci or, rarely, gram-negative bacilli. In the absence of any clue as to etiology, a combination of vancomycin and gentamicin might be particularly good coverage for streptococcal or staphylococcal infection.

8.4.2.4. Other Microorganisms

Since other microorganisms represent such a small proportion of any one expert's clinical experience, recommendations for treatment are virtually anecdotal. For that reason, these special treatment problems will be considered under the heading of special problems of microbial infection.

8.5. SPECIAL PROBLEMS OF MICROBIAL INFECTION

8.5.1. Gram-Negative Bacilli

8.5.1.1. *Pseudomonas aeruginosa*

Infections with *Ps. aeruginosa* are uncommon, the overwhelming majority occurring in drug addicts or on prosthetic heart valves. In addicts, these infections involve principally the tricuspid valve and are not distinguishable from infection with other bacteria on the basis of clinical findings.[103,126,127] The most surprising finding in these patients is their capacity to tolerate the continued presence of *Pseudomonas* in the blood with so little disability.[126,127] In some instances, fever may even transiently disappear spontaneously.[128] The relatively prolonged course of *Pseudomonas* infection in addicts may be explained by the presence of preexisting antibody, as has been demonstrated in rabbits.[129] Prompt disappearance of fever (within 2–6 days) after the start of antimicrobial therapy is usual in patients who have a good response to antimicrobial therapy, but a more delayed defervescence (18–20 days) is not incompatible with eventual cure. Disappearance of fever (9–20 days) has also been observed in patients who do not respond to antibiotics.[103]

At present, the most satisfactory antibiotic regimen for the treatment of *Pseudomonas* endocarditis has proven to be 6-week treatment with a combination of:

Carbenicillin, 30 g I.V. per day

and

Gentamicin, 8 mg/kg I.M. per day

In a series of patients with predominantly tricuspid-valve infection described by Reyes *et al.*,[103] 64% were cured with antibiotics alone and a total of 86% with medical and surgical therapy, the latter consisting of resection of the affected valve. An unusually large amount of gentamicin was used in these patients because of the failure of usual doses (3–5 mg/kg per day).[103,126] Although this was associated with frequent reversible azotemia and changes in the audiogram and electronystagmogram, clinically apparent hearing loss occurred in only one of these young addicts. Retreatment of relapses was, however, associated with greater toxicity.[103] Anicteric hepatitis due to carbenicillin was also noted in several of these patients.[103] High-dose gentamicin–carbenicillin therapy of aortic-valve *Pseudomonas* infective endocarditis (IE) in rabbits was associated with cure rates comparable to those in man.[130]

The development of azotemia requires adjustment of the amount of gentamicin administered, and carbenicillin hepatitis was an indication for the replacement of carbenicillin by polymyxin B.[103] Several patients were treated with polymyxin B or colistin (80 mg I.V. every 8 hr). It is not clear to what extent polymyxin was a useful adjunct to carbenicillin–gentamicin treatment in these patients.[103,126,408]

Pseudomonas endocarditis in addicts is sometimes complicated by simultaneous infection with other microorganisms (such as *Staph. aureus*). In these cases, the clinical picture may be more fulminant, and obviously, treatment is complicated by the necessity to include an antibiotic effective against the second microbe.[103,126] *Pseudomonas* endocarditis has also been reported as a complication of cardiac catheterization and coronary aortography.[131] A prosthetic-valve infection with *Ps. maltophila* was successfully treated with trimethoprim–sulfamethoxazole (TMP-SMZ), 3 tablets twice daily (80 mg TMP, 400 mg SMZ per tablet).[132] This latter observation suggests that a test for sensitivity of *Pseudomonas* species to TMP-SMZ should be carried out, but that with the present state of our experience, such treatment should be reserved for patients who do not respond to carbenicillin–gentamicin (? + polymyxin B). The successful treatment of addicts with tricuspid IE due to *Ps. cepacia* with TMP-SMZ has been reported,[133,134] but infections on the left side of the heart were not sterilized.[135]

8.5.1.2. *Brucella*

Endocarditis due to *Brucella* species is rare, has a high mortality, and is found in 80% of patients dying of brucellosis.[136] Curiously, it seems to be a disease found (up to the present) only in men. There are no distinguishing clinical features save for the epidemiological clues that might raise the suspicion of contact with infected animals or contaminated farm products. Although blood cultures may show growth after only a few days, they should be kept for 1 month before being confident that they are sterile.

Two patients have recently been reported who were cured after replacement of a natural aortic valve and a prosthetic mitral valve.[137,138] In both instances, cardiac surgery was carried out for hemodynamic reasons. I have had a similar patient recently who required replacement of his aortic valve.

One of the patients was treated successfully with:

Tetracycline, 2.0 g P.O. per day

Streptomycin, 2.0 g I.M. per day

Rifampin, 900 mg P.O. per day

The resected aortic valve was sterile after about 2 weeks of antibiotic treatment, including 8 days of the triple therapy outlined above. Triple therapy was continued for a total of 10 weeks.[138]

The other patient was treated with TMP-SMZ, 6 tablets a day for about 2 months and 4 tablets a day to a total of 12 months (80 mg TMP, 400 mg SMZ per tablet).[137] Two days after starting TMP-sulfa, the patient still had culturable *Brucella* in the vegetations that were removed with the prosthetic valve. Thus, cure was achieved with TMP-SMZ plus surgery despite the placement of a prosthetic valve into a contaminated operative field.

I have had a patient (male) who had his perforated aortic valve replaced, at which time vegetations contained 10^9 *Brucella* colony-forming units/gram. Treatment was begun shortly before surgery with tetracycline, and streptomycin was continued afterward until fever recurred. The patient was then given 16 tablets per day of TMP-SMZ, to which his fever responded. He continued this dosage for several months and a lower dosage for several more months for a total of 6 months. He remains asymptomatic 2 years later. Although it is difficult to define the role of the various antibiotics received by this patient, the case illustrates another cure with surgery and antibiotics as well as the ability to tolerate much larger doses of TMP-SMZ than are usually administered.

8.5.1.3. Nontyphoid Salmonellae

Salmonellae have a peculiar predilection for nonvalvular vascular endothelium. Cohen *et al.*[139] have recently reviewed the reported cases of this infection as well as their own experience and have demonstrated that in patients with nontyphoidal *Salmonella* bacteremia, there was a 25% (10/40) frequency of *Salmonella* endothelial infection in patients over age 50 whose infection was evident before admission to the hospital. Of the 10 patients in their series, 8 had preexisting valvular or coronary-artery disease.

Of patients with arteritis, the only cures were associated with surgical excision of the lesion. No patients were cured with antibiotics alone. In patients with endocarditis, cure with antibiotics alone was rare.[139]

In recent years, several patients have been described who developed *Sal-*

monella prosthetic-valve endocarditis (PVE).[140-142] One patient, treated with 20 g ampicillin I.V. per day, showed no clinical improvement until the prosthetic valve was replaced. Vegetations removed at operation were sterile, the patient having previously received 1 week of ampicillin (12 g/day) and 2 weeks of 20 g/day. The high dose of ampicillin was continued for an additional 6 weeks followed by 2.0 g/day for several months. The patient was considered cured.[140] A similar patient was treated successfully with ampicillin and gentamicin.[142] Synergy between mecillinam and ampicillin against some strains of *Salmonella* suggest future trials of this combination of antibiotics in cases where more "conventional" therapy is ineffective.[141]

8.5.1.4. *Serratia marcescens*

This infection usually occurs in addicts or in a hospital setting in debilitated patients, often under treatment with antibiotics with indwelling intravenous catheters.[143] The general problem is similar to that of infection with *Pseudomonas* species.[144]

In certain areas, there have been outbreaks of endocarditis in addicts, but in contrast to infection with *Pseudomonas,* infection is predominantly on the aortic or mitral valve with frequent valve destruction and major-vessel peripheral emboli.[145]

Most cures with antibiotics alone have been effected in addicts with tricuspid-valve involvement.[145] A combination of carbenicillin (30 g/day) and gentamicin (3–6 mg/kg per day) has been generally successful in these patients. However, the antibiotic sensitivities of *Serratia* strains are variable, and other drugs must be tested, including TMP-SMZ.[143] There are at least two patients reported with left-heart infection in whom gentamicin–carbenicillin therapy was curative.[146,147] In these two instances, the sensitivity of the infecting strain was such that serum bactericidal activity was apparent at dilutions of 1 : 16–256 with carbenicillin and conventional doses of gentamicin.

It would seem to me that the treatment problem in addicts is similar to that of *Pseudomonas* infections. In addition to paying careful attention to antibiotic sensitivities and serum bactericidal activity (SBA), consideration should be given to trials of high-dose gentamicin (8.0 mg/kg per day), despite the risks of toxicity, since the mortality with these infections is particularly high.

Serratia microorganisms have the capacity to multiply rapidly at room temperature in 5% glucose, which no doubt explains in part the importance of this bacterium in hospital infections. It is of interest that 5% glucose remains clear despite high levels of bacterial growth.[148] *Serratia* bacteria are responsible for about 6% of nosocomial bacteremias, the major sources of infection being the urinary tract, the respiratory tract (often in association with the use of intermittent positive-pressure breathing equipment), burns, surgical wounds, and phlebitis (catheter-associated).[149] It is not surprising, therefore, that PVE due to *Serratia* is not rare.[59] *Serratia* is also an important cause of post operative infection of arterial grafts.[150] Treatment in these cases as a rule requires removal and replacement of the prosthetic graft in addition to antibiotic therapy as described above. In one such case, an effort to suppress infection with bacteriophage was unsuccessful.[151]

8.5.1.5. *Escherichia coli, Proteus* Species, *Klebsiella* Species, and *Providencia*

These bacteria were exceedingly rare causes of IE prior to the advent of prosthetic-valve surgery.[66,152] Even in the most recent reviews which include the cardiac-surgery era, it is unusual for there to be more than a few patients reported from any one institution.[78,153-155] These bacteria are of interest for several reasons; since they are such common causes of bacteremia, particularly in hospitalized patients, it is often difficult to distinguish simple bacteremia with an evident primary focus from IE. This is a particular problem in the postoperative state after insertion of a prosthetic valve (see Section 8.1).[156]

It is curious that despite the frequency of bloodstream invasion with primary extravascular infections, IE is a rarity. In rabbits, fresh vegetations were found to be considerably less likely to be colonized by *E coli* than by a *Str. viridans* or *Staph. aureus*.[10] It is precisely because of this resistance to infection that it is curious how frequently previously normal heart valves are affected.[152] Involvement is usually of left-sided heart valves, and vegetations are characterized as being of unusually large size, while rarely producing valve destruction.[152]

The infecting bacteria are too diverse to be able to speak in general terms of recommended antibiotic therapy. Suffice it to say that therapy should be prolonged, at least 6 weeks, and that careful attention must be directed to the tube-dilution sensitivities of the bacteria. In general, a penicillin and an aminoglycoside should be employed, particularly where synergy is demonstrable.[146]

8.5.1.6. *Eikenella corrodens*

This peculiar microaerophilic or anaerobic gram-negative bacterium, first characterized in 1958, is generally associated with abscesses in patients with trauma or chronic disease. It is normally found in the mouth and upper respiratory tract and is usually found in association with various streptococci or staphylococci.[157] It is commonly recovered in the blood immediately after tooth extraction.[158,159] Of particular interest is the frequency with which it is responsible for infections in drug addicts who have used methylphenidate. In rabbits, *E. corrodens* produces cutaneous abscesses when associated with streptococci and injected directly into the skin. Even larger abscesses were produced when the two bacteria were mixed with methylphenidate.[157]

It has been isolated from rare patients with natural-valve endocarditis and PVE. In one instance, it was responsible for tricuspid IE (with peptostreptococcus) in an amphetamine user.[160] As a general rule, ampicillin and penicillin are effective against the organism, but minimal inhibitory concentrations (MICs) are equal to or greater than 0.2 μg/ml.[157] In one patient with mixed infection being treated with penicillin (18 million units/day), the temperature fell only when 1.0 g streptomycin/day was added.[160] It would seem that initial treatment should be for that of a "penicillin-resistant" streptococcus (see Section 8.4.2.1b) until detailed antibiotic-sensitivity studies can be carried out.

It is evident that IE with this bacterium is not easy to treat, but there are too few reported cases to make specific recommendations. There are no particular clinical features apart from its importance in addicts (who use methylphenidate) which distinguish these patients.

Experimental aortic-valve IE in rabbits with *E. corrodens* revealed the organism to be of low virulence, rarely causing death or positive blood cultures.[161] Bacteria have been demonstrated in aortic-valve vegetations in rabbits despite the inability to culture them *in vitro*.[161] A similar phenomenon had been previously observed in *Candida* IE in rabbits.[5] It has been suggested that immunofluorescent screening of "sterile" vegetations in man with antisera to certain specific microorganisms may increase the yield of etiological agents in culture-negative IE.[161]

8.5.1.7. *Campylobacter (Vibrio) fetus*

This slow-growing, gram-negative rod is a rare cause of IE, usually attacking what are believed to be normal aortic valves. Valve perforation is common, but there are no distinguishing features, save perhaps for a preceding thrombophlebitis or contact with animals. Successful treatment has been accomplished with tetracycline, chloramphenicol, or penicillin and streptomycin, according to the antibiotic sensitivities of the organism. Most cases reported in the literature which were treated successfully received tetracycline or chloramphenicol.[146,162,163]

8.5.1.8. *Hemophilus influenzae, parainfluenzae, aphrophilus,* and *paraphrophilus; Cardiobacterium hominis;* and *Actinobacillus actinomycetemcomitans*

There has been a great deal of recent interest in infections due to these "slow-growing, fastidious, gram-negative bacteria," not so much because of the overall frequency with which they cause IE, but rather because it is only in recent years that attention to bacteriological technique and classification has revealed their existence as significant causes of IE. A number of major reviews have appeared recently,[164-171] and there has been a profusion of individual case reports even since these reviews have been written. Since only 20–30 patients have been collected for each infecting bacterium (the number may have doubled by the time of this printing), it is legitimate to ask why these bacteria have excited such interest.

The peculiar growth requirements and the fact that cultures may have to be kept for several weeks are worthy of note. There is little doubt that many patients considered to have culture-negative endocarditis in the past will be diagnosed as being infected with one of these bacteria today. At the moment, the possibility must be left open as to whether there is a true increase in the frequency of these infections.

Patients with IE due to these bacteria share certain common clinical features. These organisms are found normally in the mouth and upper respiratory tract, and cases of IE have been related to prior dental procedures. In three instances, *H. aphrophilus* was cultured from the mouths of the dogs of patients with IE due to the same bacterium.(172) Infections occur predominantly in patients with underlying heart disease or prosthetic heart valves, but a high proportion—20% or more—have had normal heart valves. In four instances, *Hemophilus* infection has occurred in patients with prolapsed mitral valves and in one instance in a patient with a "floppy" valve of Marfan's syndrome.(166,173,174,175)

There is an uncommonly long delay in establishing the diagnosis, with periods of 4–6 months of symptoms being characteristic. *Cardiobacterium hominis* infections are outstanding in this regard, with patients having symptoms lasting 10 and 18 months prior to diagnosis.(164,171) Diagnoses of vasculitis with prednisone therapy have preceded correct bacteriological diagnosis, and glomerulonephritis is not uncommon, considering the few cases that have been recognized.(166,171,176)

Polymicrobial infections seemed unusually common in one series.(168) It is interesting to speculate that the finding of fastidious bacteria is easier in mixed infections where the other bacteria provide essential nutrients for *in vitro* cultivation.

There is a curious difference in sex ratio, with all infections being found predominantly in men, except for *H. parainfluenzae,* which is found predominantly in women.(164,168,177,178) As might be expected in view of the age distribution of *Hemophilus* infections in general, the age of patients infected with these bacteria was lower than that of patients with IE in general.(164,168) This trend continues in recent reports of infants and adolescents with *Hemophilus* IE not included in the aforementioned reviews.(179-182)

Infections usually occur on the left side of the heart and are frequently complicated by valve destruction and major-vessel emboli. In recent reports, 63% of patients with left-sided *H. parainfluenzae* IE had major-vessel emboli.(165) Emboli to the central nervous system are the major cause of death in these infections.(164,167) It is particularly interesting that major emboli and valve destruction have occurred toward the end of, or even after, the completion of antibiotic therapy, at a time when the infection was cured. Both complications have served as indications for replacement of the affected valves.[164,167]

It is difficult to summarize the data on antibiotic sensitivities for these bacteria. Technical difficulties in growing the microorganisms, along with variations in technique among laboratories as well as poor standardization of techniques, leave considerable doubt as to how to interpret the published results. An additional complicating factor is the finding of considerable colonial variation in tests of a single isolate.[167,168] Despite these difficulties, it is recommended that antimicrobial therapy be adjusted to the results of sensitivity testing when feasible. It is also important to take clinical response into consideration when evaluating the efficacy of therapy, but this can be misleading; sterile emboli may be associated with fever, and defervescence may be associated with continued infection within the vegetation.

It is generally recommended that ampicillin be given (12 g I.V. per day) for ampicillin-sensitive *Hemophilus* infections.[166] Penicillin is generally more active against *H. aphrophilus,*[164,169] and *H. paraphrophilus* is occasionally resistant to ampicillin.[164] It is not clear what to use in ampicillin-resistant *Hemophilus* infections and in patients with penicillin allergy.[409] Chloramphenicol if effective *in vitro,* but clinical efficacy has been unpredictable.[167,168,183,409] Vancomycin and clindamycin are usually ineffective *in vitro*. Cephalothin has been variably effective *in vivo,* despite *in vitro* sensitivity, but so has ampicillin.[167,168,177]

Geraci *et al.*[166] recommend 3 weeks of ampicillin treatment (12 g/day) for ampicillin-sensitive strains, but Chunn *et al.*[167] recommend 6–8 weeks of therapy with ampicillin, 18 g I.V. per day, in addition to gentamicin, 4.5 mg/kg I.M. per day. I am inclined toward the recommendations of Chunn and colleagues because of the high mortality of this disease, but if patients were to respond promptly to antibiotic therapy and particularly if vegetations were to disappear (by echocardiography), I would be willing to discontinue gentamicin after 3–4 weeks.

Cardiobacterium hominis has been treated successfully, usually with penicillin and streptomycin.[164] Geraci *et al.*[166] recommend penicillin or ampicillin alone for 3 weeks, as for *Hemophilus* species. I would be inclined to initiate treatment by following the recommendations given above for streptococci, according to the sensitivity to penicillin, i.e., for penicillin-sensitive (< 0.1 μg/ml) organisms:

Penicillin, 20 million units I.V. per day for 4 weeks

plus

Streptomycin, 0.5 g I.M. every 12 hr for 2 weeks

Actinobacillus actinomycetemcomitans is usually sensitive to penicillin or ampicillin and streptomycin or gentamicin. I would initiate treatment of this

TABLE 9
Antibiotic Sensitivities of Miscellaneous Gram-Negative Bacteria

Bacterium	Antibiotic sensitivities[a]	Treatment[a]	Bacteriological outcome	Ref. no.
Dialister granuliformans	—	—	Failure	187
Rothia dentocariosa	All but clindamycin	Pen, Gen	Cure	188
Moraxella nonliquefaciens	Amp, Car, Ceph, Chlor, Gent, Tet	Amp, Gen	Cure	189
Moraxella kingae	Pen, Amp, Chlor, Ceph, Ery, Kan, Tet, Meth	Pen	Cure	190
Aeromonas hydrophila	Chlor, Col, Gen, Tet, Carb	Carb, Gen	?	191
Pasteurella multocida	Pen, Amp, Tet, Chlor, Gen	Pen, Strep	Cure	192
Pasteurella pneumotropica	—	Pen	Cure	193
Pasteurella hemolytica	—	Pen, Strep	Cure	193
Salmonella typhi	Chlor, Amp	—	—	193
Streptobacillus moniliformis	—	Pen	Cure	193
Bordetella bronchiseptica	—	Pen, Strep, Tet	Cure	193
Acinetobacter	Gen, Carb, TMP-S	Gen, Car, TMP-S	Variable	193
Alcaligenes faecalis	Pen, Chlor, Strep, Tet	Pen, Chlor, Strep, Tet	Variable	193
Enterobacter	Carb, Gen, Cefamandol	—	—	193
Flavobacterium	—	—	—	193
Edwardsiella	—	—	—	193
Citrobacter	—	Ceph	Cure	193

[a] (Amp) Ampicillin; (Carb) carbenicillin; (Ceph) cephalothin; (Chlor) chloramphenicol; (Col) colistin; (Ery) erythromycin; (Gen) gentamicin; (Kan) kandamycin; (Meth) methicillin; (Pen) penicillin; (Strep) streptomycin; (Tet) tetracycline; (TMP-S) trimethoprim-sulfa.

infection with 12 g ampicillin per day for 6 weeks and gentamicin, 3–5 mg/kg per day, for 10–20 days, and adjust therapy according to antibiotic sensitivities and clinical course.[184-186]

8.5.1.9. Miscellaneous

Isolated reports of patients who have had peculiar gram-negative bacilli as causes of IE are listed in Table 9.

8.5.2. Gram-Positive Bacilli ("Diphtheroids")

There are several gram-positive bacilli that are easily confused with the skin contaminants seen in about 10% of blood cultures. These contaminants have no clinical significance.[194] Thus, diphtheroid contamination is a daily laboratory occurrence, whereas true infections with these microorganisms are relatively rare. This creates a difficult problem for a routine bacteriology laboratory. In addition, these microorganisms may be very slow-growing (several weeks), a factor which not only complicates diagnosis but also makes the interpretation of *in vitro* antimicrobial sensitivity tests very difficult.[195] In a search for sources of contamination at the time of operation in patients undergoing heart surgery, it was found that 70% of patients had a potential source of infection identified, and in over 50% of these patients, diphtheroids were the contaminating bacteria.[196] It is thus not difficult to understand the interest attached to patients with IE due to these bacteria. Particular attention must be given to the criteria for IE in these patients, since cures may represent treatment of blood-culture contaminants rather than true infections. On the other hand, the demand for surgical or autopsy verification of valve infection would undoubtedly bias our appreciation of the importance of these infections in the opposite direction.

8.5.2.1. *Listeria monocytogenes* (Sometimes formerly *Corynebacterium infantisepticum* or *parvulum*) and *Erysipelothrix monocytogenes*

IE due to *L. monocytogenes* is similar in many respects to that described for *Hemophilus* species; infections are found in the left side of the heart on what are considered to be normal or previously damaged valves (including hypertrophic myopathy) and on prosthetic valves, and rates of peripheral embolization are very high.[197-199] *Listeria* has also been responsible for infection of atrioventricular (A-V) shunts[200] and for IE in patients on long-term hemodialysis.[201] Diagnosis is often delayed because of the time necessary for the bacteria to grow *in vitro*.

Although *Listeria* infections are generally seen in infants, in patients receiving immunosuppressive medications, or in patients with underlying conditions which suppress the immune response, patients with IE do not usually fall into these categories. Patients with IE tend to be young and in good health (save for the presence of prior heart murmurs). On the other hand, in my personal experience, the 10 patients that I have seen with *Listeria* meningitis in the past 5 years have generally not (8/10) had any significant underlying disease. In a recent review of *Listeria* infections in renal-transplant patients, none (of 13) was considered to have had IE.[202] *Listeria* bacteremia may exist as an isolated entity, with recovery being recorded even in the absence of antibiotic therapy.[203] Thus, it may not be an easy matter to distinguish bacteremia from IE, in the absence of new heart murmurs, vegetations by echocardiography, or histological proof obtained at operation or autopsy.

Antibiotic sensitivities have varied considerably among different studies, but strains in general have been sensitive to penicillin G, ampicillin, and tetracycline.[198] Penicillin and aminoglycoside synergy is a frequent but not uniform finding.[204,205] Cephalosporin–aminoglycoside combinations have been shown to be effective *in vitro* and have been proposed as treatment for the patient allergic to penicillin, but evidence of their clinical efficacy is not convincing.[204-207] Another argument against the use of cephalosporins is the frequency of meningitis with *Listeria* infections and the known failure of cephalothin to prevent the development of pneumococcal meningitis when used for the treatment of pneumococcal pneumonia.

I would be inclined to initiate treatment with:

Penicillin, 20 million units I.V. per day

and

Tobramycin, 3.0 mg/kg I.M. per day

and to adjust therapy according to antibiotic sensitivities, SBA, and clinical response.

8.5.2.2. *Corynebacteria*

Aside from rare cases of IE due to toxigenic and nontoxigenic *C. diphtheriae*, the *Corynebacterium* species responsible for IE are usually not identifiable in greater detail.[60,194,195,208-211,410] About half the cases in the literature are infections that have occurred in patients with prosthetic heart valves, symptoms of infection beginning usually within 2 months of operation.[194,195] Sensitivity of these microorganisms to penicillin (and good prognosis) is the rule in patients developing infections on natural heart valves, whereas penicillin resistance (and poor prognosis) are the rule in patients with prosthetic heart valves who received prophylactic antibiotics at the time of operation.[194,195]

There are no unusual clinical features of infection save for the aforementioned difficulties in establishing the diagnosis. Although various antibiotics have been used to treat these infections, including erythromycin–fucidin or erythromycin–streptomycin combinations for penicillin-resistant strains, vancomycin is promising from studies of *in vitro* sensitivities.[194,195,410] In patients with prosthetic heart valves, surgery is as a rule necessary in addition to antibiotics to achieve cure.[194,195] Because of the persistence of transitional bacterial forms, despite antibiotic therapy, it is important to follow patients closely after diphtheroid IE, and patients with prosthetic valves in whom reoperation was not feasible should probably be kept on very long-term antibiotic suppressive therapy—at least 2 years.[195]

Diphtheroid infections are occasionally seen in patients with infected A-V shunts, in whom there has been a peculiar propensity for the development of glomerulonephritis.[212-214] In general, it has been necessary to replace the infected shunt during antibiotic therapy in order to achieve permanent cure; however, several patients have been treated successfully with intraventricular administration of antibiotics.[200] Another patient was treated "successfully" with erythromycin and rifampin, but the results of long-term follow-up after discontinuation of antibiotics are not known.[212] *Corynebacteria* have also produced IE in patients on long-term hemodialysis.[201]

8.5.2.3. *Erysipelothrix rhusiopathiae*

This is a particularly hardy microorganism, which is found in wild and domesticated animals, as well as fish. Infection in man usually begins at the site of a scratch or injury in individuals in contact with animals (erysipeloid). The skin infection is nonsuppurative and is usually self-limiting, after remissions and relapses, in 1–4 weeks.[215] Most infections are seen during the summer months. IE is a rare complication, there being about 40 cases in the world literature.[215-221] There are no distinguishing clinical characteristics apart from the epidemiology and the importance of searching for a skin lesion. By the time the patient is seen and the diagnosis of endocarditis established, the skin lesion has usually disappeared.

Therapy with 6 weeks of penicillin (20 million units I.V. per day) seems reasonable, in view of the uniform sensitivity of the microorganism to this antibiotic and its propensity to cause infection on the left side of the heart. Valve perforation and major peripheral emboli are not unusual.

8.5.2.4. *Lactobacilli*

These microorganisms are normally found in the oral, gastrointestinal, and vaginal flora. They are typical of the diphtheroid group of bacteria, often being mistaken for contaminants. They are very slow-growing (several weeks) in conventional blood cultures, due to their being microaerophilic, with preferential growth at low pH.

There are about 15 cases of IE in the literature with features that resemble those of other fastidious bacteria—frequently, a long delay in diagnosis and perhaps an increased tendency to peripheral embolization.[222-224] Although penicillin has been the most common agent used for treatment, sensitivities generally show MICs of greater than 0.2 μg/ml, and relapses are common. Vancomycin has not been effective *in vitro*.[224] In a recent study, *in vitro* bactericidal combinations included gentamicin or tobramycin with penicillin or pristinamycin, and pristinamycin with rifampin or streptomycin. The patient was treated successfully with pristinamycin and streptomycin for 6 weeks.

The phenomenon of tolerance to β-lactam antibiotics was thought to explain the slow bactericidal effect of these antibiotics *in vitro* and perhaps the unsatisfactory clinical response. Penicillin–gentamicin was bactericidal *in vitro* and was shown to be much more effective than penicillin alone in rabbit IE due to *Lactobacilli*.[70]

8.5.2.5. Miscellaneous

A single fatal case was of *Bacillus cereus* infection reported in a patient with PVE.[225] A nocardioform bacterium, *Oerskovia turbata*, has produced infection in a patient with a homograft valve prosthesis, probably due to contamination of the homograft at the time of collection.[226] Infection due to *Rothia dentocariosa* and *Actinomyces viscosus* may be confused with "diphtheroid" contamination of blood cultures.[227,228]

8.5.3. Anaerobic Bacteria

IE due to anaerobic bacteria is uncommon, there being about 40 cases reported in the literature. The majority of cases are due to *Bacteroides, Fusobacterium,* and *Clostridium* species, with isolated cases of infection due to *Spirillum* and *Megasphera*.[229-234] As is the case with other fastidious microorganisms, an important clinical feature of disease was a high frequency of major peripheral emboli.

These bacteria reside normally in the mouth, oropharynx, and gastrointestinal tract, infections or surgical procedures serving as the source of bacteremia initiating endocardial infection. Infections generally occur on previously damaged heart valves, but may also occur on normal heart valves or in drug addicts.

Treatment is satisfactory in those instances of infection with penicillin-sensitive bacteria. In cases where the infecting microorganism is resistant to penicillin, the outcome is much less favorable. Consideration should be given in these cases to treatment with carbenicillin, metronidazole, vancomycin, and rifampin, according to the *in vitro* sensitivities and clinical response of the patient.[229,231,232] Clindamycin–metronidazole combinations may also be worthy of consideration.[235] As is the case with other fastidious microorganisms, the lack of standardization of *in vitro* sensitivity tests leaves considerable doubt as to the applicability of such information to treatment. In addition, there are so few cases of anaerobic gram-negative IE that any generalization concerning therapy would be unwise.

Studies of *Bacteroides* IE in rabbits have shown differences in the biology of infections in the right side of the heart as compared with the aerobic bacteria that have been studied. Whereas the density of aerobic bacteria on the right side of the heart is less than on the left side, in the initial phase of infection (5 days), *Bacteroides fragilis* on the right side of the heart "catches up" with microbial growth on the left side.[11,236] This suggests that the lower oxygen tension on the right side of the heart favors the growth of anaerobic bacteria. On the other hand, left-sided vegetations were much more susceptible to infection than right-sided infections.[236]

The only studies of the effect of antibiotics on *Bacteroides* IE in the rabbit have been concerned with the prophylaxis of infection. These studies have demonstrated the superiority of high-dose clindamycin over other antibiotics.[237] However, it is important to emphasize that antibiotics effective in the treatment of experimental IE may be ineffective for prophylaxis under the conditions of testing.[238]

8.5.4. *Chlamydiae*

Isolated reports of IE due to *Chlamydia B* (psittacosis) and *C. trachomatis* have appeared recently.[239-243] The diagnosis is usually established postmortem or at operation to replace a perforated valve, but very rarely a positive serology leads to the correct diagnosis earlier in the evolution of the disease.[240] The disease can attack normal heart valves, and it is doubtful whether tetracycline alone (even for several months) is sufficient to eliminate the microorganism from an endocardial vegetation. Current thoughts are that the patient should remain on tetracycline(?)—indefinitely.

One should think of this possibility in patients who have had contact with birds. One group suggests that patients with known susceptibility to IE (e.g., rheumatic heart disease, prosthetic valve) be advised not to keep domestic birds.[240]

8.5.5. *Mycobacteria*

Mycobacterium chelonei has been found to contaminate porcine heart valves used as prostheses in man,[244] and two patients are reported to have developed PVE due to these *Mycobacteria,* one after having received a contaminated valve.[245,246] In both these patients, acid-fast bacilli were seen in histological studies of vegetations, but the microorganisms were not cultured. Close attention to bacteriological technique may be necessary to demonstrate these bacteria.[247]

In another patient, PVE developed in a patient who received a Bjork–Shiley valve.[248] No portal of entry was ever identified in this case. Progressive renal failure has been described in a patient with probable infection of a hemodialysis shunt.[249]

Mycobacterium fortuitum was identified as a cause of PVE in a patient with a postoperative sternal wound abscess due to this microorganism.[250] Outbreaks of postoperative wound infections due to *Myco. fortuitum* have been recorded after open-heart surgery.[250]

Mycobacteria of the *chelonei–fortuitum* group have thus been found as contaminants of porcine heart valves, but also in the dust in a hospital ward and garden soil.[248] These are very difficult infections to treat with antimicrobial agents, the organisms showing resistance to a wide spectrum of antibiotics.

Two additional patients have been reported with PVE and an infected A-V shunt.[251] In both cases, there was acid-fast microbial infection of endocardial vegetations associated with miliary spread of infection. The responsible organism was not further identified microbiologically.

8.5.6. Q Fever

Whereas Q fever usually provokes an acute, "viral-like" illness, sometimes with pneumonia, there have been patients reported sporadically who developed chronic evidence of infection and who, as part of that chronic illness, had Q fever endocarditis. Three recent reports of about 30 patients from Britain, Australia, South Africa, and the United States suggest that the problem is not at all uncommon and deserves to be looked for in any patient with a suspicion of IE in whom blood cultures are negative, particularly in the presence of liver-function abnormality and frequently with aneurysms of the base of the aorta associated with aortic regurgitation.[252-256] It has been suggested that thrombocytopenia is found in Q fever endocarditis more commonly than in other forms of endocarditis. Glomerulonephritis has also been found in patients with Q fever IE.[213,252,256,257] Placement of prosthetic heart valves is carried out for the usual hemodynamic reasons. Interestingly, the follow-up functional result of aortic-valve replacement due to Q fever IE seems better than in patients with valve replacement in IE due to other microorganisms.[258]

It is not surprising that *Rickettsiae* (or *Rickettsia*-like) microorganisms should infect the endocardium, since they invade normal endothelium (probably part of the mechanism of production of thrombocytopenia). Despite this theoretical ability to invade normal valvular endothelium, it appears that the great majority of the patients who develop Q fever endocarditis (as for other types of IE) have underlying heart disease or prosthetic heart valves.

The serological diagnosis of Q fever endocarditis is not a simple matter.

Most patients have an elevation of phase I antibody ($\geqslant 1:128$); however, titers this high have been found in totally asymptomatic patients, and proven cases have been noted where there was only elevation of phase II antibodies.[259] It has been suggested that treatment be given to patients with the clinical picture of IE who have even slight elevations of phase I antibody, even if the titer of phase II antibody is very low also.[259] Even in the absence of signs of IE, the combination of valvular heart disease and slightly elevated titers of phase I antibody is considered sufficient to initiate antibiotic treatment.[259]

Tissue diagnosis of Q fever includes microscopic examination of tissue suspension in Gimenez-stained preparations, staining of tissue with flourescein-isothiocyanate-tagged guinea pig antisera against *Coxiella burnetii,* and ultraviolet microscopy. Guinea-pig inoculation and tissue-culture techniques are also useful in identifying the microorganism.[255]

Treatment has been carried out with tetracycline, TMP-SMZ, and rifampin. The difficulty is that treatment failure, either primary or due to reseeding of vegetations from lesions in the liver or spleen, is common and there is no general standard for evaluating cure. Turck *et al.*[254] favor the use of tetracycline, 1.0 g/day, and lincomycin, 2.0 g/day. The issue as to how long to continue treatment is unsettled. One patient treated with tetracycline and lincomycin for 5 years has been without antibiotics for 4 years and 9 months and is without evidence of relapse. This is the longest survivor so far reported.[259]

8.5.7. Viruses

Despite the demonstration of the capacity of coxsackie and echoviruses to produce endocardial lesions in animals, and despite the frequency and unequivocal nature of viral myocarditis in man, there has been no convincing demonstration that viruses can establish an endothelial or valvular infection in man resembling the vegetations seen in patients with IE.[260] A single attempt to infect sterile vegetations in the rabbit with coxsackie virus B4 in a manner similar to that by which bacteria produce IE was unsuccessful.[261]

8.5.8 Fungi

IE due to fungi is a relatively new disease, the first patient being reported in 1939. In a comprehensive review of this special problem in 1978, McLeod and Remington[55] were able to analyze published and personal data from 319 patients. The subject is a difficult one from several standpoints, the first being criteria for the diagnosis. The mere finding of a positive blood culture for fungi does not constitute sufficient evidence for establishing the diagnosis of fungal IE. McLeod and Remington[55] accepted the diagnosis of fungal IE in patients in their review according to the following criteria: (1) the demonstration of fungi in endocardial tissue or (2) at least one positive blood culture with at least two of the following features: fever, new or changing murmur, valvular vegetation by echocardiography, and peripheral emboli. However, as will be discussed later, some patients who do not satisfy these criteria should probably be treated as though they had IE. The problem is quite similar to that of evaluating the importance of staphylococcal bacteremia (see Section 8.3).

The factors which increase susceptibility to fungal IE are not different from those which play a role in bacterial IE, with the exception that infection is *not found* to develop spontaneously. Patients with fungal IE have an identifiable route by which the fungi gain access to the circulation or, more specifically, the endocardium. The most common routes of access are the intravenous injections of addicts, indwelling intraveneous catheters or other intravascular devices, and cardiac surgery. In patients who develop IE under these circumstances, fungi are only a small but significant percentage of the responsible microorganisms (approximately 5% of patients with PVE and among addicts with IE).(66,262) Fungal septicemia is a frequent complication of parenteral hyperalimentation.(263)

Although a large number of fungi have been identified as casual agents in fungal IE, 90% of patients are infected with various species of *Candida* and *Aspergillus,* as well as *Histoplasma capsulatum,* among whom *Candida* species account for two thirds of infections.(55) *Candida albicans* and *Aspergillus* species are the usual pathogens after cardiac surgery, whereas non-*albicans Candida* species predominate in addicts. *Histoplasma capsulatum* was not found as a cause of IE in addicts or in patients with prosthetic heart valves in the review of McLeod and Remington(55); however, there have been three reports of endocardial infection due to this fungus after cardiac surgery, and recent reports described cases of PVE.(264,265,411) Interestingly, the nonbacterial thrombotic vegetation is said to be the only extracellular site where *Histoplasma* can grow.(266)

IE due to fungi may also be one of the manifestations of disseminated fungal infection in patients receiving immunosuppressive agents or with severe underlying diseases which depress the host's response to infection.(266) Myocardial and mural endocardial lesions are particularly frequent in these circumstances.(55,267) Finally, it is likely that the administration of antibiotics to patients plays a role in fungal infections by diminishing the normal bacterial flora, thereby allowing its replacement by fungi. There is no evidence that the administration of antibiotics either favors or is necessary for the development of fungal IE in animals.

Diagnosis of IE due to fungi may be a difficult matter. Whereas *Candida* species are regularly (about 90%) cultured from the blood of patients with IE, as mentioned earlier, the mere finding of *Candida* in the bloodstream is not sufficient evidence to establish the presence of IE, since fungemia may occur with indwelling intravenous catheters, or postoperatively, in the absence of IE.

On the other hand, IE due to *Candida* has been documented months after what has been considered transient fungemia without IE.[55,268] In one case, a patient who had developed transient fungemia during hyperalimentation returned 18 months later with evidence of IE due to *Torulopsis glabrata*.[269] This is reminiscent of the long follow-up interval (at least 1–2 years) necessary to assure the success of treatment of *Candida* (and probably other fungi) endocarditis.[270] Rubenstein et al.[269] believe that "it would seem prudent to regard every episode of fungemia as a potential endocarditis."

It has been suggested that bone-marrow cultures or cultures of arterial blood might be particularly useful in the diagnosis of fungal infection. Bone-marrow cultures are always potentially useful to detect microorganisms that have the capacity to remain alive within phagocytes (e.g., *Salmonella,* tubercle bacilli). Because of their size, it has been suggested that filtration of fungi may occur in peripheral capillary beds, thus pointing to a possible advantage of arterial cultures for detection of fungi. Hypertonic media and media employing the Castaneda principle (brain–heart infusion agar slant and brain–heart infusion broth) may also improve the yield of fungus cultures.[55]

In *Aspergillus* endocarditis in rabbits, the yield of positive blood cultures was increased by augmenting the volume of blood cultures from 1.0 ml (no blood cultures positive) to 30–40 ml (4/4 blood cultures positive).[271]

Serological tests have limited usefulness in the diagnosis of fungal IE.[55] Antibodies to *H. capsulatum* develop about 1 month after primary infection and thus may be useful diagnostically in patients in whom antibodies were not detectable at the onset of infection. The histoplasmin skin test is not useful because of the frequency of false-negative and false-positive reactions as well as its capacity to induce serum antibody formation.

Precipitins to *Candida* are found regularly in patients with *Candida* IE, but unfortuntely are also found in a significant proportion of patients after cardiac surgery and in patients with streptococcal IE, in both instances in the absence of any evidence of *Candida* infection.[55,272,273] Rising titers of *Candida* precipitins may be useful as an index of recurrent IE.[270] Precipitating antibodies to "mycelial cytoplasmic antigens" show promise of being able to distinguish superficial from invasive disease due to *Candida* infection.[268] Mannan antigens as well as chromatographic serum analysis are under study as means of detecting *Candida* infection.[55]

The clinical picture of fungal endocarditis is not distinctive, except for the high frequency of major emboli, a characteristic shared with IE due to fastidious bacteria. Approximately 80% of patients with fungal endocarditis have major embolic episodes.[55] Indeed, the fungal etiology of IE is often established by histological examination and culture of a surgically removed thrombus.

The therapy of fungal endocarditis is unsatisfactory, the majority of patients dying as a consequence of the inability to eradicate the infection. In the review of McLeod and Remington,[55] outcome of treatment was heavily dependent on whether infection was grafted upon natural valves or whether infection occurred after cardiac surgery; in the former case, 44% of patients survived, whereas in the latter, only 22% survived. The interpretation of treatment data is complicated by the need, already referred to, to follow patients for several years after presumptive cure, since clinical, surgical, and autopsy data attest to the persistence of infection for very long periods of time.

It is generally believed today that therapy of fungal endocarditis should consist of antibiotic treatment combined with surgical removal of the infected valve. There is difference of opinion, however, concerning the timing of valve replacement in patients in whom operation is not a necessity for hemodynamic reasons. McLeod and Remington[55] state that "we agree with those who consider that the risk of emboli and subsequent persistent foci of infection make prompt surgical intervention mandatory. Delay beyond a few days is rarely justified to delay surgery for the administration of antifungal drugs." On the other hand, Wain *et al.*,[274] reviewing their experience with 27 patients who developed fungal IE after homograft valve replacement, report that "9 (69%) of the 16 patients who received intensive initial chemotherapy for more than 2 weeks" had "long-term survival of 17–87 months." Reoperation was performed in nearly all the surviving patients, and those not yet reoperated at the time of writing of the report were believed to require eventual reoperation.

Survival is exceedingly uncommon in *Aspergillus* infection, being 2 of 53 patients in the review of McLeod and Remington.[55] The numbers of patients infected with fungi other than *Candida* species were too small to calculate meaningful survival rates.

The quantity of antifungal agent(s) optimal for the treatment of fungal endocarditis is not known. There may be discrepancy between results of *in vitro* sensitivity to amphotericin B and clinical effect, due in part perhaps to immunostimulatory effects of amphotericin.[275] Despite these uncertainties, amphotericin B is the first drug of choice in treating fungal endocarditis.

Although in systemic infections, it is rarely felt necessary to exceed 0.5 mg/kg per day (35 mg/day in a 70-kg patient), most authors suggest a dose of up to a maximum of about 100 mg/day in the treatment of IE.[55,274-276] Treatment is recommended for 6–8 weeks.[274-276] The dose does not have to be reduced in patients with preexisting renal-functional disturbances, but renal dysfunction is one of the major toxic effects of the drug. Medoff and Kobayashi[275] recommend discontinuing treatment for 2–5 days if glomerular filtration falls to below 20–60% of normal. Although most patients recover renal function in the months following treatment, a few remain with a 50% reduction.[275]

There is often considerable systemic toxicity which accompanies amphotericin therapy. A 50-mg vial is diluted with 10 ml sterile water and the mixture added to 500–1000 ml 5% glucose for intravenous infusion. An initial test dose of 1.0 mg is given over a period of 2–6 hr and, if tolerated, is followed by an infusion of 0.25 mg/kg the same day. By the 3rd to 4th day, the patient should receive his maintenance dose of 100 mg. Even the initial dose of 1.0 mg might produce fever, chills, and hypotension, in which case it should be lowered to 0.1 mg and then increased as tolerated.[275] The addition of 25–50 mg hydrocortisone succinate to the infusion mixture may be necessary to control the systemic symptoms. Premedication with aspirin, diphenhydramine, or prochlorperazine may also be helpful.[275]

Another effective antifungal agent, 5-fluorocytosine (5-FC), is administered orally in doses of 150 mg/kg per day (up to 12.0 g).[274,275] This drug is relatively well tolerated; hepatic toxicity (elevation of transaminase and alkaline phosphatase), nausea, vomiting, diarrhea, and bone-marrow depression are considered to be mild and reversible with reduction of dosage or stopping of the drug.[275] Intestinal perforation is listed as a rare complication of treatment. Since 5-FC is excreted by the kidney, its dosage must be reduced in the presence of reduced renal function. A proposition cited by Medoff and Kobayashi[275] is:

> 150 mg/kg in 4 divided doses if the creatinine clearance is at least 40 ml/min, reduced to 2 doses every 12 hr if the creatinine clearance is 20–40 ml/min and to 1 dose if the clearance is 10–20 ml/min.

The drug is dialyzable; therefore a single 20 mg/kg dose should be given after each dialysis to patients with renal failure.[275] Patients who could not be treated by oral administration of the drug have been treated intravenously.[274]

5-FC is not recommended as single-drug therapy for fungal endocarditis.[55] In preliminary experiments in rabbits with fungal IE, combination therapy (5-FC and amphotericin) was an advantage over amphotericin alone in *Aspergillus*, but not in *Candida*, infection.[271,277] Experience in man with combination therapy is limited; but it is considered the therapy of choice in *Candida*, cryptococcal, and perhaps torulopsis and chromomycosis infections.[275] Rifampin has also been found to act synergistically with amphotericin *in vitro*.[275]

The experimental model of *Candida* endocarditis has been carefully studied in rabbits and should serve as a good basis for future chemotherapeutic studies.[5,277-279]For example, 5-FC has proven to be surprisingly effective in the prophylaxis of *Candida* endocarditis in rabbits when given as a single injection of 75 mg/kg 40 min before fungal challenge.[65] This result was surprising, in view of the well-known resistance of experimental bacterial endocarditis to prevention with bactericidal antibiotics[238,280-282]and the ineffectiveness of 5-FC treatment of experimental *Candida* endocarditis.[277]

In addition to the fungi already discussed as being the agents most commonly isolated from patients with IE, other fungi which have been reported include: *Coccidioides immitis, Corprinus* species, *Cryptococcus neoformans,* and *Curvularia neoformans*[55]; *Paecilomyces varioti*[55,283]; *Penicillium* species, *Phialophora,* and *Phycomyces*[55]; *Rhodotorula*[55,284]; *Saccharomyces cerevisiae*[55]; *Torulopsis glabrata*[55,285]; *Trichosporon cutaneum*[286]; *Petriellidium boydii (Allescheria boydii)*[274,287,288]; and *Hormodendrum dermatitidis*.[66]

8.5.9. Pneumococci

Pneumococcal endocarditis is a rarity today. Prior to the advent of penicillin, the pneumococcus was a more frequent cause of IE than the staphylococcus.[289] When the disease was common, it was usually discovered during the course of pneumococcal pneumonia and frequently caused destruction of the aortic valve. Interestingly, type III pneumococcus, which commonly caused pneumonia, rarely caused IE, the reverse being true for types VII and XII.[289] In series of IE recently described, the pneumococcus was considered responsible for 3% of cases in 308 blood-culture-positive, non-prosthetic-valve patients.[78,153-155,290] The disease is rarely seen in infants despite the common finding (2.6%) of pneumococcal bacteremia in febrile infants seen in a walk-in clinic.[291] There are no distinctive clinical features, and the treatment is as for penicillin-sensitive streptococci (see Section 8.4.2.1a).

8.5.10. *Neisseria* Species

8.5.10.1. Gonococci

Before the development of antibiotics, gonococci were frequently the cause of IE. Kerr[292] cites the experience at Vanderbilt University where one fourth of fatal cases of IE coming to autopsy were due to gonococcal infection. IE may occur years after recognition of the initial infection, but is said to often follow arthritis.[292] The clinical picture is distinguished by a double daily temperature elevation in about half the patients and a relatively high frequency of right-heart infection, albeit the majority of infections are found on the left side of the heart.[292]

As many case reports (eight) of gonococcal IE have appeared in the past 3 years as had appeared in the previous 30 years.[293-296] Blood cultures frequently take 1–2 weeks to show growth, and cultures may be irregularly positive or negative, the latter particularly in patients with infections in the right side of the heart.[294,295] Of eight recent cases, six experienced perforated heart valves (four aortic, two pulmonary), thus confirming that the nature of the disease today is similar to that seen in the preantibiotic era.

Modern studies in man and in experimental IE in rabbits have called attention to the resistance to the bactericidal properties of serum as a feature of gonococcal strains causing sepsis of IE.[294,297] Circulating immune complexes are found in disseminated gonococcal infection without, as well as with, IE.[296] In view of the capacity of these bacteria to produce isolated infection of the pulmonary valve, a syndrome which may be difficult to diagnose clinically, consideration should be given to the possibility of gonococcal endocarditis in patients with gonococcal sepsis, even in the absence of heart murmurs and echocardiographic abnormalities.

Hepatitis may be seen in patients with gonococcal IE and has been described in rabbits with this infection.[294,297] Although liver-function abnormalities in patients with IE are more commonly due to the hepatic congestion of acute heart failure or, rarely, to infection due to *C. burnetii* (Q fever), gonococcal IE should be kept in mind as a diagnostic possibility.

8.5.10.2. Meningococci

Meningococci are a very rare cause of IE, which has been described in patients with chronic meningococcemia and in patients with prosthetic heart valves.[292,298,299] Skin rash is said to be absent in about 50% of patients with IE due to the meningococcus.[298]

8.5.10.3. Other *Neisseria* Species

Neisseria catarrhalis and other species *(flava, perflava, pharyngis)* have also been isolated from patients with IE. *Neisseria catarrhalis* infects normal heart valves and has a propensity to embolize. Treatment is as for streptococci, depending on the degree of sensitivity to penicillin[300–302] (see Section 8.4.2.1).

8.5.11. *Staphylococcus epidermidis*, Coagulase-Negative Staphylococci, and Micrococci Species

Although these bacteria are capable of producing IE in patients with natural heart valves, such cases are relatively unusual. In these instances, the bacterial strains are usually susceptible to penicillin G or B-lactamase-resistant penicillins, but on occasion are resistant to methicillin.[303–305] The prognosis for bacteriological cure is excellent, no doubt due to the relative sensitivity to the penicillins.

A more frequent problem is infection of prosthetic heart valves, of A-V shunts, and of natural heart valves in patients on chronic hemodialysis.[66,200,201,306-310] For example, *Staph. epidermidis* is the single most common microorganism recovered from patients with PVE, accounting for approximately one fourth of early (within 2 months) and late cases.[66] This is easy to understand by reference to the frequency with which it is recovered in cultures of intravenous catheter tips. Of 503 cultures, 213 revealed *Staph. epidermidis,* the next closest in frequency being *Staph. aureus,* with 78 positive cases.[311]

Among 87 patients with PVE due to *Staph. epidermidis,* collected over 15 years at 6 hospitals, methicillin resistance was noted in 53 with a cure rate of 32%, whereas the cure rate in patients with methicillin-sensitive isolates was 62%.[312] In this study, 76% of isolates contained colonies resistant to more than

100 μg/ml of methicillin or nafcillin. Vancomycin and rifampin were the only consistently effective antibiotics *in vitro*.[125]

There are no unique clinical features associated with IE due to these bacteria other than their documentation as a cause of glomerulonephritis, particularly in patients with A-V shunts.[200,307–309]

About 5% of vascular grafts become infected with these bacteria, usually in association with a skin infection in the neighborhood of the operative site.[313]

Treatment is in principle similar to that of staphylococcal IE (see Section 8.4.2.2), the choice of antibiotics being determined by the *in vitro* antibiotic sensitivities, SBA and need for surgical replacement of the prosthetic device.

8.5.12. Streptococci

A large number of different streptococci have been recovered from patients with IE. In the past, when therapy was usually decided by the name given to the microorganism, or at best based on *in vitro* disk sensitivities, it was important to know the precise name of the infecting agent so as to choose the best antibiotic agents according to separate studies of the probability of their antibiotic sensitivity. Today, this way of deciding antibiotic therapy is not acceptable. For example, *viridans* streptococci may be very resistant to penicillin (MIC > 2.0 μg/ml).[314,315] Tube-dilution sensitivities, estimations of MICs and minimal bactericidal concentrations of antibiotics, and perhaps even killing curves, as well as tests for synergy with two or more antibiotics, are essential. This is a great deal of work for a routine bacteriology laboratory, but for the moment it is necessary to have as much information of this nature as possible to guide therapy in such potentially dangerous infections. It is to be hoped that future studies will better define the information that is most useful in arriving at therapeutic decisions.

As the name of the infecting microorganism has become less critical from the standpoint of treatment, it has become more important from the point of view of understanding the pathogenesis and the epidemiology of IE. One of the most dramatic recent examples of this is the importance of identifying *Str. bovis*.

8.5.12.1. *Streptococcus bovis*

Several reports in the early 1970s emphasized the importance of distinguishing *Str. bovis,* a group D, nonenterococcal strain, from enterococci because of the increased penicillin sensitivity of *Str. bovis*. Subsequently, Klein *et al.*,[316] in 1977, encountered two patients with *Str. bovis* IE who also had carcinoma of the colon, and were stimulated to investigate a possible relation between the two diseases. These authors collected evidence that was very suggestive of an association between the two diseases and demonstrated an increased fecal carrier rate for *Str. bovis* in patients with colon carcinoma. This report was rapidly followed by similar observations by others which confirmed the findings of Klein and co-workers.[317–323] It now seems clear that any patient with *Str. bovis* endocarditis or bacteremia should have a thorough investigation for cancer, particularly of the gastrointestinal tract. The explanation for this association is not yet apparent, and the possibility exists that other streptococcal infections (such as group G) may be associated with cancer.[324,325] It is also of interest that the frequency of *Str. bovis* as a cause of IE seems to be increasing.[44]

Curiously, the original reason for wanting to identify *Str. bovis,* its increased sensitivity to penicillin in comparison with the enterococcus, can now no longer be accepted without reservation. A recent report points out that *Str. bovis* may be relatively resistant to penicillin, thus requiring a therapeutic approach identical to that described for the enterococcus.[326]

8.5.12.2. *Viridans* Streptococci

These bacteria are as a rule nontypable by Lancefield sera. They are the streptococci most frequently responsible for IE; isolates from patients consisting of *Str. sanguis, Str. mutans, Str. mitior, Str. milleri,* and *Str. salivarius,* in decreasing frequency.[327] The capacity of these bacteria to adhere to fibrin–platelet vegetations and to produce IE in man and animals has been correlated with their capacity to produce dextran as well as their ability to aggregate platelets.[327] This subject was discussed in Chapter 2.

Viridans streptococci are, as a rule, sensitive to penicillin (MIC < 0.1 μg/ml); however, as mentioned above, one cannot rely on the identification of the streptococcus to predict its sensitivity to penicillin.[315] Particularly in patients receiving antibiotics such as long-term penicillin prophylaxis, considerable resistance to penicillin may develop (MIC > 2.0 μg/ml).[314,328,329] Resistance to erythromycin has been noted in *viridans* streptococci from patients allergic to penicillin who received erythromycin for the prophylaxis of IE.[44]

The precise identification of these bacteria may be difficult. For example, in some discussions, *Str. sanguis* is considered a *viridans* streptococcus, whereas in others it is considered a member of group H.[90,327] Bacteriocin typing or other techniques may be useful in diminishing the ambiguities of classification.[330] Some authors consider *Str. bovis* a *viridans* streptococcus.[44]

As more attention is directed to identifying streptococci and examining the clinical features of infection, interesting features of epidemiology or pathogenicity become apparent. The case of *Str. bovis* has already been discussed in Section 8.5.12.1. It is of interest that *Str. milleri* has a much greater potential to produce suppurative complications than other *viridans* streptococci.[331]

The importance of *viridans* streptococci with particular nutritional requirements was considered in Section 8.2. It is important to keep in mind that the antibiotic sensitivities of bacteria with particular nutrient requirements will vary according to the availability of these special nutrients.

Streptococcus mutans is a *viridans* streptococcus which does not react with Lancefield grouping sera, but which is easily confused with group D streptococci because of the ability of many isolates to grow in the presence of 40% bile and to hydrolyze esculin and ferment mannitol.[332,333] Another feature of this streptococcus worth emphasizing is that it may appear like a diphtheroid on primary isolation from blood cultures and risks being discarded as a contaminant.[334] The classic streptococcal morphology became evident upon subculture in glucose broth.

8.5.12.3. β-Hemolytic Streptococci

Approximately 170 cases of IE due to β-hemolytic streptococci have been reported. Of the 68 cases which have been serogrouped, only 5 were group A; the remainder belonged to groups B, C, G, H, K, L, M, and O, groups B and G comprising over half the isolates.[335] Since most clinical laboratories utilize sensitivity to a bacitracin disk (0.02–0.04 unit) as the method to identify group A streptococci, it is important to emphasize that 33% of group B, 72% of group C, and 79% of group G streptococci may be sensitive to this concentration of antibiotic.[335] Furthermore, the capacity of group C and G streptococci to stimulate the production of antibody to streptolysin O is another potential source of error in determining the epidemiological significance and pathogenic potential of β-hemolytic streptococci.[324] It is of interest that streptococci belonging to groups C and L are the most common causes of spontaneous IE in the pig.[336]

Group B streptococci, originally believed to have their principal importance as pathogens in obstetrics and perinatal practice, have been emerging as an important cause of IE in adults. The rate at which cases are being reported in the literature suggests either that the bacterium is only now emerging as an important pathogen or that it is being separated from other β-hemolytic streptococci more often due to utilization of more sophisticated techniques in routine laboratory studies.[337–343]

The clinical course of IE due to group B streptococci covers the usual spectrum seen with other bacteria. The capacity for rapid valve destruction and myocardial-abscess formation has been noted. This fact together with sensitivity to penicillin, which is less than that of group A streptococci and which seems to be decreasing progressively in recent years, argue for treatment of IE due to this bacterium as described for "penicillin-resistant" streptococci (see Section 8.4.2.1b).

Group G streptococci resemble those of group B in having the potential for rapid valve destruction. Despite their sensitivity to penicillin, treatment similar to that for penicillin-resistant streptococci has been recommended in view of the tissue-destructive capacity of the bacterium.[324,325,335] In addition to stimulating the production of antibodies to streptolysin O, the M protein of type 12 group A streptococcus (a "nephritogenic" strain) has been found in the wall of group G isolates.[325] In the few reported cases of IE due to group G streptococci, no particular nephritogenicity has been observed.

Aerococcus viridans is a nonstreptococcal gram-positive coccus that has many biochemical characteristics which might lead to its identification as a *streptococcus viridans* or enterococcus.[344] It is a rare cause of IE and was sensitive to penicillin in one case.[344]

8.5.12.4. Anaerobic and Microaerophilic Streptococci

A variety of peptostreptococci and microaerophilic streptococci may cause IE. Their major interest lies in the difficulty they may present to the laboratory, since isolation may be difficult, as may the interpretation of antibiotic sensitivities.[345] The problem is similar to that of other fastidious microorganisms and to that of streptococci with special nutritional requirements.

8.6. SURGERY

When it became evident in the early 1960s that valve destruction was a common complication of infective endocarditis (IE), despite effective sterilization of the infected vegetations, and that this complication was in fact the leading cause of death in patients with IE, the replacement of these damaged valves by prostheses or valve grafts was heralded as a major therapeutic triumph. Today, the indications for cardiac surgery have been broadened to include not only the hemodynamic consequences of valve perforation, but also the treatment of recurrent embolization and antibiotic failure. At the same time, a new population of patients has emerged which is highly susceptible to developing IE at the site of the reparative surgery. The importance of the role of cardiac surgery in the management of IE is illustrated by a recent series in which, in 5 years, 31% of patients admitted with IE required valve surgery for severe congestive heart failure (CHF) (48%), uncontrolled sepsis (28%), and systemic embolization (24%).[346]

The conditions giving rise to the indications for surgical treatment were discussed in Chapter 6. In addition, those circumstances in which surgery combined with antimicrobial therapy are necessary to sterilize the infection were considered in Section 8.5. Several reviews of the role of surgery in the management of IE have been published recently.[347–351]

8.6.1. Valve Destruction—Congestive Heart Failure

The most common indication for cardiac surgery (75–95% of patients) in the management of IE is to correct the hemodynamic consequences of destruction of heart valves, almost exclusively aortic and mitral.[348,352] The immediate operative mortality is no different from that of patients without IE requiring valve replacement and is correlated directly with the degree of heart failure.[353,354] There is general agreement that the hemodynamic state takes precedence over the need to have sterilized the infection as an indication for surgery. When forced to do so, one may undertake surgery even several hours after the start of antibiotic therapy,[347,349] but naturally one would like to sterilize the infection before surgery when the hemodynamic state of the patient permits. For a given degree of heart failure, mortality is significantly higher in patients with staphylococcal and fungal infections as well as in those with infections resistant to antibiotics.[354]

Because of the risk of operating on patients with severe heart failure, it is reasonable to operate before patients reach that stage of decompensation. In general, patients with new regurgitant murmurs should be carefully observed and operation performed when heart failure shows signs of progressing despite medical therapy.[355] The difficulty is that heart failure due to destruction of a previously competent valve may progress very rapidly. Destruction of the mitral valve is less likely to lead to rapidly progressive heart failure than destruction of the aortic valve.[353,356] Proper management requires the judgment of experienced cardiologists, cardiovascular surgeons, and infectious-disease specialists. At times, CHF may progress so rapidly that hemodialysis is necessary to remove fluid prior to surgery. Recent studies point to the finding of vegetations by echocardiography as a good indicator of those patients subject to valve destruction and major emboli who will require valve surgery (See Section 8.2).

Aortic-valve replacement has been accomplished in a patient with hemophilia and in a woman who was 22 weeks pregnant.[357,358]

Rupture of the chordae tendinae of the mitral valve is another indication for surgical intervention. In one series, 8% of patients suffered this complication of IE. Surgical replacement of the mitral valve was carried out in half these patients, the clinical indication being progressive CHF.[359]

8.6.2. Antibiotic Failure

Failure to respond to antibiotics represents the second most common indication for surgery in IE (7%), occurring often in conjunction with CHF (17%).[352] This is a particular problem in drug addicts and in prosthetic-valve endocarditis

(PVE), circumstances in which infection occurs commonly with antibiotic-resistant bacteria and fungi. In PVE, antibiotics alone may be ineffective, even when the infecting microorganism is sensitive to the drugs administered, undoubtedly because of the simultaneous presence of a foreign body. The therapy and prophylaxis of experimental endocarditis with antibiotics is considerably more effective in the absence of a foreign body.[85,360]

The ability to operate successfully in patients with active infection of valvular vegetations is due to the fact that vegetations occur most often toward the free edges of the valve, thus permitting debridement of the valves and the placement of sutures in a noninfected zone of the valve ring.[361]

There is no general rule for determining when patients with IE receiving antibiotic treatment should be labeled as treatment failures. Clearly, a patient who remains febrile and continues to have positive blood cultures while receiving antibiotics is a treatment failure. On the other hand, many patients with IE continue to have fever, albeit diminished, for several weeks after antibiotics are begun. This often represents mild drug fever, which does not necessitate changing antibiotics. In other words, the judgment may be difficult. The clinical indices of the effectiveness of antibiotic treatment are considered in Chapter 9. Of course, when fever is combined with other indices compatible with persistent infection, such as CHF and embolization, the likelihood of persistent infection increases, despite negative blood cultures.

In *drug addicts* with infections of the tricuspid valves [since patients can tolerate the absence of the tricuspid for, as a rule, several months (3–18)], it has been proposed to treat refractory infection with a two-stage procedure.[362–366] In the first stage, the tricuspid valve is removed while appropriate antibiotic therapy is continued. The prosthesis is then inserted at a later time when all evidence of infection has been eliminated.

In PVE, there is difference of opinion as to when reoperation should be undertaken. For fungal endocarditis, there are those who advise prompt reoperation,[55] whereas others advise at least 2 weeks of therapy with antifungal agents (when there is evidence of suppression of infection, and when the hemodynamic status of the patient permits) before reoperation.[274]

In PVE due to bacterial infection, therapy is begun with antibiotics and continued, surgery being undertaken when there is evidence of uncontrolled infection, repeated or large emboli, or hemodynamic complications related to valve dehiscence or dysfunction[58] (see Section 10.2).

8.6.3. Peripheral Embolization

Emboli occur commonly in IE, even while patients receive effective antibiotics, and, rarely, even after completion of successful antibiotic therapy. They are one of the most dreaded complications of the disease. An embolus to a cerebral or coronary artery can be fatal or incapacitate the patient for the remainder of his life. These are unpredictable events; perhaps increased experience with echocardiography will be able to better define those patients at risk.

The decision to advise valve surgery is relatively easy when the patient has a fungal or prosthetic-valve infection which embolizes to a major vessel. Or, perhaps, also for the patient who, despite successful antibiotic therapy, embolizes and continues to have vegetations visible by echocardiography. However, cardiac surgery, even in the absence of active infection, carries a definite operative mortality (about 10%) with a variety of longer-term serious risks.[(349,353)] Thus, valve replacement is not a therapeutic procedure to be recommended lightly. It is often very difficult to weigh the relative risks in a particular patient.

A recent report describes the improved ability to visualize valvular vegetations in IE with two-dimensional echocardiography and suggests the prophylactic replacement of damaged heart valves to which are attached vegetations which "look" easily detachable.[(367)] It will require more experience to be able to determine with confidence the capacity for embolization of valvular vegetations visualized with this new technique. Conventional M-mode echo-cardiography may be very useful for identifying those patients at risk of major embolic complications (see Section 8.2).

The indications for peripheral embolectomy are beyond the scope of this discussion. Suffice it to say that coronary embolectomy has been carried out in a patient during the course of treatment for IE.[(368)] It is important to emphasize the importance of careful bacteriological and histological study of all emboli removed at operation. It may thus be possible to identify the persistence of bacterial infection or secondary infection causing the persistence (or development of new) vegetations even when blood cultures remain sterile. Many of the infections which develop as a complication of long-term intravenous antibiotic therapy are due to bacteria or fungi which are not easily detected by blood culture.

Emboli occur with particular frequency in patients with fungal IE or with valvular infections due to fastidious microorganisms (see Section 8.5).[(55,369–372)]

8.6.4. Cardiac Conduction Abnormalities

Conduction defects which develop suddenly during the course of IE may be due to metastatic infection or to the direct extension of infection from the valvular vegetations. Valve-ring abscesses are well known to be particularly associated with staphylococcal infections of natural valves or with any infection of prosthetic valves.[(361,373)]

8.6.5. Peripheral Arterial Grafts

Infection of an arterial prosthesis is virtually always an indication for its removal.[377] Antibiotics should be given as described for the treatment of IE and the infected prosthesis and any adjacent abscesses drained as soon as possible, since rupture of the graft is an ominous complication. In circumstances wherein tissue viability can be maintained in the absence of the graft, replacement can be considered after a period of antibiotic therapy, the hope being to sterilize the infected area before replacing the prosthesis. Immediate replacement of a prosthesis in a previously infected tissue bed is usually followed by infection of the new prosthesis. In these circumstances, amputation may be life-saving.

8.6.6. Purulent Thrombophlebitis

This is a rare but serious complication of intravenous therapy. About 15–25% of catheters utilized for intravenous infusions are contaminated when placed in broth culture media after removal from the patient. With semiquantitative culture techniques, it has been found that about half these represent true infection.[311,378] Catheter-related sepsis is seen only in patients with semiquantitative culture-positive catheter tips.[311] Interestingly, catheter tips cultured from patients with bacteremia due to other primary lesions are not heavily contaminated. This is consistent with experimental data in rabbits which emphasize the difficulty in initiating infection in the peripheral venous system even in the presence of a plastic catheter.[11,379]

The risk of developing sepsis increases with the duration of cannulation and varies with the type of cannula used (plastic catheter or steel needles) as well as the type of cannulation (e.g., cutdown, percutaneous, peripheral, subclavian). It is difficult to compare these risks, however, since certain procedures are more likely to be employed in the treatment of seriously ill patients. For example, total parenteral nutrition is associated with a high risk of sepsis (12%), about half the cases of which are due to *C. albicans*.[311,380–382] It is important to search for eye lesions (white retinal lesions), which may be an indication of *Candida* sepsis. even in the absence of positive blood cultures.[382] Aside from total parenteral nutrition, the risk of sepsis with intravenous cannulas varies from 0.2 to 6.5%. Arterial catheters in place for more than 4 days are positive by quantitative culture in 27% of cases and produce sepsis in 8.5% of patients (about one third of those with positive catheter cultures).[383]

It is evident that steel needles or catheters inserted percutaneously intravenously are associated with the lowest rates of septic complications, and they should be removed and, if necessary, replaced every 48–72 hours.

Purulent thrombophlebitis is a rare complication of catheter-associated sepsis, occurring in about 0.2% of patients catheterized.[311] In patients with burns, this complication is the most common source of infection in patients dying of sepsis. It has been noted in as many as 4% of burn patients.[311,327]

The diagnosis of purulent thrombophlebitis is established by detecting pus coming from the puncture site, either spontaneously or after milking of the vein peripherally. If systemic symptoms and signs of infection do not respond promptly to systemic antibiotic therapy, consideration must be given to surgical drainage of the involved vein. Local signs of inflammation may be minimal in the presence of purulent venous infection. In burn patients, surgical drainage should be carried out on an emergency basis once the infection is detected.

Noninfectious complications of percutaneous central venous catheterization have recently been summarized.[384]

8.6.7. Cardiac Catheterization and Endocardial Pacemakers

Any catheter which rests in the cavities of the heart leads to the formation of nonbacterial thrombotic vegetations (NBTVs) and a small number of these will become infected. Judging from experimental studies, the catheter need be present for only several minutes in order to produce sufficient damage to permit the initiation of IE if followed promptly by bacterial challenge.[261] In rabbits, NBTVs induced by catheters within the heart become less susceptible to infection with the passage of time.[10]

Bacteremia must be an unusual event during cardiac catheterization[385]; nevertheless, IE has been documented in close relation to cardiac catheterization.[386,387]

Despite the risks of inducing NBTV formation and IE following cardiac catheterization, these procedures (with angiography) may have considerable value, not only for the localization of infection within the heart (see Section 8.2), but also for the preoperative definition of the extent of coronary artery and vascular damage.[12,14] There is general agreement that cardiac catheterization is not indicated in unstable patients with progressive CHF due to aortic insufficiency.[12] On the other hand, in stable patients, angiography is particularly useful for the identification of valve-ring abscess and aneurysms of the sinus of Valsava.[12,14] However, in some series, embolization was a serious complication of cardiac catheterization in patients with IE.[388]

Transvenous pacemakers also serve as a rare means of inducing intravascular infection.[64,389–391] There seem to be two types of infection in such patients: hematogenous infection of intracardiac vegetations and direct extension of infection from the subcutaneous generator site.[391] In rabbits, susceptibility to hematogenous infection of catheter-induced NBTVs in the right heart decreases with the passage of time.[10] Indeed, right-heart infection in rabbits, depending on the infecting microorganism, is capable of spontaneous sterilization.[11]

In patients with transvenous pacemakers, treatment of infection may be successful without removing the pacemaker in hematogenously induced infections, a phenomenon occasionally observed in patients with PVE occurring many years after operation.[64] On the other hand, incarcerated pacemakers may have to be literally carved out of the ventricular wall in order to cure this type of infection.[389,391]

8.6.8. Miscellaneous

Two other categories of complications amenable to surgical therapy are purulent pericarditis and mycotic aneurysms and their complications, including the development of fistulae and abnormal vascular communications (and left ventricular–aortic discontinuity).[347,349,374–376]

8.7. TREATMENT OF SEPTIC ARTHRITIS AND OSTEOMYELITIS

As discussed earlier, septic bone and joint lesions occur occasionally during the course of infective endocarditis (IE) due even to bacteria (e.g., *Str. viridans*) which are normally not associated with metastatic infection.[392–398] In fact, it is likely that as technetium scanning is carried out more often in patients with bone and joint manifestations of IE, lesions will be seen much more frequently. Osteomyelitis is seen in addicts and in patients with bacteremia as a complication of intravenous cannulas.[399] The clinical differentiation of bacteremia and osteomyelitis (e.g., in an addict) from IE may be very difficult.

It is essential to obtain material to establish a bacteriological diagnosis: blood culture, biopsy, or aspiration of the bone or joint lesion. Appropriate antibiotic treatment for IE for 6–8 weeks is recommended as being satisfactory treatment for the bone and joint lesions also. It should be borne in mind that conventional radiological evidence of bone infection may be altered or may appear during the course of effective antibiotic therapy.

8.8. TREATMENT OF GLOMERULONEPHRITIS

The pathogenesis of immune-complex glomerulonephritis was discussed in Section 8.3.4.7b. Evidence is accumulating as to the potential usefulness of plasmapheresis as a means of clearing the circulation of circulating immune complexes (CICs) with consequent improvement in renal function.[257,400–402] In most instances, the glomerulonephritis seen with infective endocarditis (IE) responds promptly to effective antibiotic therapy. It is still too early to be certain of the indications for plasmapheresis, but it should certainly be considered in patients in whom CICs persist along with renal insufficiency in patients successfully treated for IE.

8.9. SPECIAL ASPECTS OF PATIENT CARE

As in the case with any heart illness, infective endocarditis (IE) is particularly disquieting to the patient. Heart trouble carries with it unambiguous overtones of a vital threat to survival, and IE is no exception. Tension and anxiety, expressed or repressed, are part and parcel of the clinical picture of IE, particularly after the patient has been told that he has an infection in the heart. This is frightening and easily leads to confusing images in his mind. It is of the utmost importance to explain carefully to the patient the nature of the illness and to give him the opportunity to express his feelings and worry. Drawing a picture of the location of the infection and emphasizing the lack of relation to heart attacks can be very helpful.

In view of the increased susceptibility to infection of the patient who has recovered from IE, it is essential to provide reassurance and specific advice about future prophylactic measures. This is particularly true for the patient who has received a prosthetic heart valve. He is likely to be discharged from the hospital from a service (surgery) that was not involved in the treatment of the original infection, and he frequently leaves believing that he no longer has to worry about antibiotic prophylaxis as he did before he got his new heart valve. In reality, however, he is probably more susceptible to developing IE than he was previously—and this susceptibility continues, as far as we know today, indefinitely.

After the patient is discharged from the hospital, the physician must be available and must take the time to investigate any symptoms that may suggest the recurrence of IE. Negative blood cultures are reassuring and help the patient in time to readjust to the variations in feelings of well-being encountered in normal living.

REFERENCES

1. Pesanti, E. L., Smith I. M.: Infective endocarditis with negative blood cultures—An analysis of 52 cases. *Am. J. Med.* **66**:43–50, 1979.
2. Editoral: Infective endocarditis with negative blood cultures. *Br. Med. J.* **2**:4, 1979.
3. Cannady, P. B., Sanford, J. P.: Negative blood cultures in infective endocarditis: A review. *South. Med. J.* **69**:1420–1424, 1976.
4. Studer, J. P., Glauser, M. P., Shapira, M.: Value of examining buffy coats for intragranulocytic micro-organisms in patients with fever. *Br. Med. J.* **1**:69–146, 1979.
5. Freedman, L. R., and Johnson, M. L.: Experimental endocarditis. IV. Tricuspid and aortic valve infection with *Candida albicans* in rabbits. *Yale J. Biol. Med.* **45**:163–175, 1972.

6. Badger, S. J., Butler, T., Kim, C. K., Johnston, K. H.: Experimental *Eikenella corrodens* endocarditis in rabbits. *Infect. Immun.* **23**:751–757, 1978.
7. Editorial: Culture-negative endocarditis. *Lancet* **2**:1164–1165, 1977.
8. Root, R. K., Metcolf, J. A.: Surface binding and enhanced killing of penicillin-treated *S. aureus* 502 A by human neutrophiles. *Clin. Res.* **27**:480A, 1979.
9. O'Keete, J. P., Gorbach, S. L.: Laboratory diagnosis of infective endocarditis, in: *Infective Endocarditis,* Rahimtoola, S. H., ed. Grune and Stratton, New York, pp. 307–325, 1978.
10. Freedman, L. R., Valone, J.: Experimental endocarditis. *Prog. Cardiovasc. Dis.* **22**:169–180, 1979.
11. Francioli, P., Freedman, L. R.: Streptococcal infection of endocardial and other intravascular vegetations in rabbits: Natural history and effect of dexamethasone. *Infect. Immun.* **24**:483–491, 1979.
12. Mills, J., Abbott, J., Utley, J. R., Ryan, C.: Role of cardiac catheterization in infective endocarditis. *Chest* **72**:576–582, 1977.
13. Harris, C. N., Dunne, E. F., Farinha, J. B., Zubiate, P., Kaye, J. H., Kaplan, M. A.: Forward angiography in the indentification of vegetations in tricuspid endocarditis. *Chest* **71**:218–220, 1977.
14. Welton, D. E., Young, J. B., Raizner, A. E., Ishimori, T., Adyanthaya, A., Miller, R. R., Chahine, R. A.: The value and safety of pre-operative cardiac catheterization during active infective endocarditis (abstract). *Am. J. Cardiol.* **43**:407, 1979.
15. Pazin, G. J., Peterson, K. L., Griff, F. W., Shaver, J. A., Ho, M.: Determination of site of infection in endocarditis. *Ann. Intern. Med.* **82**:746–750, 1975.
16. Mann, T., McLaurin, L., Grossman, W., Craige, E.: Assessing the hemodynamic severity of acute aortic regurgitation due to infective endocarditis. *N. Engl. J. Med.* **293**:108–113, 1975.
17. Pruitt, A. A., Rubin, R. H., Karchmer, A. W., Duncan, G. W.: Neurological complications of bacterial endocarditis. *Medicine* **57**:329–343, 1978.
18. Malergue, M. C., Fraisse, F., Gilbert, C., Kalmanson, D., Lecompte, Y, Witschitz, S.: Diagnostic échocardiographique des endocardites tricuspidiennes. *Arch. Mal. Coeur* **72**:641–646, 1979.
19. Mintz, G. S., Kotler, M. N., Parry, W. R.: Wide splitting of the first heart sound secondary to tricuspid valve endocarditis—A phonocardiographic echocardiographic study. *Am. J. Med.* **66**:523–527, 1979.
20. Thompson, K. R., Nanda, N. C., Gramiak, R.: The reliability of echocardiography in the diagnosis of infective endocarditis. *Radiology* **125**:473–476, 1977.
21. Ali, N., Sheikh, M. U., Andy, J. J., Roberts, W. C.: Echocardiographic observations in active infective endocarditis occurring in opiate or alcoholic addicts: A comparison of right and left-sided valvular lesions in 27 patients (abstract). *Am. J. Cardiol.* **39**:278, 1977.
22. Durack, D. T.: Experimental bacterial endocarditis. IV Structure and evolution of very early lesions. *J. Pathol.* **115**:81–89, 1975.
23. Gould, L., Freiberg, A., Lewnes, G. C., Reddy, R., Werthamer, S.: Right atrial myxoma associated with thrombocytopenia and bacterial endocarditis. *N. Y. State J. Med.* **78**:2081–2083, 1978.
24. Corrigan, E., Newhall, D., Raymond, R. D.: Left atrial myxoma—presenting as bacterial endocarditis. *Rhode Island Med. J.* **61**:410–412, 1978.
25. Rojpal, R. S., Leibsohn, J. A., Liekweg, W. G., Gross, C. M., Olinger, G. N., Rose, H. D., Bamrah, V. S.: Infected left atrial myxoma with bacteremia simulating infective endocarditis. *Arch. Intern. Med.* **139**:1176–1178, 1979.
26. Mintz, G. S., Kotler, M. N., Segal, B. L., Parry, W. R.: Comparison of two-dimensional and M-mode echocardiography in the evaluation of patients with infective endocarditis. *Am. J. Cardiol.* **43**:738–744, 1979.

27. Wann, L. S., Dillon, J. C., Weyman, A. E., Feigenbaum, H.: Echocardiography in bacterial endocarditis. *N. Engl. J. Med.* **295**:135–139, 1976.
28. Pratt, C., Whitcomb, C. Neumann, A., Mason, D. T., Amsterdam, E. A., DeMaria, A. N.: Relationship of vegetation on echogram to the clinical course and systemic emboli in bacterial endocarditis. *Am. J. Cardiol.* **41**:384, 1978.
29. Bloch, A., Stalder, H., Waldvogel, F. A., Mayor, C.: Utilité de l'echocardiographie dans le diagnostic de l'endocardite bactérienne. *Schweiz. Med. Wochenschr.* **107**:1571–1572, 1977.
30. Mintz, G. S., Kotler, M. N., Segal, B. L., Parry, W. R.: Survival of patients with aortic valve endocarditis. *Arch. Intern. Med.* **139**:862–866, 1979.
31. Strom, J., Davis, R., Frishman, W., Becker, R., Matsumoto, M., Sonnenblick, E.: The demonstration of vegetations by echocadiography in bacterial endocarditis: An indication for early surgical intervention. *Circulation* **60**:11–37, 1979.
32. Wiseman, J., Rouleau, J., Rigo, P., Strauss, H. W., Pitt, B.: Gallium-67 myocardial imaging for the detection of bacterial endocarditis. *Radiology* **120**:135, 1976.
33. Huang, J., Wong, D., Tanaka, T., Thadepoll, H., Mishkin, F.: Diagnosis of infective endocarditis in rabbits by labelled autibacterial autibody score (abstract). *Clin. Res.* **25**:377A, 1977.
34. Riba, A. L., Downs, J., Thakur, M. L., Gottschalk, A., Andriole, V. T., Zaret, B. L.: Technitium-99m stannous pyrophosphate imaging of experimental endocarditis. *Circulation* **58**:111–119, 1978.
35. Sty, J. R., Chusid, M. J.: 99m TC-pyrophosphate imaging: Bacterial endocarditis. *Pediatr. Radiol.* **8**:223–224, 1979.
36. Riba, A. L., Thakur, M. T., Gottschalk, A., Andriole, V. T., Zaret, B. L.: Imaging experimental infective endocarditis with indium-111-labelled blood cellular components. *Circulation* **59**:336–343, 1979.
37. Mallen, M. S., Hube, E. L., Brenes, M.: Comparative study of blood cultures made from artery, vein and bone marrow in patients with subacute bacterial endocarditis. *Am. Heart J.* **33**:692, 1947.
38. Freedman, L. R., Acar, J. F., Durack, D. T., Kaye, D., Waldvogel, F. A.: Infective endocarditis. *Current Chemotherapy (Proceedings of the 10th International Congress of Chemotherapy)* **1**:69–71, 1978.
39. Carey, R. B., Brause, B. D., Roberts, R. B.: Antimicrobial therapy of vitamin B_6-dependent streptococcal endocarditis. *Ann. Intern. Med.* **87**:150–154, 1977.
40. Petit, J.-C., Sicard, D.: Endocardite à streptocoque déficient cultivant en satellitisme. *Med. Malad. Infect.* **7**:506–508, 1977.
41. Carey, R. B.: Culture-negative endocarditis. *Lancet* **1**:278, 1978.
42. Roberts, K. B., Sidlak, M. J.: Satellite stretococci: A major cause of "negative" blood cultures in bacterial endocarditis? *J. Am. Med. Assoc.* **241**:2293–2294, 1979.
43. Piepkorn, M. W., Reichenbach, D. D.: Infective endocarditis associated with cell wall-deficient bacteria. *Hum. Pathol.* **9**:163–173, 1978.
44. Roberts, R. B., Krieger, A. G., Schiller, N. L., Gross, K. C.: Viridans streptococcal endocarditis: The role of various species, including pyridoxal-dependent streptococci. *Rev. Infect. Dis.* **1**:955–966, 1979.
45. Bayston, R.: Serological investigations in children with colonized Spitz–Holter valves. *J. Clin. Pathol.* **25**:718–720, 1972.
46. Bayston, R., Penny, S. R.: Excessive production of mucoid substance in staphylococcus SIIA: A possible factor in colonization of Holter shunts. *Dev. Med. Child. Neurol. Suppl.* **27**:25–28, 1972.
47. Nagel, J. G., Tuazon, C. U., Cardella, T. A., Sheagren, J. N.: Teichoic acid serologic diagnosis of staphylococcal endocarditis—Use of gel diffusion and counterimmunoelectrophoretic methods. *Ann. Intern. Med.* **82**:13–17, 1975.

48. Wheat, L. J., Kohler, R. B., White, A.: Solid-phase radioimmunoassay for detection of staphylococcal antigen in serum of rabbits with endocarditis due to *Staphylococcus aureus*. *J. Infect. Dis.* **138**:174–180, 1978.
49. Strife, C. F., McDonald, B. M., Ruley, E. J., McAdams, A. J., West, C. D.: Shunt nephritis: The nature of the serum cryoglobulins and their relation to the complement profile. *J. Pediatr.* **83**:403–413, 1976.
50. Wheat, L. J., Kohler, R. B., Tabbarah, Z., and White, A.: Circulating staphylococcal antigen in humans and immune rabbits with endocarditis due to *Staphylococcus aurens:* Inhibition of detection by preexisting antibodies. *J. Infect. Dis.* **140**:54–61, 1979.
51. Peeters, W., Mussche, M., Becaus, I., Ringoir, S.: Shunt nephritis. *Clin. Nephrol.* **9**:122–125, 1978.
52. Shanson, D. C., Hince, C.: An immunofluorescent method for detecting antibodies against viridans streptococci in *Streptococcus viridans* endocarditis. *J. Clin. Pathol.* **31**:292–293, 1978.
53. Spitzer, R. E., Stitzel, A. E., Urmson, J. R.: Is glomerulonephritis after bacterial sepsis always benign (letter)? *Lancet* **1**:871, 1978.
54. Hoppes, W. L., Smith, J. W., White, A. C.: Serological diagnosis of streptococcal endocarditis. *Clin. Res.* **24**:545A, 1976.
55. McLeod, R., Remington, J. S.: Fungal endocarditis, in: *Infective Endocarditis,* Rahimtoola, S. H., ed. Grune and Stratton, New York, pp. 211–290, 1978.
56. Maliwan, N., Reid, R., Katzen, R.: Rapid diagnosis of beta-hemolytic streptococcus group B endocarditis by buffy-coat examination and gas–liquid chromatography. *J. Clin. Pathol.* **32**:760–763, 1979.
57. Bayer, A. S., Guze, L. B.: *Staphylococcus aureus* bacteremic syndromes: Diagnostic and therapeutic update. *Dis-Month* **25**:(9), 1979.
58. Kloster, F. E.: Infective prosthetic valve endocarditis, in: *Infective Endocarditis,* Ramintoola, S. H., ed. Grune and Stratton, New York, pp. 291–305, 1978.
59. Dismukes, W. E., Karchmer, A. W.: The diagnosis of infected prosthetic heart valves: Bacteremia versus endocarditis, in: *Infections of Prosthetic Heart Valves and Vascular Grafts,* Duma, R. J., ed. University Park Press, Baltimore, pp. 61–80, 1976.
60. Wilson, W. R., Jaumin, P. M., Danielson, G. K., Giuliani, E. R., Washington, J. A., II, Geraci, J. E.: Prosthetic valve endocarditis. *Ann. Intern. Med.* **82**:751–756, 1975.
61. Arnett, E. N., Roberts, W. C.: Prosthetic valve endocarditis. *Am. J. Cardiol.* **38**:281–292, 1976.
62. Karchmer, A. W., Dismukes, W. E., Buckley, M. J., Austin, W. G.: Late prosthetic valve endocarditis clinical features influencing therapy. *Am. J. Med.* **64**:199–206, 1978.
63. Watanakunakorn, C., Baird, I. M.: *Staphylococcus aureus* bacteremia and endocarditis associated with a removable infected intravenous device. *Am. J. Med.* **63**:253–256, 1977.
64. Zeller, N. H., Lusk, R. H., Palmer, D. L.: Nonsurgical cure of endocarditis associated with a pacemaker. *Arch. Intern. Med.* **135**:580–581, 1975.
65. Demierre, G., Freedman, L. R.: Experimental endocarditis: Prophylaxis of *Candida albicans* infections by 5-fluorocystosine in rabbits. *Antimicrob. Agents Chemother.* **16**:252–254, 1979.
66. Watanakunakorn, C.: Prosthetic valve infective endocarditis. *Prog. Cardiovasc. Dis.* **22**:181–192, 1979.
67. Cohen, L., Freedman, L. R.: Damage to the aortic valve as a cause of death in bacterial endocarditis. *Ann. Intern. Med.* **55**:562–564, 1961.
68. Pulliam, L., Inokuchi, S., Hadley, W. K., Mills, J.: Penicillin tolerance in experimental streptococcal endocarditis. *Lancet* **2**:957, 1979.
69. Goldman, P. L., Petersdorf, R. G.: Significance of methicillin tolerance in experimental staphylococcal endocarditis. *Antimicrob. Agents Chemother.* **15**:802–806, 1979.

70. Bayer, A. S., Chow, A. W., Ishida, K., Guze, L. B.: Experimental infective endocarditis due to antibiotic tolerant *Lactobacillus plantarum*—Correlation of *in-vitro* susceptibility with *in-vivo* efficiency. *11th International Congress of Chemotherapy,* Abstract 1057, 1979.
71. Wilson, W. R., Geraci, J. E., Wilkowske, C. J., Washington, J. A., II: Short-term intramuscular therapy with procaine penicillin plus streptomycin for infective endocarditis due to viridans streptococci. *Circulation* **57:**1158–1161, 1978.
72. Hewitt, W. L., O'Grady, F. W., Acar, J. F., McDonald, P. J., Sande, M. A.: The rational basis for chemotherapy. *Current Chemotherapy (Proceedings of the 10th International Congress, of Chemother)* **1:**3–6, 1978.
73. Wolfe, J. C., Johnson, W. D.: Penicillin-sensitive streptococcal endocarditis—*In-vitro* and clinical observations on penicillin–streptomycin therapy. *Ann. Intern. Med.* **81:**178–181, 1974.
74. Hook, E. W., Guerrant, R. L.: Therapy of infective endocarditis, in: *Infective Endocarditis,* Kaye, D., ed. University Park Press, Baltimore, pp. 167–184, 1976.
75. Karchmer, A. W., Moellering, R. C., Jr., Maki, D. G., Swartz, M. N.: Single-antibiotic therapy for streptococcal endocarditis. *J. Am. Med. Assoc.* **241:**1801–1806, 1979.
76. Malacoff, R. F., Frank, E., Andriole, V. T.: Streptococcal endocarditis (non-enterococcal, non-group A)—Single vs combination therapy. *J. Am. Med. Assoc.* **241:**1807–1810, 1979.
77. Benn, R.: Treatment of bacterial endocarditis 1976. *Drugs* **12:**374–380, 1976.
78. Hoppes, W. L.: Treatment of bacterial endocarditis caused by penicillin-sensitive streptococci. *Arch. Intern. Med.* **137:**1122–1123, 1977.
79. Phair, J. P., Tan, J. S.: Therapy of *Streptococcus viridans* endocarditis, in: *Infective Endocarditis: An American Heart Association Symposium,* Kaplan, E. L., Tarauta, A. V., eds. American Heart Association Monograph No. 52, American Heart Association, Dallas, pp. 55–57, 1977.
80. Resnick, L., Cohen, L.: Antibiotic treatment of penicillin-sensitive streptococcal endocarditis (editorial). *J. Am. Med. Assoc.* **241:**1826–1827, 1979.
81. Bryant, R. E., Kimbrough, R. C.: Treatment of infective endocarditis, in: *Infective Endocarditis,* Rahimtoola, S. H., ed. Grune and Stratton, New York, pp. 327–360, 1978.
82. Svanbom, M., Strandell, T.: Bacterial endocarditis. II. A prospective study with clinical, laboratory and therapeutic observations. *Scand. J. Infect. Dis.* **11:**17–30, 1979.
83. Wilson, W. R., Geraci, J. E., Giuliani, E. R., Thompson, R. L., Wilkowske, C. J.: Short-term intramuscular therapy with procaine penicillin plus streptomycin for infective endocarditis due to penicillin-sensitive streptococci. *Circulation* **60:**11–36, 1979.
84. Durack, D. T., Pelletier, L. L., Petersdorf, R. C.: Chemotherapy of experimental streptococcal endocarditis. II. Synergism between penicillin and streptomycin against penicillin-sensitive streptococci. *J. Clin. Invest.* **53:**829–833, 1974.
85. Pelletier, L. L., Petersdorf, R. G., Nielson, K.: Chemotherapy of experimental streptococcal endocarditis. V. Effect of duration of infection and retained intracardiac catheter on response to treatment. *J. Lab. Clin. Med.* **87:**692–702, 1976.
86. Sande, M. A., Irwin, R. G.: Penicillin aminoglycoside synergy in experimental *Streptococcus viridans* endocarditis. *J. Infect. Dis.* **129:**572–576, 1974.
87. Edelman, R.: Controlled study of streptococcal endocarditis—A problem of feasibility (letter). *J. Am. Med. Assoc.* **242:**1612–1613, 1979.
88. Hook, E. W., III, Johnson, W. D.: Vancomycin therapy of bacterial endocarditis. *Am. J. Med.* **65:**411–415, 1978.
89. Wannamaker, L. W., Parker, M. T.: Microbiology of bacteria often responsible for infective endocarditis, in: *Infective Endocarditis: An American Heart Association Symposium,* Kaplan, E. L., Tarauta, A. V., eds. American Heart Association Monograph No. 52, Dallas, pp. 9–11, 1977.
90. Swartz, M. N.: Infective endocarditis, in: *Scientific American Medicine,* Rubenstein, E., Federman, D. D., eds. Scientific American, New York, pp. 1–25, 1979.

91. Hook, E. W., III, Roberts, R. B., Sande, M. A.: Antimicrobial therapy of experimental enterococcal endocarditis. *Antimicrob. Agents Chemother.* **8**:564–570, 1975.
92. Carrizosa, J., Kaye, D.: Antibiotic synergism in enterococcal endocarditis. *J. Lab. Clin. Med.* **88**:132–141, 1976.
93. Carrizosa, J., Kaye, D.: Penicillin and netilmicin in treatment of experimental enterococcal endocarditis. *Antimicrob. Agents Chemother.* **13**:505–508, 1978.
94. Lincoln, L. J., Weinstein, A. J., Gallagher, M., Abrutyn, E.: Penicillinase-resistant penicillins plus gentamicin in experimental enterococcal endocarditis. *Antimicrob. Agents Chemother.* **12**:484–489, 1977.
95. Westenfelder, G. O., Paterson, P. Y., Reisberg, B. E., Carlson, G. M.: Vancomycin–streptomycin synergism in enterococcal endocarditis. *J. Am. Med. Assoc.* **223**:37–40, 1973.
96. Watanakunakorn, C.: Changing epidemiology and newer aspects of infective endocarditis, in: *Advances in Internal Medicine,* Stollerman, G. H., ed. Year Book Medical Publishers, Chicago, pp. 21–47, 1977.
97. Weinstein, A. J., Lentnek, A. L.: Cephalosporin–aminoglycoside synergism in experimental enterococcal endocarditis. *Antimicrob. Agents Chemother.* **9**:983–987, 1976.
98. Abrutyn, E., Lincoln, L., Gallagher, M., Weinstein, A. J.: Cephalothin–gentamicin synergism in experimental enterococcal endocarditis. *J. Antimicrob. Chemother.* **4**:153–158, 1978.
99. Ruhen, R. W., Darrell, J. H.: Antibiotic synergism against group D streptococci in the treatment of endcarditis. *Med. J. Aust.* **2**:114–116, 1973.
100. Serra, P., Brandimarte, C., Martino, P., Carlone, S., Giunchi, G.: Synergistic treatment of enterococcal endocarditis. *Arch. Intern. Med.* **137**:1562–1567, 1977.
101. Rahal, J. J.: Antibiotic combinations: The clinical relevance of synergy and antagonism. *Medicine* **57**:179–195, 1978.
102. Calderwood, S. A., Wennersten, C., Moellering, R. C., Jr., Kunz, L. J., Krogstad, D. J.: Resistance to six aminoglycosidic aminocyclitol antibiotics among enterococci: Prevalence, evolution and relationship to synergism with penicillin. *Antimicrob. Agents Chemother.* **12**:401–405, 1977.
103. Reyes, M. P., Brown, W. J., Lerner, A. M.: Treatment of patients with Pseudomonas endocarditis with high dose aminoglycoside and carbenicillin therapy. *Medicine* **57**:57–67, 1978.
104. Sande, M. A., Johnson, M. L.: Antimicrobial therapy of experimental endocarditis caused by *Staphylococcus aureus*. *J. Infect. Dis.* **131**:367–375, 1975.
105. Sande, M. A., Courtney, K. B.: Nafcillin–gentamicin synergism in experimental staphylococcal endocarditis. *J. Lab. Clin. Med.* **88**:118–124, 1976.
106. Miller, M. H., Wexler, M. A., Steigbigel, N. H.: Single and combination antibiotic therapy of *Staphylococcus aureus* experimental endocarditis: Emergence of gentamicin-resistant mutants. *Antimicrob. Agents Chemother.* **14**:336–343, 1978.
107. Murray, H. W., Wigley, F. M., Mann, J. J., Arthur, R. R.: Combination antibiotic therapy in staphylococcal endocarditis. *Arch. Intern. Med.* **136**:480–483, 1976.
108. Haas, E. J.: Treatment of *Staphylococcus aureus* endocarditis (letter). *Arch. Intern. Med.* **137**:400–401, 1977.
109. Mann, J. J.: Treatment of *Staphylococcus aureus* endocarditis—Reply (letter). *Arch. Intern. Med.* **137**:401, 1977.
110. Watanakunakorn, C.: Prognostic factors in *Staphylococcus aureus* endocarditis and results of therapy with a penicillin and gentamicin. *Am. J. Med. Sci.* **273**:133–139, 1977.
111. Abrams, B., Sklaver, A., Hoffman, T., Greenman, R.: Single or combination therapy of staphylococcal endocarditis in intravenous drug abusers. *Ann. Intern. Med.* **90**:789–791, 1979.
112. Sande, M. A., Korzeniowski, O. M.: Comparison of nafcillin with nafcillin plus gentamicin in the treatment of addicts with *S. aureus* endocarditis. 19th Interscience Conference on Antimicrobial Agents and Chemotherapy, Abstract 362, 1979.

113. Banks, T., Fletcher, R., Ali, N.: Infective endocarditis in heroin addicts. *Am. J. Med.* **55**:444–451, 1973.
114. Sklaver, A. R., Hoffman, T. A., Greenman, R. L.: Staphylococcal endocarditis in addicts. *South. Med. J.* **71**:638–643, 1978.
115. Faville, R. J., Jr., Zaske, D. E., Kaplan, E. L., Crossley, K., Sabath, L. D., Quie, P. G.: *Staphylococcus aureus* endocarditis. *J. Am. Med. Assoc.* **240**:1963–1965, 1978.
116. Tuazon, C. U., Lin, M. Y. C., Sheagren, J. N.: *In vitro* activity of rifampin alone and in combination with nafcillin and vancomycin against pathogenic strains of *Staphylococcus aureus*. *Antimicrob. Agents Chemother.* **13**:759–761, 1978.
117. Massanari, R. M., Donta, S. T.: The efficacy of rifampin as adjunctive therapy in selected cases of staphylococcal endocarditis. *Chest* **73**:371–375, 1978.
118. Egert, J., Carrizosa, J., Kaye, D.: Comparison of methicillin, nafcillin, and oxacillin in therapy of *Staphylococcus aureus* endocarditis in rabbits. *J. Lab. Clin. Med.* **89**:1262–1268, 1977.
119. Carrizosa, J., Santoro, J., Kaye, D.: Treatment of experimental *Staphylococcus aureus* endocarditis: Comparison of cephalothin, cefazolin, and methicillin. *Antimicrob. Agents Chemother.* **13**:74–77, 1978.
120. Carrizosa, J., Kobasa, W. D., Kaye, D.: Effectiveness of nafcillin, methicillin, and cephalothin in experimental *Staphylococcus aureus* endocarditis. *Antimicrob. Agents Chemother.* **15**:735–737, 1979.
121. Bryant, R. E., Alford, R. H.: Unsuccessful treatment of staphylococcal endocarditis with cefazolin. *J. Am. Med. Assoc.* **237**:569–570, 1977.
122. Kaye, D., Hewitt, W., Remington, J. S., Turck, M.: Cefazolin and *Staphylococcus aureus* endocarditis (letter). *J. Am. Med. Assoc.* **237**:2601, 1977.
123. Bryant, R. E., Alford, R. H.: Treatment of staphylococcal endocarditis—letter. *J. Am. Med. Assoc.* **239**:1130, 1978.
124. Kaye, D., Hewitt, W., Remington, J. S., Turck, M.: Treatment of staphylococcal endocarditis—Reply. *J. Am. Med. Assoc.* **239**:1130–1131, 1978.
125. Archer, G. L., Karchmer, A. W., Dismukes, W. E.: Antibiotic susceptibility of *Staplylococcus epidermidis* isolates from patients with prosthetic valve endocarditis. 11th International Congress of Chemotherapy, Abstract 603, 1979.
126. Archer, G., Fekety, F. R., Jr., Supena, R.: *Pseudomonas aeruginosa* endocarditis in drug addicts. *Am. Heart J.* **88**:570–578, 1974.
127. Kohler, R. B., White, A.: Miscellaneous Pseudomonas disease, in: *Pseudomonas aeruginosa,* Doggett, R. G., ed. Academic Press, New York, pp. 445–494, 1979.
128. Reyes, M. P., Lerner, A. M. (letter), Alpert, J. S., Borow, K. M., Pennington, J. (reply). Pseudomonas endocarditis. *J. Am. Med. Assoc.* **241**:1576, 1979.
129. Archer, G. L., Johnston, J. L.: Effect of type-specific active immunization on the development and progression of experimental *Pseudomonas aeruginosa* endocarditis. *Infect. Immun.* **24**:167–173, 1979.
130. Archer, G. L., Fekety, F. R., Jr.: Experimental endocarditis due to *Pseudomonas aeruginosa*. II. Therapy with carbenicillin and gentamicin. *J. Infect. Dis.* **136**:327–335, 1977.
131. Witchitz, S., Gilbert, C., Withcitz, J., Gougerot, M., Vachon, F., Vic-Dupont, V.: *Pseudomonas aeruginosa* endocarditis: A report of nine cases. *Eur. J. Cardiol.* **4**:91–97, 1976.
132. Fischer, J. J.: *Pseudomonas maltophilia* endocarditis after replacement of the mitral valve: A case study. *J. Infect. Dis.* **128**(Suppl.):S771–S773, 1973.
133. Rahal, J. J., Simberkoff, M. S., Hyams, P. J.: *Pseudomonas cepacia* tricuspid endocarditis: Treatment with trimethoprim, sulfonamide and polymyxin B. *J. Infect. Dis.* **128**(Suppl.):S762–S767, 1973.
134. Neu, H. C., Garvey, G. J., Beach, M. P.: Successful treatment of *Pseudomonas cepacia* endocarditis in a heroin addict with trimethoprim–sulfamethoxazole. *J. Infect. Dis.* **128**(Suppl.):S768–S770, 1973.

135. Seligman, S. J., Madhaven, T., Alcid, D.: Trimethoprim–sufalmethoxazole in the treatment of bacterial endocarditis. *J. Infect. Dis.* **128**(Suppl.):S754–S761, 1973.
136. Perry, T. M., Belter, L. F.: Brucellosis and heart disease. 2. Fatal brucellosis, a review of the literature and report of new cases. *Amer. J. Pathol.* **36**:673–697, 1960.
137. O'Meara, J. B., Eykyn, S., Jenkins, B. S., Braimbridge, M. V., Phillips, I.: *Brucella melitensis* endocarditis: Successful treatment of an infected prosthetic mitral valve. *Thorax* **29**:377–381, 1974.
138. Pratt, D. S., Tenney, J. H., Bjork, C. M., Reller, L. B.: Successful treatment of *Brucella melitensis* endocarditis. *Am. J. Med.* **64**:897–900, 1978.
139. Cohen, P. S., O'Brien, T. F., Schoenbaum, S. C., Mederios, A. A.: The risk of endothelial infection in adults with Salmonella bacteremia. *Ann. Intern. Med.* **89**:931–932, 1978.
140. Yamamoto, N., Magidson, O., Posner, C., Mendez, A. M., Zubiate, P., Kay, J. H.: Probable Salmonella endocarditis treated with prosthetic valve replacement: A case report. *Surgery* **76**:678–681, 1974.
141. Shanson, D. C., Bridgen, W., Weaver, E. J. M.: *Salmonella enteritidis* endocarditis. *Br. Med. J.* **1**(1):612–613, 1977.
142. Avril, J. L., Berche, P., Lelguen, C. L., Daoulas-le-Bourdelles, F.: Incapacité d'une souche de *Salmonella Brandenburg* responsable d'une endocardite de recevoir des plasmides de résistance aux antibiotiques. *Med. Malad. Infect.* **7**:419–421, 1977.
143. Ball, A. P., McGhie, D., Geddes, A. M.: *Serratia marcescens* in a general hospital. *Q. J. Med. N. Ser.* **46**:63–71, 1977.
144. Yu, V. L.: *Serratia marcescens:* Historical prospective and clinical review. *N. Engl. J. Med.* **300**:887–893, 1979.
145. Mills, J., Drew, D.: *Serratia marcescens* endocarditis: A regional illness associated with intravenous drug abuse. *Ann. Intern. Med.* **84**:29–35, 1976.
146. Bryan, C. S., Marney, S. R., Alford, R. H., Bryant, R. E.: Gram-negative bacillary endocarditis. *Am. J. Med.* **58**:209–215, 1975.
147. Sands, M., Sanders, C. V.: *Serratia marcescens* endocarditis (letter). *Ann. Intern. Med.* **85**:397–398, 1976.
148. Goldmann, D. A., Maki, D. G., Bennett, J. V.: Intravenous infusion associated infections, in: *Hospital Infections,* Bennett, J. V., Brachman, P. S., eds. Little Brown, Boston, pp. 443–452, 1979.
149. Steere, A. C., Stamm, W. E., Martin, S. M., Bennett, J. V.: Gram negative rod bacteremia, in: *Hospital Infections,* Bennett, J. V., Brachman, P. S., eds. Little Brown, Boston, pp. 443–452, 1979.
150. Conn, J. H., Hardy, J. D., Chavez, C. M., Fain, W. R.: Infected arterial grafts: Experience with 22 cases with emphasis on unusual bacterial and technics. *Ann. Surg.* **171**:704–714, 1970.
151. Grimont, P.-A.-D., Grimont, F., Lacut, J.-Y., Issanchou, A.-M., Aubertin, J.: Traitement d'une endocardite à serratia par les bactériophages. *Nouv. Presse Med.* **7**:2251, 1978.
152. Carruthers, M. M.: Endocarditis due to enteric bacilli other than Salmonellae: Case reports and literature review. *Am. J. Med. Sci.* **273**:203–211, 1977.
153. Crittin, J., Waldvogel, F. A.: Endocardities bactériennes: Aspects cliniques, bactériologigues et facteurs de prognostic. *Schweiz. Med. Wochenschr.* **107**(21)(Suppl.):1–26, 1977.
154. Schnurr, L. P., Ball, A. P., Geddes, A. M., Gray, J., McGhie, D.: Bacterial endocarditis in England in the 1970's: Review of 70 patients. *Q. J. Med. N. Ser.* **46**:499–512, 1977.
155. Garvey, G. J., Neu, H. C.: Infective endocarditis—An evolving disease. *Medicine* **57**:105–127, 1978.
156. Hansing, C. E., Allen, V. D., Cherry, J. D.: *Escherichia coli* endocarditis. *Arch. Intern. Med.* **120**:472–477, 1967.
157. Brooks, G. F., O'Donoghue, J. M., Rissing, J. P., Soapes, K., Smith, J. W.: *Eikenella corrodens,* a recently recognized pathogen. *Medicine* **35**:325–342, 1977.

158. Khairat, O.: *Bacteroides corrodens* isolated from bacteremias. *J. Pathol. Bacteriol.* **94**:29–40, 1967.
159. Shinhar, E., Silver, J., Yeivin, R., Shapiro, M.: Polymicrobial endocarditis due to *Eikenella Corrdoens* and Group B streptococcus. *Isr. J. Med. Sci.* **16**:458–459, 1980.
160. Marcus, H. R., Phelps, C. M.: *Eikenella corrodens* subacute bacterial endocarditis—Mixed infection in amphetamine user. *N. Y. State J. Med.* **77**:2259–2261, 1977.
161. Badger, S. J., Butler, T., Kim, C. K., Johnston, K. H.: Experimental *Eikenella corrodens* endocarditis in rabbits. *Infect. Immun.* **23**:751–757, 1978.
162. Wozniak, R., Middleton, J., Chmel, H., de la Cruz, C., Young, R.: Gram-negative endocarditis caused by *Campylobacter fetus. South. Med. J.* **71**:1311–1312, 1978.
163. Rettig, P. J.: Campylobacter infections in human beings. *J. Pediatr.* **94**:855–864, 1979.
164. Ellner, J. J., Rosenthal, M. S., Lerner, P. I., McHenry, M. C.: Infective endocarditis caused by slow-growing, fastidious, gram-negative bacteria. *Medicine* **58**:145–158, 1979.
165. Jemsek, J. G., Greenberg, S. B., Gentry, L. O., Welton, D. E., Mattox, K. L.: *Haemophilus parainfluenzae* endocarditis: Two cases and review of the literature in the past decade. *Am. J. Med.* **66**:51–57, 1979.
166. Geraci, J. E., Wilkowske, C. J., Wilson, W. R., Washington, J. A., II: Haemophilus endocarditis—Report of 14 patients. *Mayo Clin. Proc.* **52**:209–215, 1977.
167. Chunn, C. J., Jones, S. R., McCutchan, J. A., Young, E. J., Gilbert, D. N.: *Haemophilus parainfluenzae* infective endocarditis. *Medicine* **56**:99–113, 1977.
168. Lynn, D. J., Kane, J. G., Parker, R. H.: *Haemophilus parainfluenzae* and influenzae endocarditis: A review of 40 cases. *Medicine* **56**:115–128, 1977.
169. Bieger, R. C., Brewer, N. S., Washington, J. A., II: *Haemophilus aphrophilus:* A microbiologic and clinical review and report of 42 cases. *Medicine* **57**:345–355, 1978.
170. Wormser, G. P., Bottone, E. J., Tudy, J., Hirschman, S. Z.: *Cardiobacterium hominis:* Review of prior infections and report of endocarditis on a fascia lata prosthetic heart valve. *Am. J. Med. Sci.* **276**:117–126, 1978.
171. Geraci, J. E., Griepp, P. R., Wilkowske, C. J., Wilson, W. R., Washington, J. A., II: *Cardiobacterium hominis* endocarditis—Four cases with clinical and laboratory observations. *Mayo Clin. Proc.* **53**:49–53, 1978.
172. Varghese, R., Melo, J. C., Barnwell, P., Chun, C. H., Raff, M. J.: Endocarditis due to *Hemophilus aphrophilus*—Report of a case with possible transmission from dog to man. *Chest* **72**:680–682, 1977.
173. Coker, J. E., Dworzack, D. L., Hodges, G. R., Petrie, S. C., Pugh, D. M.: The infected mitral valve—Floppy mitral valve syndrome complicated by *Haemophilus parainfluenzae* bacterial endocarditis. *J. Kans. Med. Soc.* **79**:550–552, 1978.
174. Hammond, G. W., Richardson, H., Lian, C. J., Ronald, A. R.: Two cases of Hemophilus endocarditis of prolapsed mitral valves—*Hemophilus paraphorphilus* or *parainfluenzae? Am. J. Med.* **65**:537–541, 1978.
175. DeSilva, M., Robin, S. J., Lyons, R. W., Liss, J., Rotatori, R.: *Haemophilus paraphrophilus* endocarditis in a prolapsed mitral valve. *Am. J. Clin. Pathol.* **66**:922–926, 1976.
176. Wauters, J. P., Férguson, R. K., Michaud, P. A., Knobel, P., Fontolliet, C. H.: Glomerulonephritis associated with *Hemophilus aphrophilus* endocarditis. *Clin. Nephrol.* **9**:73–76, 1978.
177. Julander, I., Lindberg, A. A., Svanbom, M.: *Haemophilus parainflueuzae*—An unconscious cause of septicemia and endocarditis. *Scand. J. Infect. Dis.* **12**:85–89, 1980.
178. Weinwurm, J. L.: Endocarditis due to two strains of *Haemophilus parainfluenzae. Can. J. Med. Technol.* **42**:109–110, 1980.
179. Dusheiko, G. M., Cassel, R.: Haemophilus endocarditis, a report of two cases. *S. Afr. Med. J.*, **54**:245–247, 1978.
180. Blair, D. C., Weiner, L. B.: Prosthetic valve endocarditis due to *Haemophilus parainfluenzae* biotype II. *Am. J. Dis. Child.* **133**:617–618, 1979.

181. Laird, W. P., Nelson, J. D., Weinberg, A. G., Huffines, F. D.: Fatal *Haemophilus influenzae* endocarditis diagnosed by echocardiography in an infant. *Pediatrics* **64:**292–295, 1979.
182. Csukás, Z., Bán, E.: *Haemophilus paraphophilius* isolated from endocarditis. *Acta Microbiol. Acad. Sci. Hung.* **25:**179–183, 1978.
183. Cooper, J. A., Lietman, P. S.: Chloramphenicol in Haemophilus endocarditis (letter). *Lancet* **2:**871, 1977.
184. Panwalker, A. P., Akalin, H. E., Zimelis, V., Jackson, G. G.: *Actinobacillus actinomycetemcomitans* endocarditis in a patient with a prosthetic aortic valve. *Infection* **5:**104–106, 1977.
185. Geraci, J. E., Wilson, W. R., Washington, J. A., II: Infective endocarditis caused by *Actinobacillus actinomycetemcomitans:* Report of four cases. *Mayo Clin. Proc.* **55:**415–419, 1980.
186. Reider, J., Wheat, J.: Endocarditis caused by *Actinobacillus actinomycetemcomitan. South. Med. J.* **72:**1219–1220, 1979.
187. Nastro, L. J., Finegold, S. M.: Endocarditis due to anaerobic gram-negative bacilli. *Am. J. Med.* **54:**482–496, 1973.
188. Pape, J., Singer, C., Kiehn, T. E., Lee, B. J., Armstrong, D.: Infective endocarditis caused by *Rothia dentocariosa. Ann. Intern. Med.* **91:**746–747, 1979.
189. Bechard, D. L., Lefroek, J. L., Tillotson, J. R.: Endocarditis caused by *Moraxella nonliquefaciens. South. Med. J.* **72:**1485–1487, 1979.
190. Miridjaman, A., Berrett, D.: Infective endocarditis caused by *Moraxella Kingae. West. J. Med.* **129:**344–346, 1978.
191. Davis, W. A., II, Kane, J. G., Garagusi, V. F.: Human Aeromonas infections: A review of the literature and a case report of endocarditis. *Medicine* **57:**267–277, 1978.
192. Lehamann, V., Knutsen, S. B., Ragnhildstveit, E., Skagseth, E., Solberg, C. O.: Endocarditis caused by *Pasteurella multocida. Scand. J. Infect. Dis.* **9:**247–248, 1977.
193. Cohen, P. S., Maquire, J. H., Weinstein, L.: Infective endocarditis caused by gram-negative bacteria: A review of the literature, 1945–1977. *Prog. Cardiovasc. Dis.* **22:**205–242, 1980.
194. Van Scoy, R. E., Cohen, S. N., Geraci, J. E., Washington, J. A., II: Coryneform bacterial endocarditis. *Mayo Clin. Proc.* **52:**216–219, 1977.
195. Gerry, J. L., Greenough, W. B., III: Diphtheroid endocarditis: Report of nine cases and review of literature. *Johns Hopkins Med. J.* **139:**61–68, 1976.
196. Hornick, R. B.: Source of contamination in open heart surgery, in: *Infection of Prosthetic Heart Valves and Vascular Grafts,* Duma, R. J., ed. University Park Press, Baltimore, pp. 81–99, 1976.
197. Bassan, R.: Bacterial endocarditis produced by *Listeria monocytogenes. Am. J. Clin. Pathol.* **63:**522–527, 1975.
198. Bayer, A. S., Chow, A. W., Guze, L. B.: *Listeria monocytogenes* endocarditis: Report of a case and review of the literature. *Am. J. Med. Sci.* **273:**319–323, 1977.
199. Pitcher, D., Mary, D.: *Listeria monocytogenes* endocarditis in hypertrophic cardiomyopathy. *Br. Med. J.* **1:**961, 1978.
200. Wald, S. L., McLaurin, R. L.: Shunt-associated glomerulonephritis. *Neurosurgery* **3:**146–150, 1978.
201. Leonard, A., Raij, L., Shapiro, F. L.: Bacterial endocarditis in regularly dialyzed patients. *Kidney Int.* **4:**407–422, 1973.
202. Schröter, G. P. J., Weil, R., III: *Listeria monocytogenes* infection after renal transplantation. *Arch. Intern. Med.* **137:**1395–1399, 1977.
203. Armstrong, D.: *Listeria monocytogenes,* in: *Principles and Practice of Infectous Diseases,* Mandell, G. L., Douglas, R. G., Jr.: Bennett, J. E., eds. John Wiley, New York, pp. 1626–1633, 1979.
204. Saravolatz, L. D., Burch, K. H., Madhavan, T., Quinn, E. L.: Listerial prosthetic valve endocarditis. *J. Am. Med. Assoc.* **240:**2186–2187, 1978.
205. Kaplan, J., Stollenwerk, A.: *Listeria monocytogenes* endocarditis (letter). *Arch. Intern. Med.* **137:**1484, 1977.

206. Holshouser, C. A., Ansbacher, R., McNitt, T., Steele, R.: Bacterial endocarditis due to *Listeria monocytogenes* in a pregnant diabetic. *Obstet. Gynecol.* **51**:9s–10s, 1978.
207. Clark, R. A.: Bacterial endocarditis caused by *Listeria monocytogenes. West. J. Med.* **126**:403–405, 1977.
208. Davidson, S., Rotem, Y., Bogkowski, B., Rubenstein, E.: *Corynebacterium diphtheriae* endocarditis. *Am. J. Med. Sci.* **271**:351–353, 1976.
209. Guard, R. W.: Non-toxogenic *Corynebacterium diphtheriae* causing subacute bacterial endocarditis: Case report. *Pathology* **11**:533–535, 1979.
210. Rasmussen, V., Bremmelgaard, A., Korner, B., Hauns, S., Rasmussen, E.: Acute *Corynebacterium endocarditis* causing aortic valve destruction—Successful treatment with antibiotics and valve replacement. *Scand. J. Infect. Dis.* **11**:89–92, 1979.
211. Jootar, P., Gherunpong, V., Saitanu, K.: *Corynebacterium pyogenes* endocarditis—Report of a case with necropsy and review of the literature. *J. Med. Assoc. Thailand* **61**:596–601, 1978.
212. Bolton, W. K., Sande, M. A., Normansell, D. E., Sturgill, B. C., Westervelt, F. B.: Ventriculojugular shunt nephritis with *Corynebacterium bovis. Am. J. Med.* **59**:417–423, 1975.
213. Uff, J. S., Evans, D. J.: 11. Glomerular disease in infective endocarditis, in: Proceedings of the Pathological Society of Great Britain and Ireland. *J. Med. Microbiol.* **10**:Pi, 1977.
214. O'Regan, S., Makker, S. D.: Shunt nephritis: Demonstration of diphtheroid antigen in glomeruli *Amer. J. Med. Sci.* **278**:161–165, 1979.
215. Borchardt, K. A., Sullivan, R. W., Blumberg, R. S., Gelber, R. H., Botch, V., Crull, S., Ullyot, D. J.: *Erysipelothrix rhusiopathiae* endocarditis. *West. J. Med.* **127**:149–151, 1977.
216. Guenel, J., Freland, C., Lucas, J.: Septicémie à *Erysipelothrix rhusiopathiae* avec endocardite—Discussion à propos de 2 nouveaux cas. *Ouest Med.* **30**:1473–1478, 1977.
217. Freland, C.: Les infections à *Erysipelothrix rhusiopathiae*—Revue générale à propos de 31 cas de septicémies avec endocardites reléves dans la litérature. *Pathol. Biol.* **25**:345–352, 1977.
218. Park, C. H., Poretz, D. M., Goldenberg, R.: Erysipelothrix endocarditis with cutaneous lesion. *South. Med. J.* **69**:1101–1103, 1976.
219. James, O., Morgan, O., Adam, M., Schallibaum, E.: *Erysipelothrix insidiosa* endocarditis—A report of two cases in Jamaica. *West Indian Med. J.* **25**:265–268, 1976.
220. Baird, P. J., Benn, R.: Erysipelothrix endocarditis. *Med. J. Aust.* **2**:743–745, 1975.
221. Muirhead, N., Reid, T. M. S.: *Erysipelothrix rhusiopathiae* endocarditis. *J. Infect.* **2**:83, 1980.
222. Tenenbaum, M. J., Warner, J. F.: *Lactobacillus casei* endocarditis (letter). *Ann. Intern. Med.* **82**:539, 1975.
223. Isenberg, D.: Lactobacillus infective endocarditis. *Proc. R. Soc. Med.* **70**:278–281, 1977.
224. Dupont, B., Lapresle, C.: Maladie d'Osler à lactobacille. *Nouv. Presse Med.* **6**:3627–3628, 1977.
225. Block, C. S., Levy, M. L., Fritz, V. U.: *Bacillus cereus* endocarditis. *S. Afr. Med. J.* **53**:556–557, 1978.
226. Reller, L. B., Maddoux, G. L., Eckman, M. R., Pappas, G.: Bacterial endocarditis caused by *Oerskovia turbata. Ann. Intern. Med.* **83**:664–666, 1975.
227. Gutschik, E.: Case report: Endocarditis caused by *Actinomyces viscosus. Scand. J. Infect. Dis.* **8**:271–274, 1976.
228. Schafer, F. J., Wing, E. J., Norden, C. W.: Infectious endocarditis caused by *Rothia dentocariosa. Ann. Intern. Med.* **91**:747–748, 1979.
229. Nastro, L. J., Finegold, S. M.: Endocarditis due to anaerobic gram-negative bacilli. *Am. J. Med.* **54**:482–496, 1973.
230. Felner, J. M., Dowell, V. R., Jr.: Anaerobic bacterial endocarditis. *N. Engl. J. Med.* **283**:1188–1192, 1970.
231. Seggie, J.: Fusobacterium endocarditis treated with metronidazole. *Br. Med. J.* **1**:960–961, 1978.

232. Al-Ibrahim, M. S., Holzman, R. S.: Treatment of Bacteroides endocarditis with carbenicillin. *Am. J. Med. Sci.* **273:**105–107, 1977.
233. McIntosh, C. S., Vickers, P. J., Isaacs, A. J.: Spirillum endocarditis. *Postgrad. Med. J.- 51:645–648, 1975.*
234. Brancaccio, M., Legendre, G. G.: *Megasphaera elsdenii* endocarditis. *J. Clin. Microbiol.* **10:**72–74, 1979.
235. Busch, D. F., Sutter, V. L., Finegold, S. M.: Activity of combinations of antibiotics against *Bacteroides fragilis. J. Infect. Dis.* **133:**321–328, 1976.
236. Carrizosa, J., Tanphaichitra, D., Levison, M. E.: Experimental *Bacteroides fragilis* endocarditis in rabbits. *Infect. Immun.* **15:**871–973, 1977.
237. Goldman, P. L., Durack, D. T., Petersdorf, R. G.: Effect of antibiotics on the prevention of experimental *Bacteroides fragilis* endocarditis. *Antimicrobial Agents Chemother.* **14:**755–760, 1978.
238. Durack, D. T., Peterdorf, R. G.: Chemotherapy of experimental streptococcal endocarditis. I. Comparison of commonly recommended prophylactic regimens. *J. Clin. Invest.* **52:**592–598, 1973.
239. Ward, C., Sagar, H. J., Cooper, D., Ward, A. M.: Insidious endocarditis caused by *Chlamydia psittaci. Br. Med. J.* **4:**734–735, 1975.
240. Dick, D. C., McGregor, C. G. A., Mitchell, K. G., Sommerville, R. G., Wheatley, D. J.: Endocarditis as a manifestation of Chlamydia B infection (psittacosis). *Br. Heart J.* **39:**914–916, 1977.
241. Van der Bel-Kahn, J. M., Watanakunakorn, C., Menefee, M. G., Long, H. D., Dicter, R.: *Chlamydia trachomatis* endocarditis. *Am. Heart J.* **95:**627–636, 1978.
242. Editorial: Chlamydial endocarditis. *Lancet* **1:**132, 1980.
243. Regan, R. J., Dathan, J. R. E., and Treharne, J. D.: Infective endocarditis with glomerulonephritis associated with cat *Chlamydia (C. psittaci)* infection. *Br. Heart J.* **42:**349–352, 1979.
244. Laskowski, L. F., Marr, J. J., Spernoga, J. F., Frank, N. J., Barner, H. B., Kaiser, G., Tyras, D. H.: Fastidious mycobacteria grown from porcine prosthetic-heart-valve cultures. *N. Engl. J. Med.* **297:**101–102, 1977.
245. Levy, C., Curtin, J. A., Watkins, A., Marsh, B., Garcia, J., Mispireta, L.: *Mycobacterium chelonei* infection of porcine heart valves. *N. Engl. J. Med.* **297:**667–668, 1977.
246. O'Rourke, F., Shanahan, M. X., Harkness, J. L.: Endocarditis with an acid-fast organism after porcine heart-valve replacement (letter). *Lancet* **2:**686, 1978.
247. Matthews, P. R. J., McDiarmid, A.: Endocarditis with acid-fast organism after porcine heart-valve replacement (letter). *Lancet* **2:**844, 1978.
248. Altmann, G., Horowitz, A., Kaplinsky, N., Frankl, O.: Prosthetic valve endocarditis due to *Mycobacterium chelonei. J. Clin. Microbiol.* **1:**531–533, 1975.
249. Becker, G. J., Walker, R. G., Dziukas, L. J., Harvey, K. J., Valentine, R., Kincaid-Smith, P.: Renal infection with *Mycobacterium chelonei. Aust. N. Z. J. Med.* **10:**44–47,1980.
250. Narasimhan, S. L., Austin, T. W.: Prosthetic valve endocarditis due to *Mycobacterium fortuitum. Can. Med. Assoc.* **119:**154–155, 1978.
251. Wainwright, J.: Tuberculous endocarditis—A report of 2 cases. *S. Afr. Med. J.* **56:**731–733, 1979.
252. Rosman, M. S., Lubbe, W. F., Hayden, M., Basson, N., Uys, C. J.: Q fever endocarditis, a report of two cases. *S. Afr. Med. J.* **53:**296–300, 1978.
253. Wilson, H. G., Neilson, G. H., Galea, E. G., Stafford, G., O'Brien, M. F.: Q fever endocarditis in Queensland. *Circulation* **53:**680–684, 1976.
254. Turck, W. P. G., Howitt, G., Turnberg, L. A., Fox, H., Longson, M., Matthews, M. B., Das Gupta, R.: Chronic Q fever. *Q. J. Med. N. Ser.* **45:**193–217, 1976.
255. Kimbrough, R. C., Ormsbee, R. A., Peacock, M., Rogers, W. R., Bennets, R. W., Raaf, J., Krause, A., Gardner, C.: Q Fever endocarditis in the United States. *Ann. Intern. Med.* **91:**400–402, 1979.

256. Marquez, A. U. Junyent, J. M., Arara, V. V., Saqué, A. P., Cardellach, F., Lopez, F. N., Revert, L., Ròzman Y. C.: Endocarditis por *Coxiella burnetti* forma crónica de la fiebre Q: A propòsito de un caso. *Med. Clin. (Barcelona)* **73**:242–246, 1979.
257. Hall, G. H., Hart R. J. C., Davies, S. W., George, M., Head, A. C.: Glomerulonephritis associated with *Coxiella burnetti* endocarditis (letter). *Br. Med. J.* **2**:275, 1975.
258. Hossack, K. F., Neilson, G. H.: Excercise testing following aortic valve replacement for aortic incompetence due to Q fever endocarditis and bacterial endocarditis (abstract). *Aust. N. Z. J. Med.* **6**:184, 1976.
259. Turck, W. P. G.: Observations on Q fever endocarditis (letter). *Am. Heart J.* **96**:564–565, 1978.
260. Lerner, A. M.: Myocarditis and pericarditis, in: *Principles and Practice of Infectious Diseases*, Mandell, G. L., Douglas, R. G., Jr., Bennett, J. E., eds. John Wiley, New York, pp. 711–723, 1979.
261. Durack, D. T., Beeson, P. B., Petersdorf, R. G.: Experimental bacterial endocarditis. III. Production and progress of the disease in rabbits. *Br. J. Exp. Pathol.* **54**:142–151, 1973.
262. Reisberg, B. E.: Infective endocarditis in the narcotic addict. *Prog. Cardiovasc. Dis.* **22**:193–204, 1979.
263. Curry, C. R., Quie, P. G.: Fungal septicemia in patients receiving parenteral hyperalimentation. *N. Engl. J. Med.* **285**:1221–1225, 1971.
264. Canlas, M. S., Dillon, M. L., Jr.: *Histoplasma capsulatum* endocarditis: Report of a case following heart surgery. *Angiology* **28**:454–463, 1977.
265. Alexander, W. J., Mowry, R. W., Cobbs, C. G., Dismukes, W. E.: Prosthetic valve endocarditis caused by *histoplasma capsulatum*. *J. Am. Med. Assoc.* **242**:1399–1400, 1979.
266. Meleny, H. E., cited by Kerr [(292)] (p. 78).
267. Walsh, T. J., Hutchins, G. M.: Aspergillus mural endocarditis. *Am. J. Clin. Pathol.* **71**:640–644, 1979.
268. Case Records of the Massachusetts General Hospital: Case 27-1979. *N. Engl. J. Med.* **301**:34–42, 1979.
269. Rubenstein, E., Noriega, E. R., Simberkoff, M. S., Holzman, R., Rahal, J. J.: Fungal endocarditis: Analysis of 24 cases and review of the literature. *Medicine* **54**:331–344, 1975.
270. Galgiani, J. N., Stevens, D. A.: Fungal endocarditis: Need for guidelines in evaluating therapy—Experience with two patients previously reported. *J. Thorac. Cardiovasc. Surg.* **73**:293–296, 1977.
271. Carrizosa, J., Kohn, C., Levison, M. E.: Experimental Aspergillus endocarditis in rabbits. *J. Lab. Clin. Med.* **86**:746–753, 1975.
272. Iannini, P. B., Everett, E. D., Pappas, G., LaForce, F. M.: *Candida precipitins* as a diagnostic aid in Candida endocarditis. *J. Am. Med. Assoc.* **236**:2518–2520, 1976.
273. Bacon, P. A., Davidson, C., Smith, B.: Antibodies to Candida and autoantibodies in subacute bacterial endocarditis. *Q. J. Med. N. Ser.* **43**:537–550, 1974.
274. Wain, W., Thompson, R., Ahmed, M., Yacoub, M.: The role of chemotherapy in the management of fungal endocarditis following homograft valve replacement. *Postgrad. Med. J.* **55**:629–631, 1979.
275. Medoff, G., Kobayashi: G. S.: Strategies in treatment of septenia fungal infections. *N. Engl. J. Med.* **302**:145–155, 1980.
276. Weinstein, L., Schlesinger, J.: Treatment of infective endocarditis—1973, in: *Progress in Cardiovascular Diseases*, Vol. XVI, Sonnenblick, E. H., ed. Grune and Stratton, New York, pp. 275–302, 1973.
277. Sande, M. A., Bowman, C. R., Calderone, R. A.: Experimental *Candida albicans* endocarditis: Characterization of the disease and response to therapy. *Infect. Immun.* **17**:140–147, 1977.
278. Calderone, R. A., Rotondo, M. F., Sande, M. A.: *Candida albicans* endocarditis: Ultrastructural studies of vegetation formation. *Infect. Immun.* **20**:279–289, 1978.

279. Al-Doory, Y., Paasch, L. H., Zook, B. C., Rhorer, R. G.: Pathological studies in experimental candida endocarditis. *Jpn. Heart J.* **20**:427–440, 1979.
280. Southwick, F. S., Durack, D. T.: Chemotherapy of experimental streptococcal endocarditis. III. Failure of a bacteriostatic agent (tetracycline) in prophylaxis. *J. Clin. Pathol.* **27**:261–264, 1974.
281. Pelletier, L. L., Durack, D. T., Petersdorf, R. G., Nielson, K.: Chemotherapy of experimental streptococcal endocarditis. IV. Further observations on prophylaxis. *J. Clin. Invest.* **56**:319–330, 1975.
282. Durack, D. T., Starkebaum, M. K., Petersdorf, R. G.: Chemotherapy of experimental endocarditis. VI. Prevention of enterococcal endocarditis. *J. Lab. Clin. Med.* **90**:171–179, 1977.
283. McClellan, J. R., Hamilton, J. D., Alexander, J. A., Wolfe, W. G., Reed, J. B.: *Paecilomyces varioti* endocarditis on a prosthetic aortic valve. *J. Thorac. Cardiovasc. Surg.* **71**:472–475, 1976.
284. Naveh, Y., Friedman, A., Merzbach, D., Hashman, N.: Case reports: Endocarditis caused by rhodotorula successfully treated with 5 fluorocytosine. *Br. Heart J.* **37**:101–104, 1975.
285. Cornere, B. M.: *Torulopsis glabrata* endocarditis (letter). *Am. J. Clin. Pathol.* **71**:737, 1979.
286. Marier, R., Zakhireh, B., Downs, J., Wynne, B., Hammond, G. L., Andriole, V. T.: *Trichosporon cutaneum* endocarditis. *Scand. J. Infect. Dis.* **10**:255–256, 1978.
287. Roberts, F. J., Allen, P., Maybee, T. K.: *Petriellidium boydii (Allescheria boydii)* endocarditis associated with porcine valve replacement (letter). *Can. Med. Assoc. J.* **117**:1250–1252, 1977.
288. Davis, W. A., Isner, J., Bracery, A., Roberts, W. C., Garagusi, V. F.: Disseminated *Petriellidium boydii* and pacemaker endocarditis. *Am. J. Med.* **69**:929–932, 1980.
289. Ruegsegger, J. M.: Pneumococcal endocarditis. *Am. Heart J.* **56**:867–877, 1958.
290. Svanbom, M., Strandell, T.: Bacterial endocarditis. I. A prospective study of etiology, underlying factors and foci of infection. *Scand. J. Infect. Dis.* **10**:193–202, 1978.
291. Tolaymat, A., Rhatigan, R. M., Levin, S.: Pneumococcal endocarditis in infants. *South. Med. J.* **72**:448–451, 1979.
292. Kerr, A.: *Subacute Bacterial Endocarditis.* Charles C. Thomas, Springfield, Illinois, 343 pages, 1955.
293. Condie, F, Handsfield, H. H., Taylor, J. W., Klopfenstein, L.: Death due to gonococcal endocarditis—Washington State. *Morbid. Mortal. Weekly Rep.* **28**:261, 1979.
294. John, J. F., Nichols, J. T., Eisenhower, E. A., Farrar, W. E.: Gonococcal endocarditis. *Sexually Transm. Dis.* **4**:84–88, 1977.
295. Dzindzio, B. S., Meyer, L. R., Osterholm, R., Hopeman, A., Woltjen, J., Forker, A. D.: Isolated gonococcal pulmonary valve endocarditis: Diagnosis by echocardiography. *Circulation* **59**:1319–1324, 1979.
296. Cooke, D. B., Arensberg, D., Felner, J. M., Rimland, D., Lesser, L. M.: Gonococcal endocarditis in the antibiotic era. *Arch. Intern. Med.* **139**:1247–1250, 1979.
297. Kaspar, R. L., Drutz, D. J.: Perihepatitis and hepatitis as complications of experimental endocarditis due to *Neisseria gonorrhoeae* in the rabbit. *J. Infect. Dis.* **136**:37–42, 1977.
298. Dennis, J., Edwards, L. D., Fisher, T. N., Makeever, L:. Endocarditis on a Bjork–Shiley mitral prosthesis due to *Neisseria meningitidis*. *Scand. J. Thorac. Cardiovasc. Surg.* **11**:205–209, 1977.
299. Fass, R. J., Saslaw, S.: Chronic meningococcemia. *Arch. Intern. Med.* **130**:943–946, 1972.
300. Gay, R. M., Sevier, R. E.: *Neisseria sicca* endocarditis: Report of a case and review of the literature. *J. Clin. Microbiol.* **8**:729–732, 1978.
301. Pollock, A. A., Holzman, R. S.: *Neisseria catarrhalis* endocarditis. *Ann. Intern. Med.* **85**:206–207, 1976.
302. Douer, D., Danziger, Y., Pinkhas, J.: *Neisseria catarrhalis* endocarditis (letter). *Ann. Intern. Med.* **86**:116, 1977.

303. Keys, T. F., Hewitt, W. L.: Endocarditis due to micrococci and *Staphylococcus epidermidis*. *Arch. Intern. Med.* **132**:216–220, 1973.
304. Bernardet, P., Auvergnat, J.-C., Donzear, J.-P., Suc, C., Sabot, G., Sassi, J.-L.: Endocardites bactériennes à *Staphylococcus epidermidis*. *Nouv. Presse Med.* **8**:1671–1673, 1979.
305. Williams, D. N., Peterson, P. K., Verhoef, J., Laverdiere, M., Sabath, L. D.: Endocarditis caused by coagulase-negative Staphylococci. *Infection* **7**:5–9, 1979.
306. Schoenbaum, S. C., Gardner, P., Shillito, J.: Infections of cerebro-spinal fluid shunts: Epidemiology, clinical manifestations and therapy. *J. Infect. Dis.* **131**:543–552, 1975.
307. Labrune, B., Levy, M., Bauby, C., Gubler, M.-C., Mallet, R.: Les glomerulonephrites secondaires aux derivations ventriculo-atriales ("shunt nephritis"). *Arch. Fr. Pediatr.* **30**:793–808, 1973.
308. Stickler, G. B., Shin, M. H., Burke, E. C., Holley, K. E., Miller, R. H., Segar, W. E.: Diffuse glomerulonephritis associated with infected ventriculoatrial shunt. *N. Engl. J. Med.* **279**:1077–1082, 1968.
309. Verhoef, J., Peterson, P. K., Williams, D. N., Laverdiere, M., Sabath, L. D.: Atrio-ventricular shunt infections and endocarditis due to *Staphylococcus epidermidis*. *Zentralbl. Bakteriol. Hyg. Parasitenkd. Abt. 1: Orig Infektionskr.* **A241**:95–100, 1978.
310. Old, D. C., McNeill, G. P.: Endocarditis due to *Micrococcus sedentarius incertae sedis*. *J. Clin. Pathol.* **32**:951–952, 1979.
311. Rhame, F. S., Maki, D. G., Bennett, J. V.: Intravenous cannula-associated infections, in: *Hospital Infections*, Bennett, J. V., Brachman, P. S., eds. Little, Brown, Boston, pp. 433–442, 1979.
312. Karchmer, A. W., Dismukes, W. E., Johnson, W. D., Jr., Wilson, W. R., Archer, G. L., Sande, M. A.: *Staphylococcus epidermidis* prosthetic valve endocarditis. 11th International Congress of Chemotherapy and 19th Interscience Conference on Antimicrobial Agents and Chemotherapy, 1979, Abstract 365.
313. Liekweg, W. G. J., Levinson, S. A., Greenfield, L. J.: Infections of vascular grafts: Incidence, anatomic location, etiologic agents, morbidity and mortality, in: *Infections of Prosthetic Heart Valves and Vascular Grafts*, Duma, R. J., ed. University Park Press, Baltimore, pp. 239–251, 1977.
314. Penicillin-resistant Viridans streptococcal endocarditis—North Carolina. *Morbid. Mortal. Weekly Rep.* **28**:327–333, 1979.
315. Bourgault, A.-M., Wilson, W. R., Washington, J. A., II: Antimicrobial susceptibilities of species of Viridans Streptococci. *J. Infect. Dis.* **140**:316–321, 1979.
316. Klein, R. S., Recco, R. A., Catalano, M. T., Edberg, S. C., Casey, J. I., Steigbigel, N. H.: Association of *Streptococcus bovis* with carcinoma of the colon. *N. Engl. J. Med.* **297**:800–802, 1977.
317. Noble, C. J., Uttley, A. H. C., Falk, R. H., Richardson, P. J.: *Streptococcus bovis* endocarditis and colonic cancer (letter). *Lancet* **1**:766, 1978.
318. Brooks, R. J., Ravreby, W. D., Keusch, G., Bottone, E.: More on *Streptococcus bovis* endocarditis and bowel carcinoma (letter). *N. Engl. J. Med.* **298**:572, 1978.
319. Levy, B. S., Von Reyon, C. F., Arbeit, R. D., Friedland, J., Crumpacker, C.: More on *Streptococcus bovis* endocarditis and bowel carcinoma (letter). *N. Engl. J. Med.* **298**:572–573, 1978.
320. Murray, H. W., Roberts, R. B.: *Streptococcus bovis* bacteremia heralding serious gastrointestinal disease. 17th ICAAC, 1977, Abstract 376.
321. Ponge, B., Launois, J. P.: Association cancer digestif et endocardite subaigüe. *Nouv. Presse Med.* **8**:2201, 1979.
322. Dorra, M., Dechy, H., Dournon, E., Le Mercier, Y., Coulbois, J., Lang, F.: Association d'endocardites à streptocoques D avec des cancers digestifs—Remarques critiques sur la notion de la portée. *Nouv. Presse Med.* **8**:3174, 1979.

323. Dunham, W. R., Simpson, J. H., Feest, T. G., Cruickshank, J. G.: *Streptococcus bovis* endocarditis and colorectal disease. *Lancet* **1:**421–422, 1980.
324. Wasilauskas, B. L.: Subacute bacterial endocarditis caused by Group G hemolytic Streptococcus. *Am. J. Dis. Child.* **131:**1416–1417, 1977.
325. Bouza, E., Meyer, R. D., Busch, D. F.: Group G streptococcal endocarditis. *Am. J. Clin. Pathol.* **70:**108–111, 1978.
326. Savitch, C. B., Barry, A. L., Hoeprich, P. D., Infective endocarditis caused by *Streptococcus bovis* resistant to the lethal effect of penicillin G. *Arch. Intern. Med.* **138:**931–934, 1978.
327. Scheld, W. M., Sande, M. A.: Endocarditis and intravascular infections, in: *Principles and Practice of Infectious Diseases,* Mandell, G. L., Douglas, R. G., Bennett, J. E., eds. John Wiley, New York, pp. 653–690, 1979.
328. Parillo, J. E., Borst, C. G., Lt., Mazur, M. H., Iannini, P., Lt. Cd., Klempner, M. S., Moellering, R. C., Jr., Anderson, S. E., Cd.: Endocarditis due to resistant viridans Streptococci during oral penicillin chemoprophylaxis. *N. Engl. J. Med.* **300:**296–300, 1979.
329. Burch, K., Quinn, E. L., Romig, D., Cox, F., Fisher, E., Madhavan, T.: Penicillin-resistant viridans streptococcus endocarditis related to the administration of penicillin G or carbenicillin and alterations in mouth flora. *Henry Ford Hosp. Med. J.* **23:**3–8, 1975.
330. Upton, G. W., Dalton, H. P., Kolstad, R. A.: Bacteriocin typing of streptococcal isolates from endocarditis. *J. Clin. Microbiol.* **5:**517–520, 1977.
331. Masur, H., Murray, H. W., Gross, K., Roberts, R. B.: *Streptococcus milleri:* A viridans streptococcus causing significant pyogenic infection. *17th Interscience Conference on Antimicrobial Agents and Chemotherapy,* 1977, *Abstract 375.*
332. Smith, J. P., Marymont, J. H., Schweers, J. H.: Subacute bacterial endocarditis due to *Streptococcus mutans. Am. J. Med. Technol.* **43:**429–432, 1976.
333. Horodniceanu, T., Delbos, F., Chabbert, Y. A.: Caractéristiques des socuhes de *Streptococcus mutans* isolées d'endocardites subaigües et sensibilité aux antibiotiques. *Ann. Microbiol.* **128A:**205–216, 1977.
334. Emmerson, A. M., Eykyn, S.: *Streptococcus mutans* endocarditis—A trap for the unwary (letter). *Br. Med. J.* **1:**905, 1977.
335. Blair, D. C., Martin, D. B.: Beta hemolytic streptococcal endocarditis: Predominance of non-group a organisms. *Am. J. Med. Sci.* **276:**269–277, 1978.
336. Jones, J. E. T.: Bacterial endocarditis in the pig with special reference to streptococcal endocarditis. *J. Comp. Pathol.* **90:**11–28, 1980.
337. Vilde, J.-L., Roujeau, J.-C., Bure, A., Verliac, F., Bastin, R.: Infections graves et septicémies à streptocoque du groupe B chez l'adulte—A propos de 4 observations, dont une endocardite tricuspidienne compliquée de glomerulonéphrite. *Sem. Hop. Paris* **50:**355–362, 1974.
338. John, J. F., Jr., Cook, F. V.: Endocarditis associated with disseminated group B streptococcal infection. *Amer. J. Med. Sci.* **274:**197–201, 1977.
339. Hager, W. D., Speck, E. L., Mathew, P. K., Boger, J. N., Wallace, W. A.: Endocarditis with myocardial abscesses and pericarditis in an adult—Group B streptococcus as a cause. *Arch. Intern. Med.* **137:**1725–1728, 1977.
340. Reid, T. M. S.: Group B streptococcal endocarditis. *Scot. Med. J.* **22:**13–15, 1977.
341. Lerner, P. I., Gopalakrishna, K. V., Wolinsky, E., McHenry, M. C., Tan, J. S., Rosenthal, M.: Group B streptococcus *(S. agalactiae)* bacteremia in adults: Analysis of 32 cases and review of the literature. *Medicine* **56:**457–473, 1977.
342. Murcia, A., Lyons, R. W.: Group B streptococcus endocarditis in a prosthetic valve. *Arch. Intern. Med.* **138:**1304–1306, 1978.
343. Jemsek, J. G., Gentry, L. O., Greenberg, S. B.: Malignant Group B streptococcal endocarditis associated with saline-induced abortion. *Chest* **76:**965–967, 1979.
344. Untereker, W. J., Hanna, B. A.: Endocarditis and osteomyelitis caused by *Aerococcus viridans. Mt. Sinai J. Med.* **43:**248–252, 1976.

345. Gorbach, S. L.: Other anaerobic bacteria, in: *Principles and Practice of Infectious Diseases*, Mandell, G. L., Douglas, R. G., Bennett, J. E., eds. John Wiley, New York, pp. 1893–1899, 1979.
346. Boyd, A. D., Spencer, F. C., Isom, O. W., Cunningham, J. N., Reed, G. E., Acinapura, A. J., Tice, D. A.: Infective endocarditis—An analysis of 54 surgically treated patients. *J. Thorac. Cardiovasc. Surg.* **73:**23–30, 1977.
347. Okies, J. E., Starr, A.: Cardiac surgery in infective endocarditis, in: *Infective Endocarditis*, Rahimtoola, S. H., ed. Grune and Stratton, New York, pp. 361–377, 1978.
348. Stinson, E. B.: Surgical treatment of infective endocarditis. *Prog. Cardiovasc. Dis.* **22:**145–168, 1979.
. 349. McAnulty, J. H., Rahimtoola, S. H.: Surgery for infective endocarditis. *Clin. Cardiol.* **242:**77–79, 1979.
350. Editorial: Surgical treatment of infective endocarditis. *Lancet* **1:**194–195, 1979.
351. Rapaport, E.: Editorial: The changing role of surgery of the management of infective endocarditis. *Circulation* **58:**598–599, 1978.
352. Black, S., O'Rourke, R. A., Karliner, J. S.: Role of surgery in the treatment of primary infective endocarditis. *Am. J. Med.* **56:**357–368, 1974.
353. Wilson, W. R., Danielson, G. K., Giuliani, E. R., Washington, J. A., II, Jaumin, P. M., Geraci, J. E.: Cardiac valve replacement in congestive heart failure due to infective endocarditis. *Mayo Clin. Proc.* **54:**223–226, 1979.
354. Richardson, J. V., Karp, R. B., Kirklin, J. W., Dismukes, W. E.: Treatment of infective endocarditis: A 10-year comparative analysis. *Circulation* **58:**589–597, 1978.
355. Borges, J. S., Roberts, R. B., Johnson, W. D.: Bacterial endocarditis: Valve replacement in aortic insufficiency. *Ann. Intern. Med.* **79:**757–758, 1973.
356. Becker, R. M., Frishman, W., Frater, R. M.: Surgery for mitral valve endocarditis. *Chest* **75:**314–319, 1979.
357. Brockman, S. K., Aprill, S. N., Rabiner, F. S.: Aortic valve replacement in hemophilia—Report of a case. *J. Am. Med. Assoc.* **222:**660–661, 1972.
358. Nazarian, M., McCullough, G. H., Fielder, D. L.: Bacterial endocarditis in pregnancy—Successful surgical correction. *J. Thorac. Cardiovasc. Surg.* **71:**880–883, 1976.
359. Bastin, R., Le Heuzy, J. Y., Frottier, J., Vilde, J. L., Bricaire, F., Kernbaum, S., Verliac, F.: Endocardite bactérienne et insuffisance mitrale avec rupture de cordages. *Med. Malad. Infect.* **9:**603–608, 1979.
360. Heraief, E., Glauser, M., Freedman, L. R.: Vancomycin prophylaxis of streptococcal endocarditis in rats, in: *Current Chemotherapy and Infectious Disease (Proceedings of the 11th International Congress of Chemotherapy and 19th Interscience Conference on Antimicrobial Agents and Chemotherapy,* American Society of Microbiology, Washington, D.C., pp. 911–913, 1980.
361. Roberts, W. C.: Characteristics and consequences of infective endocarditis (active or healed or both) learned from morphologic studies, in: *Infective Endocarditis*, Rahimtoola, S. H., ed. Grune and Stratton, New York, pp. 55–123, 1978.
362. Sethia, B., Williams, B. T.: Tricuspid valve excision without replacement in a case of endocarditis secondary to drug abuse. *Br. Heart J.* **40:**579–580, 1978.
363. Simberkoff, M. S., Isom, W., Smithivas, T.: Noriega, E. R., Rahal, J. J.: Two-stage tricuspid valve replacement for mixed bacterial endocarditis. *Arch. Intern. Med.* **133:**212–216, 1974.
364. Wright, J. S., Glennie, J. S.: Excision of tricuspid valve with later replacement in endocarditis of drug addiction. *Thorax* **33:**518–519, 1978.
365. Arneborn, P., Björk, V. O., Rodriguez, L., Svanbom, M.: Two-stage replacement of tricuspid valve in active endocarditis. *Br. Heart J.* **39:**1276–1278, 1977.
366. Reller, L. B.: Valve resection for endocarditis (letter). *Ann. Intern. Med.* **90:**277–278, 1979.

367. Egeblad, H., Wennevold, A., Berning, J., Lauridsen, P.: Mitral valve replacement in infective endocarditis as prophylaxis against embolism: Identification of patients at risk by 2-dimensional echocardiogarphy. *Eur. J. Cardiol.* **10:**369–373, 1979.
368. Pfeifer, J. F., Lipton, M. J., Oury, J. H., Angell, W. W., Hultgren, H. N.: Acute coronary embolism complicating bacterial endocarditis: Operative treatment. *Am. J. Cardiol.* **37:**920–922, 1976.
369. Montague, N. T., Sugg, W. L.: Candida endocarditis with femoral emboli. *J. Thorac. Cardiovasc. Surg.* **67:**322–327, 1974.
370. Gladstone, J. L., Friedman, S. A., Cerruti, M. M., Jomain, S. L.: Treatment of candida endocarditis and arteritis. *J. Thorac. Cardiovasc. Surg.* **71:**835–838, 1976.
371. Gulmen, S., Anderson, W. R.: Candida endocarditis with distal aortic embolization. *Minn. Med.* **60:**469–471, 1977.
372. Collins, G. J., Rich, N. M., Hobson, R. W., Anderson, C. A., Green, D.: Multiple mycotic aneurisms due to candida endocarditis. *Ann. Surg.* **186:**136–139, 1977.
373. Weinstein, L., Rubin, R. H.: Infective endocarditis—1973, in: *Progress in Cardiovascular Diseases,* Vol. XVI, No. 3, Sonnenblick, E. H., ed., Grune and Stratton, New York, pp. 239–274, 1973.
374. Danielson, G. K., Titus, J. L., DuShane, J. W.: Successful treatment of aortic valve endocarditis and aortic root abacesses by insertion of prosthetic valve in ascending aorta and placement of bypass grafts to coronary arteries. *J. Thorac. Cardiovasc. Surg.* **67:**443–449, 1974.
375. Pitlik, S., Cohen, L., Melamed, R., Rosenfeld, J.: Mural endocarditis associated with recurrent false aneurysm of the left ventricle. *Chest* **71:**227–229, 1977.
376. Frantz, P. T., Murray, G. F., Benson, R. W.: Surgical management of left ventricular aortic discontinuity complicating bacterial endocarditis. *Ann. Thorac. Surg.* **29:**1–7, 1980.
377. Lindenauer, S. M.: Surgical treatment of infected grafts, in: *Infections of Prosthetic Heart Valves and Vascular Grafts,* Duma, R. J., ed. University Park Press, Baltimore, pp. 287–302, 1977.
378. Maki, D. G., Jarrett, F., Sarafin, H. W.: A semiquantitative culture method for indentification of catheter-related infection in the burn patient. *J. Surg. Res.* **22:**513–520, 1977.
379. Garrison, P., Freedman, L. R.: Experimental endocarditis. I. Staphylococcal endocarditis in rabbits resulting from placement of a polyethylene catheter in the right side of the heart. *Yale J. Biol. Med.* **42:**394–410, 1970.
380. Goldmann, D. A., Maki, D. G.: Infection control in total parenteral nutrition. *J. Am. Med. Assoc.* **223:**1360–1364, 1973.
381. Dillon, J. D., Jr., Schaffner, W., Van Way, C. W., III, Meng, H. C.: Septicemia and total parenteral nutrition—Distinguishing catheter-related from other septic episodes. *J. Am. Med. Assoc.* **223:**1341–1344, 1973.
382. Montgomerie, J. Z., Edwards, J. E., Jr.: Association of infection due to *Candida albicans* with intravenous hyperalimentation. *J. Infect. Dis.* **137:**197–201, 1978.
383. Band, J. D., Maki, D. G.: Infections caused by arterial catheters used for hemodynamic monitoring. *Am. J. Med.* **67:**735–741, 1979.
384. McGoon, M. D., Benedetto, P. W., Greene, B. M.: Complications of percutaneous central venous catherization: A report of two cases and review of the literature. *Johns Hopkins Med. J.* **145:**1–6, 1979.
385. Sande, M. A., Levison, M. E., Lukas, D. S., Kaye, D.: Bacteremia associated with cardiac catheterization. *N. Engl. J. Med.* **281:**1104–1106, 1969.
386. Sipes, J. N., Thompson, R. L., Hook, E. W.: Prophylaxis of infective endocarditis: A reevaluation *Annu. Rev. Med.* **28:**371–391, 1977.

387. Rubin, S. J., Lyons, R. W., Murcia, A. J.: Endocarditis associated with cardiac catheterization due to a gram-positive coccus designated *Micrococcus mucilaginosus incertae sedis*. *J. Clin. Microbiol.* **7**:546–549, 1978.
388. Delaye, J., Beaune, J., Pourchaire, J., Loire, R.: Gonin, A.: Les risques de l'exploration hémodynamique dans l'endocardite infectieuse. *Coeur Med. Interne* **15**:533–540, 1976.
389. Garcia, R., Hakimi-Naini, M.: Bacterial endocarditis and incarceration of a transvenous pacemaker. *Henry Ford Hosp. Med. J.* **23**:135–140, 1975.
390. Ward, C., Naik, D. R., Jonstone, M. C.: Tricuspid endocarditis complicating pacemaker implantation demonstrated by echocardiography. *Br. J. Radiol.* **52**:501–502, 1979.
391. Bryan, C. S., Sutton, J. P., Saunders, D. E., Longaker, D. W., Smith, C. W.: Endocarditis related to transvenous pacemakers. *J. Thorac. Cardiovasc. Surg.* **75**:758–762, 1978.
392. Leonard, A., Raij, L., Shapiro, F. L.: Bacterial endocarditis in regularly dialyzed patients. *Kidney Int.* **4**:407–422, 1973.
393. Storck, D., Jeanmaire, H., Geitner, S., Kuntz, J. L., Herrmann, P.: Endocarditis bactériennes revelées par des manifestations rhumatismales. *J. Med. Strasbourg* **8**:537–540, 1977.
394. Choubrac, P., Mathé, G., Haas, C., Crickx, B., Robin, P.-M., Dyan, A., Dubois, G.: Spondylodiscites révélatrices d'endocardites bactériennes. *Ann. Med. Interne* **127**:117–121, 1976.
395. Acar, J.-F., Durin, R., Deloux, G., Barthalon, M., Guibert, J.: A propos de deux cas de spondylodiscites révélatrices d'une endocardite à *Streptocoque viridans*. *Gaz. Med. Fr.* **81**:2351–2356, 1974.
396. Good, A. E., Hague, J. M., Kauffmann, C. A.: Streptococcal endocarditis initially seen as septic arthritis. *Arch. Intern. Med.* **138**:805–806, 1978.
397. Rodriguez, C., Ryckewaert, A., Dryll, A.: Manifestations articulaires et musculaires des endocardites bactériennes. *Nouv. Presse Med.* **7**:4111–4114, 1978.
398. Mund, D. J.: Pyogenic vertebral osteomyelitis—Manifestation of bacterial endocarditis. *N. Y. State J. Med.* **80**:980–982, 1980.
399. Musher, D. M., Thorsteinsson, S. B., Minuth, J. N., Luchi, R. J.: Vertebral osteomyelitis—Still a diagnostic pitfall. *Arch. Intern. Med.* **136**:105–110, 1976.
400. Baglin, A., Normand, J.-P., Tancrède, C., Callard, P., Brunet, A., Fritel, D.: Anurie prolongée au cours d'une endocardite bactérienne. *Ann. Med. Interne.* **126**:241–250, 1975.
401. Pertschuk, L. P., Vuletin, J. C., Sutton, A. L., Velazquez, L. A.: Demonstration of antigen and immune complex in glomerulonephritis due to *Staphylococcus aureus*. *Am. J. Clin. Pathol.* **66**:1027, 1976.
402. McKenzie, P. E., Taylor, A. E., Woodroffe, A. J., Seymour, A. E., Chan, Y.-L., Clarkson, A. R.: Plasmapheresis in glomerulonephritis. *Clin. Nephrol.* **12**:97–108, 1979.
403. Holloway, Y., Dankert, J., Hess, J.: Penicillin tolerance and bacterial endocarditis. *Lancet* **1**:589, 1980.
404. Pelletier, L. L.: Treatment of experimental *Staphyloccus aureus* endocarditis: Effect of methicillin tolerance. *Clin. Res.* **28**:376A, 1980.
405. Savitch, C. B., Pulliam, L., Cooper, R., Mills, J.: β-Lactam tolerance among strains of viridans streptococci recovered from patients with endocarditis previously treated with antimicrobials. 20th ICAAC, 1980, Abstract 355.
406. Pelletier, L. L., Petersdorf, R. G.: Infective endocarditis: A review of 125 cases from the University of Washington Hospitals, 1963–1972. *Medicine* **56**(4):287–313, 1977.
407. Sande, M. A., Scheld, W. M.: Combination antibiotic therapy of bacterial endocarditis. *Ann. Intern. Med.* **92**:390–395, 1980.
408. Diaz, C. R., Fossieck, B. E., Parker, R. H.: Pseudomonas endocarditis: Cure with carbenicillin and polymyxin B. *South. Med. J.* **70**:869–871, 1977.

409. Smith, P. W., Chambers, W. A., Walker, C. A.: Ampicillin resistant *Haemophilus parainfluenzae* endocarditis. *Am. J. Med. Sci.* **278:**173–176, 1979.
410. Murray, B. E., Karchmer, A. W., Moellering, R. C., Jr.: Diphtheroid prosthetic valve endocarditis. *Am. J. Med.* **69:**838–848, 1980.
411. Bradsher, R. W., Wickre, C. G., Savage, A. M., Harston, W. E., Alford, R.: *Histoplasma capsulatum* endocarditis cured by amphotericin B combined with surgery. *Chest* **78:**791–795, 1980.

9

Indices of Effectiveness of Treatment

9.1. CLINICAL

Evidence of clinical improvement after the institution of effective antibiotic treatment is usually not dramatic. Patients may have prompt normalization of temperature, in which case they might feel very much better quickly. On the other hand, although fever usually does subside within 2–4 days, this subsidence is gradual, and dramatic response is not the rule. Persistence of fever may indicate ineffective antibiotic therapy or a drug reaction. In some patients, persistent low-grade fever will continue as long as the patient receives antibiotics. Reappearance of fever after an afebrile interval may indicate embolization (pulmonary or arterial), infectious complications of prolonged intravenous therapy, reseeding of the bloodstream from a peripheral abscess, or drug reaction. Rarely, persistence of fever may be an indication of the presence of concomitant underlying disease such as lymphoma or myxoma.

Gastrointestinal symptoms (ileus, abdominal discomfort, vomiting) may take several days to a week to disappear. The spleen may decrease in size concomitant with a decrease in fever. Occasionally, splenectomy is necessary to remove a metastatic focus of infection in the spleen.[1–3]

The continued appearance of petechiae and embolization is not uncommon during the first week of effective treatment. These complications of the disease become less frequent with sterilization of the vegetations, but they may occur even many months after successful treatment. The same is true of the glomerulonephritis due to circulating immune complexes (CICs). There is usually evidence of prompt and progressive improvement in renal function and urinary findings, but rarely, patients have been reported with persistent renal disease, probably due to persistence of CICs. Steroid therapy has been reported useful for the management of this post-infective endocarditis (IE) immune-complex disease and plasmapheresis has been recommended for treatment of glomerulonephritis (see Section 8.8).

Blood cultures usually become negative within a few days of starting effective antibiotic therapy. Persistence of positive blood cultures beyond the 2nd or 3rd day should lead to the strong suspicion that either the antibiotics which were ordered were not given, or they were inactivated by other medications in the infusion solution, or they were ineffective. Of course, prompt defervescence of fever and disappearance of bacteria from the bloodstream do not mean that the antibiotics being administered will result in long-term cure. Suppression of infection with bacteriostatic antibiotics or persistence of infection in an abscess or in relation to a foreign body (prosthetic valve) despite theoretically correct bactericidal antibiotics will result in temporary amelioration of the signs and symptoms of IE only to have a return of fever (perhaps with a negative blood culture) immediately after antibiotics are discontinued or after a delay of days, weeks, or months. Indolent microorganisms, such as those found in prosthetic-valve endocarditis, may lie dormant for many months before becoming clinically evident, and as mentioned in Section 8.5.8, the treatment of fungal *(Candida)* endocarditis cannot be considered successful until several years have elapsed after the completion of therapy without recurrence of disease.

9.2. LABORATORY

9.2.1. Serum Bactericidal Activity

There is experimental evidence pointing to a role for serum bactericidal activity (SBA) in determining the capacity of bacteria to multiply within intravascular vegetations (see Section 4.1). *Escherichia coli, Neisseria,* gonococci, the *Pseudomonas aeruginosa* are capable of establishing IE in the rabbit only if they are resistant to the bactericidal effect of normal serum.[4–6] In addition, a strain of *E. coli* in which susceptibility to the SBA was induced by treatment with rifampin lost its capacity to produce IE in rabbits.[7]

The outcome of antibiotic treatment of IE (*Streptococcus mitis* and *Str. sanguis*) in experimental animals has been directly correlated with SBA brought about by the presence of antibiotics in the serum.[8,9] On the other hand, the outcome of treatment of staphylococcal IE in rabbits with different antimicrobial agents did not correlate with the bactericidal activity in the serum.[10,11]

The correlation between SBA and IE in man is far from established. It is well known that gram-negative bacteria recovered from the bloodstream are predominantly serum-resistant strains. In a series of patients with *Pseudomonas* IE, 28 of 30 strains were serum-resistant.[12] On the other hand, clinical response to infection in these patients was not correlated with the SBA effect of serum during treatment with antibiotics.[13]

Bryan *et al.*[14] found that an SBA titer of at least 1:8 was a useful guide in the treatment of IE due to gram-negative bacteria and was useful as well for adjusting antibiotic dosage in the face of antibiotic toxicity.

With the more common streptococcal infections in man, it is as a rule an easy matter to administer quantities of antibiotics which induce SBA equal to or greater than 1:8. But these infections are virtually always sterilized by antibiotics. In staphylococcal and enterococcal IE, it is not unusual to *not* be able to achieve this kind of SBA in serum and yet achieve cure of infection.

Most experts consider the test of limited usefulness, and yet for the practicing physician it is comforting to know that the antibiotics being administered do produce a bactericidal effect which is demonstrable *in vitro*.[15,16] The issue as to whether peak or trough bactericidal activity is the most important is unresolved.

Most, perhaps all, of the difficulty with the test is the lack of standardization of methods employed.[16–19] Some of the difficulties have to do with the variability among strains of bacteria and the difficulty in establishing uniform methods for their cultivation *in vitro*, a problem similar to that of determining the minimal inhibitory concentration (MIC) of antibiotics for fastidious microorganisms. Curiously, *in vitro*, the MIC may change with change in the temperature of incubation of the bacteria. The extent and direction of change vary with the bacteria and the antibiotic.[31]

My personal procedure is to measure peak (30 min after injection) and trough (before the next injection) levels of SBA and to adjust dosages and antibiotic combinations in order to achieve a satisfactory bactericidal effect within the limits of toxicity of the antibiotics being administered. If, on the other hand, there is a satisfactory clinical response in a patient in whom "effective" SBA cannot be achieved (without producing antibiotic toxicity), I rely on clinical indices of response, taking into consideration the general clinical experience in treatment as described in Chapter 8.

9.2.2. Other Studies

It happens not infrequently that patients with IE have very little fever or have only a gradual fall in temperature with antibiotic therapy. Under these circumstances, it is useful to examine other indices in addition to SBA which can give an indication of the effectiveness of antibiotic therapy. For example, the development of reticulocytosis in patients with anemia or a fall in the titers of rhumatoid factor or CICs can be useful indices of the suppression of the intravascular infection. The normalization of an elevated peripheral white blood count and the disappearance of red cells from the urine can also serve as reassurance that the infectious process is under control. In the case of *Candida* infection, a decrease in the titer of *Candida* precipitins may serve as a useful guide to the progress of the infection.[20] In patients thought to have been successfully treated for *Candida* endocarditis or who have had "transient candidemia," it is recommended that *Candida* precipitins be monitored at first monthly (perhaps for 6 months), then at 3– and 6-month intervals for several years.[21]

It is not known, however, to what extent these biological indices indicate true sterilization of infection or whether they would not occur just as rapidly with a diminution in the number of bacteria in the vegetation or a suppression of their level of metabolic activity as might be accomplished with bacteriostatic antibiotics.

9.3. BACTERIOLOGY OF SURGICALLY REMOVED VEGETATIONS

The ability, in recent years, to surgically remove damaged heart valves and vegetations has provided an unprecedented opportunity to study bacteriologically and histologically the outcome of antibiotic therapy after varying periods of treatment. Nevertheless, there are few reports in which such studies have been described. Unfortunately, the bacteriological techniques were all qualitative, thus making interpretation difficult, particularly in view of the universally reported discrepancy between histological and culture results. Furthermore, in no instances were sufficient details concerning antibiotic therapy given to be able to comment about the advantages or disadvantages of specific antimicrobial regimens.

Despite these limitations, it is of interest to review the data. In two of the studies, little can be said other than that bacteria can be identified in vegetations even after weeks of antibiotic therapy. Because of the localization of vegetations to the free edge of the valve cusp, surgery was usually successful (without infection of the prosthesis) despite the identification of microorganisms in the vegetations.[22,23] Indeed, in one analysis, the presence of bacteria (by strain or culture) in vegetations was not correlated with duration of treatment, and neither was correlated with outcome of surgery.[24] In three other studies, an effort was made to correlate duration of treatment with bacteriological finding.[25–27] In one of these reports, streptococci (non-group D) were visible histologically in 12 of 17 patients including 4 of 6 operated 6–30 months after the conclusion of treatment. Cultures were positive in 2 of 4 patients within 15 days of treatment (1 of the streptococci was resistant to the antibiotics administered).[27] In another study, streptococci were neither cultured from nor seen in vegetations from 3 patients 4–6 weeks after completion of antibiotic therapy.[26] However, within 10 days of the onset of treatment (with sterilization of the blood culture in all instances), streptococci were seen in 4 of 4 patients and cultured in 2 of them.[26]

The results for enterococci, staphylococci, and other microorganisms were often positive for both culture and histology. Of course, in the presence of uncontrolled infection, vegetations were uniformly positive by both techniques.

A third study, similar to the other two except that it included heart-valve examination at autopsy, revealed positive gram stains in the majority of patients and positive cultures in about one third, when vegetations were examined after up to 4 weeks of antibiotic therapy.[25]

These studies are difficult to interpret, particularly in view of what is known from experiments in rabbits. It was shown several years ago that valvular vegetations in which *Candida albicans* were easily seen with conventional stains could be sterile with usual cultural techniques.[28] Furthermore, in rabbits with IE due to *Eikenella corrodens*, despite the recovery of a mean of $10^{5.3}$ colony-forming units/g vegetation, bacteria were not seen by Gram stain, but were easily visualized by immunofluorescent staining.[29] In a patient treated with antibiotics, bacteria were visualized in a heart-valve vegetation by scanning and transmission electron microscopy despite negative results of bacteriological cultures.[30]

Evidently, microorganisms may be visible but not culturable and vice versa with conventional histological and microbiological techniques. Undoubtedly, dead bacteria may persist in vegetations for varying intervals of time.

In summary, the best hope of being able to learn about the effectiveness of antibiotics and the risk of cardiac surgery in such patients is to perform the following studies:

1. Quantitative bacteriology of the vegetations.
2. Routine histology with microbial stains and perhaps electron microscopy.
3. Immunofluorescent studies in cases where the microorganism recovered preoperatively from the bloodstream is used as the antigen to prepare antisera (or perhaps with the use of pooled cross-reacting antigens).

It is evident that one must be cautious in drawing general conclusions about the efficacy of antibiotics from studies of vegetations from patients requiring surgical replacement of severely damaged valves. It is not known whether antibiotics are less effective in sterilizing such vegetations as compared with vegetations on valves which are hemodynamically intact.

REFERENCES

1. Lingeman, C. J., Smith, E. B., Battersby, J. S., Behnke, R. H.: Subacute bacterial endocarditis—Splenectomy in cases refractory to antibiotic therapy. *Arch. Intern. Med.* **97**:309–314, 1956.
2. Godeau, P., Wechsler, B., Herreman, G., Balafrej, M., Bletry, O., Squalli, S.: Rupture de rate au cours des endocardites bactériennes: 2 observations. *Nouv. Presse Med.* **8**:2811–2814, 1979.
3. Gonin, A., Berthou, J. D., Simonin, C., Delaye, J. C., Roques, J. C., Dufoix, V.: Ruptures spontanées de rate au cours de l'endocardite infectieuse—A propos de 3 nouvelles observations. *Lyon Med.* **229**(12):1269–1271, 1973.

4. Durack, D. T., Beeson, P. B.: Protective role of complement in experimental *Escherichia coli* endocarditis. *Infect. Immun.* **16**:213–217, 1977.
5. Archer G., Fekety, F. R., Jr.: Experimental endocarditis due to *Pseudomonas aeruginosa*. I. Description of a model. *J. Infect. Dis.* **134**:1–7, 1976.
6. Kaspar, R. L., Drutz, D. J.: Perihepatitis and hepatitis as complications of experimental endocarditis due to *Neisseria gonorrhoeae* in the rabbit. *J. Infect. Dis.* **136**:37–42, 1977.
7. Alexander, W. J., Curtiss, R., III, Bradac, J. A., Cobbs, C. G.: Rifampin modifies serum susceptibility of *E. coli* and its virulence in rabbit endocarditis model (abstract). *Clin. Res.* **26**:26A, 1978.
8. Pulliam, L., Inokuchi, S., Hadley, W. K., Mills, J.: Penicillin tolerance in experimental streptococcal endocarditis. *Lancet* **2**:957, 1979.
9. Carrizosa, J., Kaye, D.: Antibiotic concentrations in serum, serum bactericidal activity, and results of therapy of streptococal endocarditis in rabbits. *Antimicrob. Agents Chemother.* **12**:479–483, 1977.
10. Egert, J., Carrizosa, J., Kaye, D.: Comparison of methicillin, nafcillin, and oxacillin in therapy of *Staphylococcus aureus* endocarditis in rabbits. *J. Lab. Clin. Med.* **89**:1262–1268, 1977.
11. Carrizosa, J., Santoro, J., Kaye, D.: Treatment of experimental *Staphylococcus aureus* endocarditis: Comparison of cephalothin, cefazolin, and methicillin. *Antimicrob. Agents Chemother.* **13**:74–77, 1978.
12. Reyes, M. P., Riad El-Khatib, M., Brown, W. J., Smith, F., Lerner, A. M.: Synergy between carbenicillin and an aminoglyocoside (gentamicin or tobramycin) against *Pseudomonas aeruginosa* isolated from patients with endocarditis and sensitivity of isolates to normal human serum. *J. Infect. Dis.* **140**:192–202, 1979.
13. Reyes, M. P., Brown, W. J., Lerner, A. M.: Treatment of patients with Pseudomonas endocarditis with high dose aminoglycoside and carbenicillin therapy. *Medicine* **57**:57–67, 1978.
14. Bryan, C. S., Marney, S. R., Alford, R. H., Bryant, R. E.: Gram-negative bacillary endocarditis. *Am. J. Med.* **58**:209–215, 1975.
15. O'Keate, J. P., Gorbach, S. L.: Laboratory diagnosis of infective endocarditis, in: *Infective Endocarditis,* Rahintoola, S. H., Ed. Grune and Stratton, New York, pp. 307–325, 1978.
16. Bryant, R. E., Kimbrough, R. C.: Treatment of infective endocarditis, in: *Infective Endocarditis,* Rahintoola, S. H., Ed. Grune and Stratton, New York, pp. 327–360, 1978.
17. Pien, F. D., Williams, R. D., Vosti, K. L.: Comparison of broth and human serum as the diluent in the serum bactericidal test. *Antimicrob. Agents Chemother.* **7**:113–114, 1975.
18. Stratton, C. W., Reller, L. B.: Serum dilution test for bactericidal activity. I. Selection of a physiology diluent. *J. Infect. Dis.* **136**:187–195, 1977.
19. Reller, L. B., Stratton, C. W.: Serum dilution test for bactericidal activity. II. Standardization and correlation with antimicrobials assays and susceptibility tests. *J. Infect. Dis.* **136**:196–204, 1977.
20. McLoed, R., Remington, J. S.: Fungal endocarditis, in: *Infective Endocarditis,* Rahimtoola, S.H., Ed. Grune and Stratton, New York, pp. 211–290, 1978.
21. Seeling, M. S., Golberg, P., Kozinn, P. J., Berger. A. R.: Fungal endocarditis: Patients at risk and their treatment. *Postgrad. Med. J.* **55**:632–641, 1979.
22. Bastin, R., Vilde, J. L., Frottier, J., Lejeune, A.: La chirurgie cardiaque dans les endocardites a la periode infectieuse *Coeur—No. Special:* Journées internationales de cardiologie conascrées aux remplacements valvulaires, Oct. 1974, Deauville.
23. Stinson, E. B., Griepp, R. B., Vosti, K., Copeland, J. G., Shumway, N. E.: Operative treatment of active endocarditis. *J. Thorac. Cardiovasc. Surg.* **71**:659–665, 1976.
24. Stinson, E. B.: Surgical treatment of infective endocarditis. *Prog. Cardiovasc. Dis.* **22**:145–168, 1979.
25. Olsen, E. G. J.: Endomyocardial fibrosis and Löffler's endocarditis parietalis fibroplastica. *Postgrad. Med. J.* **53**:538–540, 1977

26. Boyd, A. D., Spencer, F. C., Isom, O. W., Cunningham, J. N., Reed, G. E., Acinapura, A. J., Tice, D. A.: Infective endocarditis—An analysis of 54 surgically treated patients. *J. Thorac. Cardiovasc. Surg.* **73**:23–30, 1977.
27. Christol, D., Witchitz, S., Duval, J., Guyonnaud, C. D., Bouton, C., Garnier, I.: Etude anatomique et bactériologique des pièces de valvulectomie chez les malades ayant une endocardite bactérienne. *Nouv. Presse Med.* **6**:1355–1358, 1977.
28. Freedman, L. R., Johnson, M. L.: Experimental endocarditis. IV. Tricuspid and aortic value infection with *Candida albicans* in rabbits. *Yale J. Biol. Med.* **45**:163–175, 1972.
29. Badger, S. J., Butler, T., Kim, C. K., Johnston, K. H.: Experimental *Eikenella corrodens* endocarditis in rabbits. *Infect. Immuno.* **23**:751–757, 1978.
30. McGowan, D. A.: Scanning electron microscopy of heart-valve vegetations. *Lancet* **2**:822, 1977.
31. Mackowiak, P. A., Cohen, R. L.: The effect of physiological hyperthermia on minimal inhibitory concentrations (MICs). 20th ICAAC, Sept. 1980, Abstract 399.

10

Outcome of Treatment

10.1. MEDICAL

Despite the availability of chemotherapeutic agents capable of sterilizing endocardial vegetations, infective endocarditis (IE) remains a disease with a high mortality. How high depends on the location of the infection, the nature of the infecting microorganism, and the expertness with which the major cause of death, valve destruction, is recognized and treated surgically.

In addition to the causes of death associated with complications of the active infection, there is also an important mortality during the years following bacteriological cure which depends on the underlying cardiac or noncardiac disease on which IE was grafted as well as the amount of cardiac, neurological, or renal–vascular damage suffered during the acute phase of the illness. There is also a well-known increased susceptibility of developing IE in subjects who have recovered from previous episodes. Because of the large number of factors known to influence mortality, it is difficult to speak of the mortality of IE without dividing the data into so many groups that the numbers are insufficient to obtain meaningful figures.

For example, as has been mentioned several times, infections on the right side of the heart have a much better prognosis than those on the left. Infections are more easily sterilized and the hemodynamic consequences of valve destruction much less severe on the right side of the heart.[1] In addition, the vast majority of patients with right-heart IE seen today are drug addicts in whom the pathogenesis of infection is probably different than in other patients with IE. So it is that any consideration of outcome of treatment of IE must take into consideration the location of the infection.

The complications of IE and the principal causes of death were discussed in Section 6.6. It is sufficient to reemphasize that persistent infection is a rare cause of death in streptococcal IE, but a common one in IE due to fungi, gram-negative bacilli, and staphylococci.

Since the major cause of death in IE in the antibiotic era is congestive heart failure (CHF) due to valve destruction, it is of the greatest importance to learn more about the factors that influence the local destructive process. Up to now, the focus of experimental studies in rabbits and of therapeutic trials in man has been primarily on sterilization of the infection. On the other hand, many patients go for long periods of time with active IE without destroying the affected valve, whereas other patients seem to develop aortic insufficiency shortly after developing the symptoms of infection. Although this difference in clinical evolution may be due in part to the invasive properties of different microorganisms, it is not clear that this is the sole or even the most important factor determining the outcome of treatment.

Furthermore, prosthetic-valve surgery, although life saving for the patient with acute CHF due to valve perforation, is not without risk of complications of its own. Clearly, future improvements in the mortality (and morbidity) of IE will depend upon our capacity to prevent valve destruction (and embolization).

10.2. SURGICAL

The surgical treatment of valve destruction due to IE is the most important advance in the treatment of this disease since the introduction of antibiotics. When it became evident, about 20 years ago, that valve destruction was the most common cause of death in patients with IE in the antibiotic era, it was evident that replacement of the damaged valve with a prosthesis held the prospect of preventing the lethal consequences of this hemodynamic catastrophe.[2] This promise has been largely fulfilled.

CHF due to valve destruction is the major indication for valve replacement in IE, the other major but less frequent indications being uncontrolled infection and repeated embolization (see Section 8.6). Studies of the outcome of valve replacement have demonstrated without question that the immediate mortality associated with surgery is directly proportional to the degree of heart failure present at the time of operation.[3–5] In a review published in 1974, reviewing 235 cases of cardiac surgery in IE, reflecting surgical experience almost exclusively prior to 1970, the major indication for valve replacement was *intractable* heart failure, and immediate mortality was 25%.[3] In the more recent series, the overall mortality was 10%, but the majority of patients operated were categorized as class II (New York Heart Association) CHF.[4] The mortality in patients with aortic-valve replacement and intractable (class IV) CHF remains 22%.[4] Thus, it is evident that mortality is less in patients with less severe CHF. It is generally agreed that the great majority of patients with valve destruction due to IE who develop CHF will in the long run require valve replacement. The only question is when (see Section 8.6).

A recent suggestion that all patients with staphylococcal IE be treated surgically irrespective of the presence of CHF or other indications for surgery does not seem warranted on the basis of the data presented.[5]

The complications of treatment by artificial valve replacement, in addition to heart failure and intractable infection, include embolic phenomena (including coronary emboli), valve dehiscence, valve-ring or myocardial abscesses, heart block, and dissection of the aorta, as well as the complications of long-term anticoagulant therapy. Another important risk to be borne in mind is susceptibility to developing IE, which, as far as is known at present, continues indefinitely. The need for prophylactic antibiotic administration prior to dental and other procedures (e.g., urological) in these patients cannot be overemphasized.

In patients operated upon for IE, it has been possible in two recent series to calculate the long-term survival. Patients who left the hospital having been operated during the acute phase of IE had a 5-year survival of about 66%, whereas those operated after healing of IE had a 5-year survival of 72%.[6] These figures are comparable to those of another series, in which it is pointed out, however, that of the 5-year survivors, 15% had class III or IV CHF and about one fourth had late paravalvular leaks, one fourth of whom required reoperation.[5]

Although these represent global figures and do not take into consideration such factors as the age of the patients, presence of underlying disease, and the infecting microorganism, they are useful as an overall guide. It must also be borne in mind that patients treated medically also have a need for late heart-valve surgery, 25% in 5 years in one series.[5] This will vary, obviously, according to the criteria for operation in the early phase of illness. In one series, the actuarial experience over a 5-year period, after hospital discharge, of patients who were medically treated during the period of active cardiac surgery was similar to that of those who had been operated.[5] In the pre-cardiac-surgery era, the 5-year survival for patients with IE discharged from the hospital with a heart murmur of aortic insufficiency was about 50%, declining about 17% annually for the first 2 years and less than 4% per year thereafter.[7]

The surgical treatment of late prosthetic-valve endocarditis (PVE) carries a variable mortality risk, in some series perhaps similar to that of the surgical treatment of IE occurring on natural valves.[5,8] On the other hand, the mortality from early PVE is about 70%, a reflection, no doubt, of the antibiotic resistance of the microorganisms and the precarious hemodynamic state of the patients.[5,8]

In still another series, there was no significant difference in mortality between early and late PVE, which was, in each case, about 70%.[9] This series illustrates, once again, the bacteriological similarity between early and late infections and emphasizes the importance of early surgical valve replacement in nonstreptococcal infections of prosthetic valves.

The development of infection in a vascular graft is ominous, the overall mortality being about 50% for aortofemoral and iliofemoral grafts and somewhat lower for femoropopliteal grafts (9–36% depending on the series), related no doubt to the ease of diagnosis of the latter.[10]

Patients with aortoiliofemoral and femoropopliteal grafts usually present with wound infections, whereas patients with aortoilial grafts present usually with sepsis, hemorrhage, or gastrointestinal bleeding.[10] In these patients, prognosis is best for those in whom the infected grafts are excised promptly. Under these circumstances, there is an amputation rate of about 50% in patients with femoropopliteal grafts, but zero mortality.[10]

REFERENCES

1. Freedman, L.R., Valone, J.: Experimental endocarditis. *Prog. Cardiovasc. Dis.* **22:**169–180, 1979.
2. Cohen, L., Freedman, L.R.: Damage to the aortic valve as a cause of death in bacterial endocarditis. *Ann. Intern. Med.* **55:**562–564, 1961.
3. Black, S., O'Rourke, R.A., Karliner, J.S.: Role of surgery in the treatment of primary infective endocarditis. *Am. J. Med.* **56:**357–368, 1974.
4. Wilson, W.R., Danielson, G.K., Giuliani, E.R., Washington, J.A., II, Jaumin, P.M., Geraci, J.E.: Cardiac valve replacement in congestive heart failure due to infective endocarditis. *Mayo Clin. Proc.* **54:**223–226, 1979.
5. Richardson, J.V., Karp, R.B., Kirklin, J.W., Dismukes, W.E.: Treatment of infective endocarditis: A 10-year comparative analysis. *Circulation* **58:**589–597, 1978.
6. Stinson, E.B.: Surgical treatment of infective endocarditis. *Prog. Cardiovasc. Dis.* **22:**145–168, 1979.
7. Kaye, D.: Cure rates and long-term prognosis, in: *Infective Endocarditis,* Kaye, D., ed. University Park Press, Baltimore, pp. 201–211, 1976.
8. Watanakunakorn, L.: Prosthetic valve endocarditis. *Prog. Cardiovasc. Dis.* **22:**181–192, 1978.
9. Masur, H., Johnson, W.D., Jr.: Prosthetic valve endocarditis. *J. Thorac. Cardiovasc. Surg.* **80:**31–37, 1980.
10. Liekweg, W.G., Jr., Levinson, S.A., Greenfield, L.J.: Infections of vascular grafts: Incidence, anatomic location, etiologic agents, morbidity and mortality, in: *Infections of Prostatic Heart Valves and Vascular Grafts,* Duma, R.J., ed. University Park Press, Baltimore, pp. 239–251, 1977.

11

Complications of Treatment

The complications of correct treatment of intravascular infections are those that one would expect with long-term high-dose antibiotic therapy. The physician must be particularly alert to the development of vestibular disturbances (20–30% of patients treated with recommended regimen for enterococcal endocarditis) due to streptomycin therapy and to discontinue streptomycin after 4 weeks when this is detected.

Many (if not all) of the antibiotics recommended are nephrotoxic, and one can only speculate as to the role of antibiotic therapy in many of the renal lesions being documented today with immunofluorescent techniques. Similarly, febrile drug reactions are common and may complicate the evaluation of the patient's response to treatment. I have seen two instances of agranulocytosis developing during treatment with penicillin. Similar patients have been reported by others.[1] Changing antibiotics was accompanied by gradual recovery. There seemed to be no adverse effect of the agranulocytosis on the evolution of the infection, which, after all, is already in a state of "localized agranulocytosis."

The administration of antibiotics in the quantities recommended implies the administration of significant amounts of cations: approximately 30 meq potassium/20 million units potassium penicillin G, 25 meq sodium/10 g nafcillin, and 140 meq sodium/30 g carbenicillin. These quantities of cations can be clinically significant in altering the water and electrolyte balance of patients at risk of developing congestive heart failure and renal insufficiency as well as in patients with hypertension.

Patients subjected to long-term intravenous therapy, usually with plastic catheters, are of course subject to all the hazards of this treatment: breaking off and embolization of catheters, localized infection, and sepsis. Catheter-induced sepsis can of course graft another microorganism on an already infected intravascular vegetation. One must exercise the greatest caution in the placement and care of these catheters—they have been known to produce infective endocarditis.

REFERENCE

1. Colvin, B., Rogers, M., Layton, C.: Case report: Benzylpenicillin-induced leucopenia—Complication of treatment of bacterial endocarditis. *Br. Heart J.* **36**:216–219, 1974.

Appendix

AHA Committee Report: Prevention of Bacterial Endocarditis

Bacterial endocarditis remains one of the most serious complications of cardiac disease. The morbidity and mortality remain significant despite advances in antimicrobial therapy and cardiovascular surgery. This infection occurs most often in patients with structural abnormalities of the heart or great vessels. Effective measures for prevention of this infection by physicians and dentists are highly desirable.

Dental treatment, or surgical procedures or instrumentation involving the upper respiratory tract, genitourinary tract, or lower gastrointestinal tract, may be associated with transitory bacteremia. Bacteria in the bloodstream may lodge on damaged or abnormal valves such as are found in rheumatic or congenital heart disease or on endocardium near congenital anatomic defects, causing bacterial endocarditis or endarteritis. However, it is not possible to predict specific patients with structural heart disease in whom this infection will occur, nor the specific causal event.

Prophylaxis is recommended in those situations most likely to be associated with bacteremia since bacterial endocarditis cannot occur without a preceding

This report was prepared by the Committee on Prevention of Rheumatic Fever and Bacterial Endocarditis of the American Heart Association and is reprinted, with permission, from News from the American Heart Association, *Circulation* **56**(1):139A–143A, 1977. The committee members are Edward L. Kaplan, M.D., Chairman; Bascom F. Anthony, M.D.; Alan Bisno, M.D.; David Durack, M.B., D.Phil.; Harold Houser, M.D.; H. Dean Millard, D.D.S.; Jay Sanford, M.D.; Stanford T. Shulman, M.D.; Max Stillerman, M.D.; Angelo Taranta, M.D.; Nanette Wenger, M.D.

bacteremia. Certain patients (e.g., those with prosthetic heart valves) appear to be at higher risk to develop endocarditis than are others (e.g., those with mitral valve prolapse syndrome). Likewise, certain dental (e.g., extractions) and surgical (e.g., genitourinary tract surgery) procedures appear to be much more likely to initiate significant bacteremia than are others. These factors, although difficult to quantitate, have been considered in developing these recommendations.

Since there have been no controlled clinical trials, adequate data for comparing various methods for prevention of endocarditis in man are not available. However, an experimental animal model permitting consistent induction of bacterial endocarditis with microorganisms which often cause the infection in man has allowed experimental evaluation of both prophylaxis and treatment. Data from these studies, although derived from animal rather than clinical investigations, represent the only direct information on the efficacy of prophylaxis that is presently available. This information has influenced formulation of the current recommendations. The significant morbidity and mortality associated with infective endocarditis and the paucity of conclusive clinical studies emphasize the need for continuing research into the epidemiology, pathogenesis, prevention, and therapy of infective endocarditis.

When selecting antibiotics for bacterial endocarditis prophylaxis one should consider both the variety of bacteria that is likely to enter the bloodstream from any given site and those organisms most likely to cause this infection. Certain species of microorganisms cause the majority of cases of infective endocarditis, and their antimicrobial sensitivity patterns have been defined. The present recommendations are based on a review of available information about the organisms responsible for endocarditis including their *in vivo* and *in vitro* sensitivity to specific antibiotics and the pharmacokinetics of these drugs.

In general, *parenteral administration* of antibiotics provides more predictable blood levels and is preferred when practical, especially for patients thought to be at high risk. Optimal prophylaxis requires close cooperation between physicians, and between physicians and dentists.

DENTAL PROCEDURES AND UPPER RESPIRATORY TRACT SURGICAL PROCEDURES

Patients at risk to develop infective endocarditis should maintain the highest level of oral health to reduce potential sources of bacterial seeding. Even in the absence of dental procedures, poor dental hygiene or other dental disease such as periodontal or periapical infections may induce bacteremia. Patients without natural teeth are not free from the risk of bacterial endocarditis. Ulcers caused by ill-fitting dentures should be promptly cared for since they may be a source of bacteremia.

Antibiotic prophylaxis is recommended with *all* dental procedures (including routine professional cleaning) that are likely to cause gingival bleeding. Chemoprophylaxis for dental procedures in children should be managed in a similar manner to the way in which it is handled in adults. Although not a procedure, one exception to this is the spontaneous shedding of deciduous teeth; there are no data to suggest a significant risk of bacteremia accompanying this common event.

Devices which utilize water under pressure to clean between teeth, and dental flossing, may improve dental hygiene, but they also have been shown to cause bacteremia. However, bacterial endocarditis associated with the use of these devices has not been reported. Present data are insufficient to make firm recommendations with regard to their use in patients susceptible to endocarditis. However caution is advised in their use by patients with cardiac defects, especially when oral hygiene is poor.

Several studies suggest that *local gingival degerming* immediately preceding a dental procedure provides some degree of protection against bacteremia. However, use of this technique is controversial, since gingival sulcus irrigation itself could theoretically induce bacteremia. If local degerming is employed, it should be used only as an adjunct to antibiotic prophylaxis.

Since alpha hemolytic streptococci (e.g., viridans streptococci) are the organisms most commonly implicated in bacterial endocarditis following dental

TABLE A1
Prophylaxis for Dental Procedures and for Surgical Procedures of the Upper Respiratory Tract

Procedures	Most congenital heart disease[a]; rheumatic or other acquired valvular heart disease; idiopathic hypertrophic subaortic stenosis; mitral valve[b] prolapse syndrome with mitral insufficiency	Prosthetic heart valves[c]
All dental procedures that are likely to result in gingival bleeding[d]	Regimen A or B	Regimen B
Surgery or instrumentation of the respiratory tract[e]	Regimen A or B	Regimen B

[a] For example, ventricular septal defect, tetralogy of Fallot, aortic stenosis, pulmonic stenosis, complex cyanotic heart disease, patent ductus arteriosus, or systemic to pulmonary artery shunts. Does *not* include uncomplicated secundum atrial septal defect.

[b] Although cases of infective endocarditis in patients with mitral valve prolapse syndrome have been documented, the incidence appears to be relatively low and the necessity for prophylaxis in all of these patients has not yet been established.

[c] Some patients with a prosthetic heart valve in whom a high level of oral health is being maintained may be offered oral antibiotic prophylaxis for routine dental procedures except the following: parenteral antibiotics are recommended for patients with prosthetic valves who require extensive dental procedures, especially extractions, or oral or gingival surgical procedures.

[d] Does not include shedding of deciduous teeth or simple adjustment of orthodontic appliances.

[e] For example, tonsillectomy, adenoidectomy, bronchoscopy, and other surgical procedures of the upper respiratory tract involving disruption of the respiratory mucosa (see the text).

procedures, antibiotic prophylaxis should be specifically directed toward them. Certain procedures on the upper respiratory tract (e.g., tonsillectomy or adenoidectomy, bronchoscopy—especially with a rigid bronchoscope—and surgical procedures involving respiratory mucosa) also may cause bacteremia. Since bacteria entering the bloodstream after these procedures usually have similar antibiotic sensitivities to those recovered following dental procedures, the same regimens are recommended.

Table A1 contains suggested regimens for chemoprophylaxis for dental procedures, or surgical procedures and instrumentation of the upper respiratory tract. The order of listing does not imply superiority of one regimen over another although parenteral administration is favored when practical. The committee also favors the combined use of penicillin and streptomycin or the use of vancomycin in the penicillin allergic patient (Regimen B) in those patients felt to be at high risk (e.g., prosthetic valves).

REGIMENS FOR DENTAL PROCEDURES AND SURGERY OF THE UPPER RESPIRATORY TRACT

Regimen A—Penicillin

1. Parenteral–Oral Combined

Adults: Aqueous crystalline penicillin G (1,000,000 units intramuscularly) mixed with *procaine penicillin G* (600,000 units intramuscularly). Give 30 minutes to 1 hour prior to procedure and then give penicillin V (formerly called phenoxymethyl penicillin) 500 mg orally every 6 hours for 8 doses.*

Children†: *Aqueous crystalline penicillin G* (30,000 units/kg intramuscularly) mixed with *procaine penicillin G* (600,000 units intramuscularly). Timing of doses for children is the same as for adults. For children less than 60 lb, the dose of penicillin V is 250 mg orally every 6 hours for 8 doses.*

2. Oral

Adults: Penicillin V (2.0 gm orally 30 minutes to 1 hour prior to the procedure and then 500 mg orally every 6 hours for 8 doses).*

* In unusual circumstances or in the case of delayed healing, it may be prudent to provide additional doses of antibiotics even though available data suggest that bacteremia rarely persists longer than 15 minutes after the procedure. The physician or dentist may also choose to use the parenteral route of administration for all of the doses in selected situations.

† Doses for children should not exceed recommendations for adults for a single dose or for a 24-hour period.

Children†: *Penicillin V* (2.0 gm orally 30 minutes to 1 hour prior to procedure and then 500 mg orally every 6 hours for 8 doses.* For children less than 60 lb use 1.0 gm orally 30 minutes to 1 hour prior to the procedure and then 250 mg orally every 6 hours for 8 doses).*

Children†: *Vancomycin* (20 mg/kg intravenously over 30 minutes to 1 hour).** Timing of doses for children is the same as for adults. *Erythromycin* dose is 10 mg/kg every 6 hours for 8 doses.*

For Patients Allergic to Penicillin

Use *either Vancomycin* (see Regimen B)

or

Adults: Erythromycin (1.0 gm orally 1½–2 hours prior to the procedure and then 500 mg orally every 6 hours for 8 doses).*

Children: Erythromycin (20 mg/kg orally 1½–2 hours prior to the procedure and then 10 mg/kg every 6 hours for 8 doses).*

Regimen B—Penicillin plus Streptomycin

Adults: Aqueous crystalline penicillin G (1,000,000 units intramuscularly)

mixed with

Procaine penicillin G (600,000 units intramuscularly)

plus

Streptomycin (1 gm intramuscularly).

Give 30 minutes to 1 hour prior to the procedure; then penicillin V 500 mg orally every 6 hours for 8 doses.*

Children†: *Aqueous crystalline penicillin G* (30,000 units/kg intramuscularly)

mixed with

Procaine penicillin G (600,000 units intramuscularly)

plus

Streptomycin (20 mg/kg intramuscularly). Timing of doses for children is the same as for adults. For children less than 60 lb, the recommended oral dose of penicillin V is 250 mg every 6 hours for 8 doses.*

For Patients Allergic to Penicillin

Adults: Vancomycin (1 gm intravenously over 30 minutes to 1 hour). Start

† Doses for children should not exceed recommendations for adults for a single dose or for a 24-hour period.

* In unusual circumstances or in the case of delayed healing, it may be prudent to provide additional doses of antibiotics even though available data suggest that bacteremia rarely persists longer than 15 minutes after the procedure. The physician or dentist may also choose to use the parenteral route of administration for all of the doses in selected situations.

** For vancomycin the total dose for children should not exceed 44 mg/kg/24 hours.

initial vancomycin infusion ½ to 1 hour prior to procedure; then *erythromycin* 500 mg orally every 6 hours for 8 doses.*

GENITOURINARY TRACT AND GASTROINTESTINAL TRACT SURGERY OR INSTRUMENTATION

Bacteremia may be caused by surgery or instrumentation of the genitourinary tract (especially urethral or prostatic manipulations, including urethral catheterization whether the urine is infected or not). It may also accompany surgery and instrumentation of the lower gastrointestinal tract and of the gallbladder, and may be associated with obstetrical infections such as septic abortion or peripartum infection. Documented cases of bacterial endocarditis have been recorded following these procedures and antibiotic prophylaxis to prevent this infection should be employed.

Endocarditis following uncomplicated vaginal delivery is extremely rare; the necessity for antibiotic prophylaxis has not been firmly established. Likewise, upper gastrointestinal endoscopy (without biopsy), percutaneous liver biopsy, proctoscopy, sigmoidoscopy, barium enema, pelvic examination, dilatation and curettage of the uterus, and uncomplicated insertion or removal of intrauterine devices (IUDs)—although occasionally associated with bacteremia—have only very rarely, if ever, been associated with development of infective endocarditis. Based upon currently available evidence, they do not require antibiotic prophylaxis in most patients with underlying heart disease. However, since the patient with a prosthetic valve appears to be at especially high risk, it may be wise to administer antibiotic prophylaxis with these procedures. This empiric recommendation is based more upon concern than definitive data.

Enterococci (e.g., *Streptococcus fecalis*) are frequently responsible for endocarditis following genitourinary tract and gastrointestinal tract surgery or instrumentation. Although bacteremia and even sepsis with gram-negative bacteria may follow instrumentation of the genitourinary tract or gastrointestinal tract, these organisms only rarely cause bacterial endocarditis. Thus, antibiotic prophylaxis to prevent endocarditis following these procedures should be directed primarily against enterococci. Because these procedures are usually performed in a hospital or clinic, parenteral antibiotics are recommended.

Suggested antibiotic regimens for gastrointestinal and genitourinary tract surgery and instrumentation are shown below.

* In unusual circumstances or in the case of delayed healing, it may be prudent to provide additional doses of antibiotics even though available data suggest that bacteremia rarely persists longer than 15 minutes after the procedure. The physician or dentist may also choose to use the parenteral route of administration for all of the doses in selected situations.

REGIMENS FOR GASTROINTESTINAL AND GENITO-URINARY TRACT SURGERY AND INSTRUMENTATION*

Adults: Aqueous crystalline penicillin G (2,000,000 units intramuscularly or intravenously)

or

Ampicillin (1.0 gm intramuscularly or intravenously)

plus

Gentamicin [1.5 mg/kg (not to exceed 80 mg) intramuscularly or intravenously]

or

Streptomycin (1.0 gm intramuscularly)

Give initial doses 30 minutes to 1 hour prior to procedure. If gentamicin is used then give a similar dose of gentamicin and penicillin (or ampicillin) every 8 hours for two additional doses.† If streptomycin is used then give a similar dose of streptomycin and penicillin (or ampicillin) every 12 hours for two additional doses.†

Children‡: Aqueous crystalline penicillin G (30,000 units/kg intramuscularly or intravenously)

or

Ampicillin (50 mg/kg intramuscularly or intravenously)

plus

Gentamicin (2.0 mg/kg intramuscularly or intravenously)

or

Streptomycin (20 mg/kg intramuscularly)

Timing of doses for children is the same as for adults.†

For Those Patients Who Are Allergic to Penicillin†

Adults: Vancomycin (1.0 gm intravenously given over 30 minutes to 1 hour) plus *Streptomycin* (1.0 gm intramuscularly). A single dose of these antibiotics

* In patients with significantly compromised renal function, it may be necessary to modify the dose of antibiotics used. Some of these doses may exceed manufacturer's recommendations for a 24 hour period. However, since they are only recommended for a 24 hour period in most cases, it is unlikely that toxicity will occur.

† During prolonged procedures, or in the case of delayed healing, it may be necessary to provide additional doses of antibiotics. For brief outpatient procedures such as uncomplicated catheterization of the bladder one dose may be sufficient.

‡ For those *patients receiving continuous oral penicillin for secondary prevention of rheumatic fever*, alpha hemolytic streptococci which are relatively resistant to penicillin are occasionally found in the oral cavity. While it is likely that the doses of penicillin recommended in Regimen A are sufficient to control these organisms, the physician or dentist may choose one of the suggestions in Regimen B or may choose oral erythromycin.

begun 30 minutes to 1 hour prior to the procedure is probably sufficient, but the same dose may be repeated in 12 hours.†

*Children‡: Vancomycin*** (20 mg/kg given intravenously over 30 minutes to 1 hour) plus *Streptomycin* (20 mg/kg intramuscularly). Timing of doses for children is the same as for adults.†

CARDIAC SURGERY

Patients undergoing cardiac surgery utilizing extracorporeal circulation—especially those requiring placement of prosthetic heart valves or needing prosthetic intravascular or intracardiac materials—are at risk to develop infective endocarditis in the perioperative and postoperative periods. Because the morbidity and mortality of infective endocarditis in such patients are high, maximal preventive efforts are indicated, including the use of prophylactic antibiotics.

Early postoperative infective endocarditis following these surgical procedures is most often due to *Staphylococcus aureus* (coagulase positive) or *Staphylococcus epidermidis* (coagulase negative). Streptococci, gram negative bacteria, and fungi are less frequently responsible. No single antibiotic regimen is effective against all these organisms. Furthermore, the prolonged use of broad spectrum antibiotics may itself predispose to superinfection with unusual or highly resistant microorganisms. Therefore, antibiotic prophylaxis at the time of open heart surgery should be directed primarily against staphylococci and should be of short duration. The choice of antibiotic should be influenced by each individual hospital's antibiotic sensitivity data, but *penicillinase resistant penicillins* or *cephalosporin antibiotics* are most often selected. Antibiotic prophylaxis should be started shortly before the operative procedure and usually is continued for no more than three to five days postoperatively to reduce the likelihood of emergence of resistant microorganisms. The physician or surgeon should consider the effects of cardiopulmonary bypass on serum antibiotic levels and time the doses accordingly.

Careful preoperative dental evaluation is recommended so that any required dental treatment can be carried out *several weeks prior* to cardiac surgery when-

† Doses for children should not exceed recommendations for adults for a single dose or for a 24-hour period.

‡ For those *patients receiving continuous oral penicillin for secondary prevention of rheumatic fever,* alpha hemolytic streptococci which are relatively resistant to penicillin are occasionally found in the oral cavity. While it is likely that the doses of penicillin recommended in Regimen A are sufficient to control these organisms, the physician or dentist may choose one of the suggestions in Regimen B or may choose oral erythromycin.

** For vancomycin the total dose for children should not exceed 44 mg/kg/24 hours.

ever possible. Such measures may decrease the incidence of late postoperative endocarditis (occurring later than 6–8 weeks following surgery) which is often due to the same organisms which are responsible for causing infective endocarditis in the unoperated patient.

STATUS FOLLOWING CARDIAC SURGERY

Following cardiovascular surgery the same precautions should be observed that have been outlined for the unoperated patient undergoing dental, gastrointestinal, genitourinary, and other procedures. As far as is known, the risk of endocarditis probably continues indefinitely; it appears particularly significant in patients with prosthetic heart valves. Exceptions are patients with an uncomplicated secundum atrial septal defect repaired by direct suture without a prosthetic patch, and patients who have had ligation and division of a patent ductus arteriosus; these patients do not appear to be at increased risk of developing endocarditis. For these two defects, prophylaxis for prevention of infective endocarditis is not necessary following a healing period of six months after surgery. Although prophylactic antibiotics are often given intraoperatively, there is no evidence to suggest that patients who have undergone coronary artery operations are at risk to develop endocarditis in the months and years following surgery unless there is another cardiac defect present; prophylactic antibiotics to protect against endocarditis are not needed in these postoperative patients.

OTHER INDICATIONS FOR ANTIBIOTIC PROPHYLAXIS TO PREVENT ENDOCARDITIS

In susceptible patients chemoprophylaxis to prevent endocarditis is also indicated for surgical procedures on *any infected or contaminated tissues,* including incision and drainage of abscesses. Antibiotic prophylaxis for the indicated dental and surgical procedures should also be given to those patients who have had a documented previous episode of infective endocarditis, even in the absence of clinically detectable heart disease.

Indwelling vascular catheters, especially those which reside in one of the cardiac chambers, present a continual danger. Particular care should be given to maintaining the sterility of these catheters and to avoiding unnecessarily prolonged use.

Indwelling transvenous cardiac pacemakers appear to present a low risk of endocarditis; however dentists and physicians may choose to employ prophylactic antibiotics to cover dental and surgical procedures in these patients. The same recommendations apply to renal dialysis patients with implanted arteriovenous shunt appliances. Although no firm recommendation can be made on the basis of current information, antibiotic prophylaxis for prevention of bacteremia provoked by dental and surgical procedures also deserves consideration in patients with ventriculoatrial shunts placed to relieve hydrocephalus since there are documented cases of infective endocarditis in these patients.

Prophylactic antibiotics are *not* required in diagnostic cardiac catheterization and angiography since, with standard techniques, the occurrence of endocarditis following these procedures has proven to be extremely uncommon.

It is important to recognize that antibiotic doses used to prevent recurrences of acute rheumatic fever ("secondary" rheumatic fever prophylaxis) are *inadequate* for the prevention of bacterial endocarditis (see reference). Special attention should be paid to these patients and appropriate antibiotics should be prescribed *in addition* to the antibiotic they are receiving for prevention of group A beta hemolytic streptococcal infections (the addition of an aminoglycoside to appropriate doses of penicillin, or the use of erythromycin or vancomycin).

WARNING

The committee recognizes that it is not possible to make recommendations for all possible clinical situations. Practitioners should exercise their clinical judgment in determining the duration and choice of antibiotic(s) when special circumstances apply. Furthermore, since endocarditis may occur despite antibiotic prophylaxis, physicians and dentists should maintain a high index of suspicion in the interpretation of any unusual clinical events following the above procedures. Early diagnosis is important to reduce complications, sequelae, and mortality.

SELECTED REFERENCES

1. American Heart Association Committee on Prevention of Rheumatic Fever: Prevention of rheumatic fever. *Circulation* **55:**1, 1977.
2. Durack, D.T., Petersdorf, R.G.: Chemotherapy of experimental streptococcal endocarditis. I. Comparison of commonly recommended prophylactic regimens. *J. Clin. Invest.* **52:**592, 1973.
3. Durack, D.T., Starkebaum, M.S., Petersdorf, R.G.: Chemotherapy of experimental streptococcal endocarditis. VI. Prevention of enterococcal endocarditis. *J. Lab. Clin. Med.* **90:**71, 1977.
4. Editorial: Prophylaxis of bacteria endocarditis: Faith, Hope, and Charitable Interpretations. *Lancet* **I:**519, 1976.
5. Everett, E.D., Hirschman, J.V.: Transient bacteremia and endocarditis prophylaxis: A review. *Medicine* **56:**61, 1977.
6. Finland, M.: Current problems in infective endocarditis. *Mod. Concepts Cardiovasc. Dis.* **41:**53, 1972.
7. Parker, M.T., Ball, L.C.: Streptococci and aerococci associated with systemic infection in man. *J. Med. Microbiol.* **9:**275, 1976.

8. Pelletier, L.L., Jr., Durack, D.T., Petersdorf, R.G.: Chemotherapy of experimental streptococcal endocarditis. IV. Further observations on prophylaxis. *J. Clin. Invest.* **56:**319, 1975.
9. Sande, M.A., Levison, M.E., Lukas, D.S., Kaye D.: Bacteremia associated with cardiac catheterization. *N. Engl. J. Med.* **281:**1104, 1969.
10. Sande, M.A., Johnson, W.D., Hook, E.W., Kaye D.: Sustained bacteremia in patients with prosthetic cardiac valves. *N. Engl. J. Med.* **286:**1067, 1972.
11. Scopp, I.W., Orvieto, L.D.: Gingival degerming by povidone-iodine irrigation: Bacteremia reduction in extraction procedures. *J. Am. Dent. Assoc.* **83:**1294, 1971.
12. Sipes, J.N., Thompson, R.L., Hook E.W.: Prophylaxis of infective endocarditis: A reevaluation. *Annu. Rev. Med.* **28:**371, 1977.
13. Sullivan, N.M., Sutter, V.L., Mims, M.M., Marsh, V.H., Finegold, S.M.: Clinical aspects of bacteremia after manipulation of the genitourinary tract. *J. Infect. Dis.* **127:**49, 1973.

BOOKS

1. *Infective Endocarditis—An American Heart Association Symposium,* Kaplan, E.L., Taranta, A.V. American Heart Association Monograph Series No. 52, American Heart Association, Dallas, Texas, 1977.
2. *Infective Endocarditis,* edited by Donald Kaye, University Park Press, Baltimore, Maryland 1976.
3. *Subacute Bacterial Endocarditis,* by Andrew Kerr, Jr., Charles C Thomas, publisher, Springfield, Illinois 1955.

Index

MIX
Papier aus verantwortungsvollen Quellen
Paper from responsible sources
FSC® C105338
FSC
www.fsc.org

If you have any concerns about our products,
you can contact us on
ProductSafety@springernature.com

In case Publisher is established outside the EU,
the EU authorized representative is:
Springer Nature Customer Service Center GmbH
Europaplatz 3, 69115 Heidelberg, Germany

Printed by Libri Plureos GmbH
in Hamburg, Germany